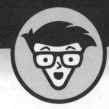

Dad's Guide to Pregnancy

3rd Edition

by Matthew M.F. Miller and Sharon Perkins

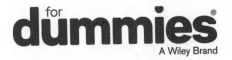

for dummies®
A Wiley Brand

Dad's Guide to Pregnancy For Dummies®, 3rd Edition

Published by: **John Wiley & Sons, Inc.**, 111 River Street, Hoboken, NJ 07030-5774, www.wiley.com

Copyright © 2022 by John Wiley & Sons, Inc., Hoboken, New Jersey

Published simultaneously in Canada

For general information on our other products and services, please contact our Customer Care Department within the U.S. at 877-762-2974, outside the U.S. at 317-572-3993, or fax 317-572-4002. For technical support, please visit https://hub.wiley.com/community/support/dummies.

Wiley publishes in a variety of print and electronic formats and by print-on-demand. Some material included with standard print versions of this book may not be included in e-books or in print-on-demand. If this book refers to media such as a CD or DVD that is not included in the version you purchased, you may download this material at http://booksupport.wiley.com. For more information about Wiley products, visit www.wiley.com.

Library of Congress Control Number: 2022934308

ISBN 978-1-119-86715-9 (pbk); ISBN 978-1-119-86716-6 (ebk); ISBN 978-1-119-86717-3 (ebk)

SKY10033765_032422

Contents at a Glance

Table of Contents

CHAPTER 14: Survival Tips for Bumps, Boo-Boos, and More 295

Introduction

Welcome to impending fatherhood! Being a dad is better than you can ever imagine and far less scary than you probably believe it to be. One of the main reasons we wrote this book was to empower men to get actively involved in every aspect of the childbirth process, as well as the care, feeding, and nurturing of newborns. Most dads-to-be have only an elementary idea of what parenthood is going to be like, and their excitement mixes liberally with sheer terror and trepidation. We hope this book will spare you some of that fear and concern by giving you the knowledge you need to feel confident.

In the not-so-distant past, men were removed from the processes of pregnancy, labor and delivery, and even most aspects of raising children. On TV, fathers have long been portrayed as bumbling, emotionally distant fools incapable of changing diapers, getting kids to go to bed, or handling any of the routine tasks that mothers seem to do with ease. In reality, today's dad is confident, capable, and totally in love with his children — and not afraid to let it show. Not that it all comes easily and naturally. Learning how to support your pregnant partner and, subsequently, to care for a newborn takes time, effort, and education.

Most men in the world become fathers at some point, and most enter the experience without much knowledge of how babies develop, how to be a supportive partner, or what their role should be in the process. But not you. Because you're reading this book, you'll be prepared for just about anything and know exactly what it takes to be an equal partner on the pregnancy (and parenting) journey.

About This Book

This book answers all the burning questions you have about the impact your partner's pregnancy will have on your life. Of course, we tell you how your sex life will change because we know that's near the top of your list. We also explain everything you ever wanted to know about how a fetus develops, what it's like to live with a pregnant woman, and how your pocketbook will be hit by adding a new member (or members) to your family.

Additionally, we delve a little into what to expect the first six months or so after the baby arrives. We walk you through the ins and outs of feeding, changing diapers, dealing with common illnesses and emergencies, and staying sane and true to yourself through it all.

As you read this book, you'll notice a few things:

>> We use *he* and *she* interchangeably throughout because we don't know whether your baby is a boy or a girl.

>> We use the term *medical practitioner* when we talk about anyone medical because we don't know whether you're working with a doctor or midwife, a pediatrician or a nurse practitioner.

>> We call your partner *your partner* because that's what she is, in every sense.

>> We sprinkle shaded boxes throughout the text. They contain information that's interesting but not essential to the topic at hand, so feel free to skip over them if you're pressed for time.

Basically, after reading this book, you'll feel completely prepared for fatherhood. You won't actually *be* completely prepared, because no one ever is, but you'll at least feel like you are until the baby comes.

Foolish Assumptions

Expectant dads are often the forgotten partner in the new family-to-be, and they need all the understanding they can get. If you're reading this, we assume you fall into at least one of the following categories:

>> You're an expectant dad.

>> You're hoping to become an expectant dad.

>> You're already a father but looking to learn new tricks for the next go-round.

>> You know an expectant dad and want to get into his head and understand why he's behaving the way he is.

Icons Used In This Book

Icons are another handy tool you can use as you work your way through this book. If you find the tips really helpful, for instance, you can skim through and search for that icon. Following are the icons we use in this book:

REMEMBER

The Remember icon sits next to information we hope stays in your head for more than two minutes.

TIP

The Tip icon gives helpful insider info that may take years to learn on your own.

WARNING

Whenever we use a Warning icon, you'd better sit up and take notice, because not heeding our warning could be disastrous for you or your loved ones.

Beyond the Book

You can find a little more helpful related information at https://www.dummies.com, where you can peruse this book's Cheat Sheet. To get this handy resource, go to the website and type *Dad's Guide to Pregnancy For Dummies Cheat Sheet* in the Search box.

Where to Go from Here

This is where we tell you to go read the book, already!

Although you can start absolutely any place and get the benefit of our expertise, if your partner isn't yet pregnant or is newly pregnant, we suggest starting at the beginning and reading right on through. It will calm your nerves, we promise.

If you're the last-minute type of guy and you're reading this book just a few months (or weeks!) before the impending birth, you can certainly skip the first trimester stuff (at least this time around) and start wherever makes the most sense for you.

And if you got this book at the beginning of the pregnancy but never got around to opening it until now, when baby has his first case of sniffles, that's okay too — we still have plenty of valuable information for you. Pregnancy is the start of the adventure, but the fun continues long after.

1

You're Going to Be a Dad (Yes, You)

Think about whether the time is right to consider adding someone new to your household.

Confront your fears and feelings about how having a baby will change your life.

Take stock of your readiness to become a parent, with all that parenthood entails financially, emotionally, and even physically.

Review Conception 101 to fill in the gaps in your baby-making knowledge.

Decide to make the necessary lifestyle changes to ensure success in the pregnancy department.

Deal with not being able to be physically present during pregnancy and childbirth.

Chapter **1**

Welcome to Dad Land

Apparently, congratulations are in order: Either you're going to be a father sometime within the next nine months or you're in the planning stages of becoming a dad. Either way, you've come to the right place. You'll face no bigger life decision than choosing to become a parent. (And no bigger jolt than being told baby is coming if you didn't expect it!) The best gift you can give to your soon-to-be child is confidence, and the only way to feel confident before becoming a parent is to prepare yourself for the journey that lies ahead.

Perhaps you're already floored by equal doses of joy and fear, which is a good sign that you recognize the magnitude of the change, but fear not — you're up for the challenge of fatherhood. Emotions run deep when confronted with the prospect of raising a child, mainly because it's a huge commitment and responsibility that, unlike a job, never has off-hours. Babies are expensive, con-fusing, and time consuming, and for many fathers, they represent the end of a carefree "youth" that extends well into adulthood.

Experiencing a jumble of feelings is normal, and the more you take those emotions to heart and explore what fatherhood means to you — and what kind of father you want to be — the easier the transition will be when baby arrives.

The Glorious, Frightening, Mind-Boggling World of Fatherhood

What exactly does it mean to be a father? The answer depends on the kind of father you want to be for your child. In recent years, movies, TV shows, and even commercials have begun to transition from the bumbling, know-nothing father of yore to the modern dad who's just as comfortable changing a diaper as he is fixing a car. Fathers today range from traditional to equal partners in every aspect of parenting.

Most parents today don't adhere to the traditional masculine and feminine roles that your parents and grandparents grew up with. Women work, men work, and caring for the home — inside and out — is both partners' responsibility. Today, fatherhood is a flexible word that's defined by how involved you want to be in the rearing of your child, but the more involved you are in your child's upbringing, the more likely she is to be a well-adjusted, loving, and confident person.

A father? Who, me?

Yes, you. As strange as it sounds, you're going to be a father. A great one at that, because just through the mere act of reading this book, you're taking the proverbial bull by the horns and doing your homework to find out what it takes to be a good dad from day one. As they say, anyone can be a father, but it takes someone special to be a dad.

Even if you've never held a baby before, don't let self-doubt rule the day. Being a good father isn't about knowing everything about everything; it's about loving and caring for a baby to the best of your abilities. So don't be afraid. Yes, that's easier said than done, but being fearful of what lies ahead doesn't change the fact that you've got a baby on the way, however far off that little bundle's arrival may be.

TIP

If the thought of fatherhood scares you, you need to get used to the label, and the more you say and internalize it, the more it will become you. Start by saying the words "I'm going to be a father" out loud a few times. Maybe even look into a mirror while you say it. You may feel silly, but that's a small price to pay for a major confidence boost. (Besides, the only person who will see you is you!)

Reacting to a life-changing event

Turning into a tearful, slobbering mess upon finding out that you're going to be a father isn't unusual. Nor is throwing up, feeling faint, laughing, swearing, or any of the normal, healthy reactions people have upon receiving life-altering information.

REMEMBER

If your reaction isn't 100 percent positive, that's okay, too. Just remember that your partner likely won't be particularly thrilled if you get upset, defensive, or angry when she tells you she's expecting. If you're feeling angry or scared, do your best to react to the news with calmness and class. You'll have plenty of time to revisit any concerns or frustrations after you give the situation some time to sink in.

Some dads-to-be go into fix-it mode upon hearing the news, ready and eager to crunch budget numbers, baby-proof the entire home in a single night, begin making college plans 18 years in advance, and so on. Feeling like you need to get everything in order before baby arrives is normal, but remember that you can't do it all in a day. Take some time to celebrate before you dive into the practical side of life with baby. (For more advice on handling the big news, refer to Chapter 4.)

Dealing with fatherhood fears

Even men who've been lucky enough to be surrounded by positive male role models find themselves doubting whether they have what it takes to be a dad. It's like the fear of starting a new job amplified by 100. Part of being a good father is taking the time to confront these fears so that when baby comes, you don't parent with fear. Following are some of the common fear-based questions men ask themselves in regard to fatherhood:

>> Am I ready to give up my present life (free time, flexibility, freedom) to be a dad?

>> Will I have time for my pastimes and friends?

>> Will I ever sleep again?

>> Is this the end of my marriage and sex life as I know it?

>> Do we have enough money to raise a child?

>> Do I know enough about kids to be a good dad?

>> Am I mature enough to be a good role model for my child?

>> What if the baby comes and I don't love him?

Your head may be spinning with all the questions you ask yourself, and although you can't answer them all right away, you need to address them at some point. However, plenty of men have felt unprepared and unwilling to become fathers and turned out to be great dads, so don't despair if your initial answers to the preceding questions are mostly negative.

Parenthood involves a lot of sacrifice, but it doesn't have to sound the death knell for your identity or happiness. Talk with your partner, a trusted friend, or a therapist — anyone who will listen to you and support your concerns without getting defensive — about the questions you have. You'll find that some of your fears have no basis in reality and that others — such as the fear of losing yourself and your free time — require you to reprioritize your time and energy.

WARNING

Regardless of what your fears may be, don't let them fester. No man is an island, and you can't effectively deal with all those emotions by yourself. Starting an open dialogue with your partner keeps you both on the same page, which is a good start toward making you two an effective parenting duo.

Debunking six common myths

Many of the concerns or fears you may have about fatherhood likely originated from the long-standing myths of what a father's role should be in his child's life. Not all that long ago, men stood in the waiting room at the hospital during delivery and returned to work the next day. Nowadays, the landscape of fatherhood is vastly different, leaving the modern dad wondering where he fits in the parenting scheme.

The following sections outline some of the most common misconceptions about fatherhood. We debunk these myths to help you understand how to be a more-involved father.

Myth #1: Only the mom-to-be should have input about labor and delivery

Though the focus is on your partner — she is, after all, the one carrying your child — you also matter, and you have the right to voice your opinions along the way. Throughout the pregnancy, share what you're experiencing and let her know what scares you. She has a lot to think through and worry about, too, but the more you deal with those issues together, the stronger your relationship will become.

If you have thoughts and opinions about what kind of delivery option you're most comfortable with, share those with her as well. Although ultimately you need to let your partner pick the childbirth option that's best for her, she deserves to know your feelings on the matter. Getting involved in the decision-making process isn't just your right — it's the right thing to do. (Check out Chapter 9 to start getting informed on birthing options and the many decisions you'll need to make.)

Myth #2: Men aren't ideal caretakers for newborns

Boobs are generally the issue at the forefront of this myth. No, you can't breast-feed your child or know what it's like to give birth. Because a lot of fathers don't have that initial connection, they wonder what exactly they're supposed to do.

Mother and baby are attached to each other for nine months, but after baby arrives, it's open season on bonding and caretaking. When your partner isn't breast-feeding, hold, rock, and engage in skin-to-skin contact with your baby whenever possible. Changing diapers, bathing, and changing clothes are just a few of the activities you can do to get involved. And the more involved you get, the less likely you are to feel left out of the equation. Chapter 11 provides tips for caring for your new baby so you can feel confident in your abilities.

Myth #3: You'll never have sex or sleep ever again

Good things come to those who wait, and you'll have to wait. Sex won't happen for at least six to eight weeks following delivery, and even then you have a long road back to normalcy. For many couples, a normal sex life after childbirth isn't as active as it once was, but you can work with your partner to make sure both of your needs are being met.

One need that will deter your sex life — and override the sex need — is sleep. Babies don't sleep through the night. They wake up hungry and demand an alert parent to feed them, burp them, and soothe them back to sleep. Some babies begin sleeping through the night at six months; other kids don't until the age of 3. The good news is that they all do it eventually, and when you begin to understand your baby's patterns, you'll be able to figure out a routine that allows you to maximize the shut-eye you get every day.

Myth #4: Active fathers can't succeed in the business world

Unless work is the only obligation you've ever had in your adult life, you're probably used to juggling more than one thing. Fathers who are active in the community or fill their schedules with copious hours of hobbies have to reevaluate their priorities. Family comes first, work comes second, and with the support of a loving partner and a few good babysitters, you can continue on your career trajectory as planned.

In fact, being a dad may just make you a more effective worker. Having so many demands on your time can make you better at time management and maximizing your workday. Focus on work at work and home at home and you'll succeed in both arenas.

Myth #5: You're destined to become your father

Destiny is really just a code word for the tendency many men have to mimic their father's behaviors, good or bad. If you didn't like an aspect of your father's parenting or don't want to repeat a major mistake that he perpetrated, talk about it with your partner. The more you talk about it, the less likely you are to repeat that mistake because you'll engage your partner as a support system working with you to help you avoid it.

TIP

At the same time, don't forget to replicate and celebrate the things your father did right. You'll be chilled to the bone the first time you say something that your father used to say, but remember that repeating the good actions isn't a bad thing. Don't try to be different from your father "just because." Identify what he did that was right and what was wrong and use that as a blueprint for your parenting style.

Myth #6: You'll fall in love with baby at first sight

Babies aren't always so beautiful right after being born, but that's to be expected, given what they've just gone through to enter the world. Don't feel guilty if you look at your baby and aren't immediately enamored with her (them). Emotions are difficult to control, and for some fathers — and even mothers — falling head over heels for your baby may take some time.

Childbirth is a long, intense experience (as we describe in Chapter 10), so allow yourself adequate time to rest and get to know the new addition to your family. If you suffer from feelings of regret or extreme sadness, or if you experience thoughts of harming yourself or the baby, seek immediate medical assistance.

Becoming a Modern Dad

Dads today are involved in every aspect of a child's life. They're no longer relegated to teaching sports, roughhousing, and serving as disciplinarians. Modern fatherhood is all about using your strengths, talents, and interests to shape your relationship and interactions with your child.

Modern dads change diapers, feed the baby, wake up in the middle of the night to care for a crying child, and take baby for a run. They don't "baby-sit" their children; they're capable parents, and no job falls outside the realm of their capabilities. Though all that involvement does mean you'll put in far more effort and time than previous generations, it also means that you're bridging the gap of emotional distance that used to be so prevalent in the father-child experience.

The sections that follow (and the chapters in Part 4) offer information and advice on making changes and stepping into the practical role of daddy.

Changes in your personal life

If what you fear most is losing the freedom to spend as much time as you want engaging in leisure activities, then you're in for some life-altering sacrifices. Babies require you to say no to a lot of commitments that the prebaby you would have been eager to engage in. Don't make a lot of outside-the-home plans that you consider optional, at least at first.

For the first six months, going out at night is challenging, especially if your partner is breast-feeding and/or you don't live near family. However, as your baby ages, leaving him with a babysitter becomes more feasible and less stressful.

Perhaps what you fear the most is the impact baby will have on your relationship with your partner. This fear is valid, given that you'll scarcely find time for the two of you to be alone. But that doesn't mean you won't have time to connect.

TIP

Just because going out as a couple is tough to manage doesn't mean you can't have ample one-on-one time. Plan stay-in dates that start at baby's bedtime. Order food or make an elegant dinner, queue up a movie, or play your favorite board game. Try not to talk about baby. Rather, focus on each other and talk about topics that interest you both.

Changes in your professional life

Depending on the requirements of your job, your daily routine may go completely unchanged aside from the uptick in yawns due to late-night feedings and fussiness. Thoughts of your new family may make focusing difficult, especially when you first return to work following any paternity leave or vacation time you take. It won't be long, though, before you settle back into a normal routine, and work just may become the one arena of your life that provides a respite from parenting duties.

Workaholics, however, find themselves at a crossroads. Some choose to cut back on hours spent at the office, whereas others, hopefully with the full support of their partners, proceed with business as usual. There's no right or wrong way to balance a demanding job with a new baby as long as you and your partner are comfortable with the arrangement and you spend enough quality time with your child.

What is quality time? It's time you spend with your child, focusing *on* your child. Some people say quality time has nothing to do with the quantity of time you spend with your child, but we feel that it's affected by the amount of time you devote to your child. Give as much as you can because the old adage is true — they grow up so fast. Your smartphone will still be there when baby goes to bed.

Some dads even leave the workforce altogether or take work-at-home positions to provide full-time childcare for their newborn.

If you choose this route, make sure to check out Chapter 14, which notes some important considerations of being a stay-at-home daddy.

Lifestyle changes to consider

Bad habits are hard to break, but when you have the added stress of a baby, those habits can be even harder to conquer. That said, you're about to have a child — a sponge that will soak up your every word and action — so it's time to clean up your act. Following are a few lifestyle alterations to consider making so you can lead by example without reservation:

>> **Control your anger and censor your potty mouth.** Kids learn how to treat and interact with others at a very young age. Start revising your behavior now and get used to swearing less, before your kid picks up some foul-mouthed communication habits.

>> **Develop routines.** Be it running errands, cooking, making phone calls, or paying the bills, get systems in place to ensure that everything gets done with the least amount of stress. Knowing who does what when keeps you on track when baby throws a wrench into everything.

>> **Eat healthier.** Your partner needs to be extremely diligent about eating pregnancy-positive foods, so use this time as an opportunity to get your diet in order. Soon enough, you'll be cooking for three, and if you're already in the habit of preparing healthy foods, you'll have no trouble providing proper nutrition to your child.

>> **Lose weight.** If you're considerably overweight, you're more susceptible to illness and a shortened life span. Furthermore, children of obese parents are more likely to be obese. Kids learn nutrition and lifestyle habits from their parents, so set a good example and give your child a fair shot at a long, healthy life.

>> **Organize and de-clutter your home.** Create a safe, livable place for your new addition, which also helps decrease the amount of stress in your life.

>> **Quit smoking/drinking too much/taking recreational drugs.** Secondhand smoke increases the risk of illness for your child and the likelihood that she'll become a smoker as an adult. Frequent overconsumption of alcohol makes you

less likely to be a responsible parent capable of making good, safe decisions for baby. In fact, alcohol and drugs often lead to harmful and neglectful decisions that can land you in legal trouble and your child in the foster care system.

>> **Spend less money on nonessential items.** Teaching kids fiscal responsibility is just as important as teaching them social responsibility. Plus, kids aren't cheap, so stop spending $50 per week on lattes and comic books and start banking your savings to provide a sound, secure future for your family.

>> **Start an exercise regimen.** Physically active, healthy parents get less run down and are less susceptible to illness. Plus, you want to live a long life with your children.

Bringing baby into a turbulent world

Our modern life seems to get more complex by the day, from politics and social media to pandemics and increasingly erratic natural disasters — now might seem like a particularly scary time to bring a baby into the world. If you're concerned, remember you're not alone. Millennials are waiting longer to get married, buy a home, and have children. There's never a "right" time to have a baby — when you're ready, the rest of the noise won't matter as much. Your decision to have a child is separate from the chaos that has always been and will always be, and as long as you provide a safe, happy home, your baby will be happy and healthy, too. The best thing you can do is be honest with your partner about any concerns you have and decide together how you want to raise your child. It's never too soon to start discussing the world you want for your child and to figure out how you can facilitate providing that world.

Also, during pregnancy (and beyond!) it's absolutely okay to take a break from social media, to unfollow people and pages that cause stress, and to take a break from podcasts and cable news. Sure, it might feel like sticking your head in the sand, but a stress-free and happy pregnancy is your number-one job. Anything that stands in the way of that can be excised or paused in your life for as long as you both desire.

Deciding to Take the Plunge (or Not)

Deciding the right time in life to have a baby isn't an easy task, especially because circumstances change on a seemingly daily basis. However, family planning is an essential step that can minimize what ifs, frustrations, and regrets. After you have a baby, you can't take it back. Knowing when you're ready to be parents and then trying to conceive means that when you actually *do* get pregnant, the timing will be right. Or at least as right as any time can be, considering you have such little control over life's variables.

Determining whether you're ready

How does it feel when you know you want to be a father? And how can you know when you're actually ready to start trying for a baby? Those questions have no simple answers because the feeling is different for everyone, but suffice it to say, you'll know when you know.

One sign to look for is a prolonged interest and fascination with the babies of friends and family members. Some women jokingly refer to their growing desire for a baby as *baby fever,* and many men experience similar feelings. The desire to procreate, to have your genes carried on in the species, can be powerful. Just make sure it's a desire that lasts more than a day.

Also, make sure you take the time to analyze the impact baby will have on your life. If you're in the final two years of a college program, waiting to have a child may be in your best interest. If you're unemployed, perhaps you want to put off trying until you find a job you like that can support a family.

REMEMBER

Just because you're ready doesn't make now the right time. Don't decide to have a baby on an impulse. Think about the impact a child will have on your time, money, and home, and if you don't see any major obstacles, then by all means, proceed. Obviously, you can choose to proceed even if having a baby now doesn't make sense on every level, but first make sure you can provide a loving, safe home and can pay for all the things baby needs to thrive.

Telling your partner you're ready

You can tell your partner anytime and anyplace that you're ready to take the plunge into parenthood, but however you broach the subject, remember that she may not be as ready as you. A good way to introduce the topic is by asking her questions about her feelings on when is the right time to have a baby.

Let her know how excited you are, but also let her know that you've thought about the finances and logistics of having a baby, too. Fatherhood involves a lot more than choosing a name and a nursery theme. A big part of feeling ready is knowing that your partner isn't just enamored with the idea of a child but is also prepared for the practicalities of responsibly starting a family.

You don't have to outline every aspect of how and why you're ready, but do treat the idea with respect and let your partner know you're sincere by proving that you've actually thought it through.

Telling your partner you're not ready

If your partner is already pregnant, do not under *any* circumstances tell her you're not ready. If, however, the two of you are simply exploring the idea of having a child, now is the perfect time to speak your piece and let her know that you're just not prepared for fatherhood.

Reasons for not being ready vary from practical (not enough money or time) to logistical (still in school or caring for a sick parent) to selfish (not ready to share the Xbox). No reason is wrong, but if your partner is ready for a baby, don't expect her to be fully supportive of your rationale.

REMEMBER

Regardless, don't agree to have a child before you're up for the challenge just so your partner doesn't get angry with you. Be honest, because once she's pregnant, you can't do anything to change the situation. If you're uncertain now, be honest and speak up!

Being patient when one of you is ready (and the other isn't)

Being on different pages can be an uncomfortable position for any couple, especially when it comes to the kid issue. Men have long been saddled with the Peter Pan label whenever they announce they aren't ready to "grow up" and have kids. Women are unfairly chastised for choosing career over family if they aren't ready to have a child.

Everyone has his reasons for wanting or not wanting to have a baby, and every one of them is valid — at least to the person who isn't ready. We don't recommend attempting to persuade your partner, or vice versa, to have a baby. Having a child with someone who isn't ready is setting up your relationship — and your relationship with the child — for failure.

TIP

If one of you isn't ready, try to work out a timeline as to when the wary party will be ready. If you can't set a definitive date, choose a time to revisit the topic. Check in with each other at least every six months. Nagging the other person isn't a good idea, but if it's something one of you wants, then you should continue to work toward a solution.

Seek counseling at any point if you and your partner fight about the issue frequently or if one of you decides that you never want children. Couples who are at an impasse about whether to have children often need the guidance of a trained professional.

Dealing with an unexpected pregnancy

Unplanned pregnancies aren't uncommon, and for the majority of people in a committed relationship, adjusting to the surprising news is often no more than a minor bump in the road. If you unexpectedly find out that you're going to be a dad, don't get angry with your partner. Blaming the other person is easy when emotions run high, but don't forget how you got into this situation in the first place. It does, indeed, take two.

Birth control and family planning are the responsibility of both the man and the woman, and accidents sometimes happen. The best thing you can do in this instance is to talk with your partner about your options and start making a plan for how to give that child the best life you possibly can. Having a child unexpectedly isn't the end of the world, and you don't have to feel ready to have a baby to be a good father.

Welcoming long-awaited pregnancies

Getting pregnant isn't always as easy as they make it look in the movies, as the millions of infertile couples know all too well. (And if you and your partner are dealing with infertility, head to Chapter 2 for help.) Finding out that you're pregnant after a long wait brings a mixed bag of emotions, most of which are joyful.

If you and your partner have been struggling to get pregnant, you likely feel relieved that you're about to get the gift you've been working so hard to find, but don't be surprised if you have difficulty adjusting to life outside of the infertility world. After months and years of scheduled sex, countless doctor visits, and innumerable disappointments, not everyone transitions into the pregnancy phase with ease.

You also may struggle with extreme fear because of previous mis-carriages, close calls, and years of frustration with the process. Allow yourselves the opportunity to gripe, complain, worry, and grieve for a process that took a lot of patience and energy. Frus-trations that were bottled up for the sake of optimism may finally surface, which is absolutely healthy.

REMEMBER

Just because you've finally achieved your goal doesn't make all the feelings of sadness and frustration suddenly disappear. If you and/or your partner have trouble letting go of the feelings that gripped you during your fertility struggle, you can find count-less support groups, online communities, and blogs that provide both of you a place to talk about what you've been through. You can also learn transition tips from others who've been through the same thing. Moving forward does get easier, but it can take time — and a heaping helping of support.

Peering into the Pregnancy Crystal Ball

When you get used to the idea of being a father, you may won-der what comes next. For the uninitiated, first-time dad, the nine months of pregnancy are a whirlwind of planning, worrying, parties, nesting, name searching, doctor visits, and information gathering as you move toward baby's birth. In the following sec-tions we lay out what you can expect in each *trimester* (a period of three months).

First trimester

In the first trimester, which encompasses the first three months of pregnancy, your partner will likely suffer from a host of common pregnancy symptoms immortalized and caricatured in numerous movies and TV shows, such as nausea, (food aversions), intense sleepiness, (fatigue), unexplained tears, and baffling cravings for the oddest food combinations imaginable.

Because your baby's major organs form during this time, he's most susceptible to injury from environmental factors, such as certain medications ingested by your partner. He's also growing in a way he never will again. By the end of the first trimester, your baby grows to be about 3 or 4 inches long and weighs approximately 1 ounce.

By the time he reaches the end of the first three months, your baby's arms, legs, hands, and feet are fully formed, and he's able to open and close his fists. The circulatory and urinary systems are fully functional, meaning that, yes, he urinates into the amniotic fluid on a daily basis. Secondary body parts, such as fingernails, teeth, and reproductive organs, begin developing.

Want more information on the miracle that is the first trimester? Head to Chapter 4 for all the minute details.

On the practical side, don't forget to take a look at your medical insurance and make sure you understand your benefits.

Second trimester

During the second trimester, most of your partner's early pregnancy symptoms, such as extreme fatigue, disappear, but she finally begins to look like the pregnant person she is. She may begin struggling with the not-so-fun aspects of carrying another human being around, such as weight gain. She may also exhibit characteristics you associate more with your grandmom than your partner, such as forgetfulness.

This is also the pregnancy period when the fun stuff begins. Around 18 to 20 weeks, your partner has the ultrasound that can determine the baby's sex — if you choose to find out and if the baby allows the ultrasound technician a clear view. It's also the time when you register for your baby shower, prepare the nursery, weed through countless baby names, attend birthing classes, and think about baby-proofing your house.

By the end of the second trimester, your baby is roughly 14 inches long and weighs about 2 pounds. Her skin is still translucent, but her eyes are beginning to open and close. Your partner is also likely to start feeling movements and even baby's tiny hiccups. Check out Chapter 5 to find out more about the second trimester.

Third trimester

Assuming all goes according to plan and your baby bakes until he's full term (meaning he isn't born before 37 weeks) or later, the third trimester can be one of the longest three-month periods of your — and your partner's — life. Your partner begins to feel uncomfortable as her ever-increasing abdominal girth makes it difficult to move and sleep normally, and you both get antsy about the impending arrival.

REMEMBER

To make the most of the time, you and your partner need to take care of business by doing the following:

>> Picking a pediatrician who you're comfortable with and who has a similar parenting philosophy as you and your partner

>> Crafting your birth plan (and hiring a doula if you want one)

>> Getting your maternity and paternity leave squared away

>> Creating a phone tree to announce baby's arrival

>> Finishing up any odd projects around the house that need to be done prior to baby's arrival

During the third trimester, your baby is fully developed and focused on growing larger and stronger for life on the outside. See Chapter 8 for the full details.

REMEMBER

The third trimester is also the last time for many, many years that you and your partner exist solely as a couple, so be sure to take the time to indulge yourselves in the things you love to do together. (take your "babymoon" but don't plan travel after 36 weeks in pregnancy). Life may feel like it's on pause for at least the first six months of baby's existence, so get out now and enjoy the freedom of childlessness. Soon enough, your life will be a lot more complicated and busy — and happy, too. Very, very happy.

WHILE YOU WERE GESTATING: CREATING A PREGNANCY TIME CAPSULE

Because the first few weeks of pregnancy are likely to be rather uneventful, now is a good time to start a time capsule for the year your baby will be born. Many years down the road, when your child is an adult, it will be a touching, informative look back at the time when she entered the world. For you and your partner, it will be a fun, celebratory action to kick off the pregnancy festivities.

Keep movie ticket stubs, takeout menus, a newspaper from the day you found out your partner was pregnant (as well as clippings of the most important headlines of the year), favorite ads, magazine clippings, and so on. Include pop culture elements that define the year as well as some of your favorite things.

As you choose names, add the list of all potential names to the time capsule. When you choose a paint color for the nursery, put in the paint color card. Any decision you and your partner make for the baby is a good candidate for inclusion. It may seem silly now, but in 20 years it will be the best gift you can give your child.

Chapter **2**

Your Conception Primer

You may have spent years trying not to get pregnant, so the change from not trying to trying can be rather unsettling. Having trouble with something even the most clueless people manage to do effortlessly can cause you to lose sleep at night and can turn sex into a job. Getting pregnant is hard work . . . sometimes.

In this chapter, we tell you how to make the getting-pregnant process painless *and* fun — even if it takes longer than you expected.

Sperm, Meet Egg: Baby Making 101

Getting pregnant requires that several key players be on the field at the right time: namely, good sperm, a mature egg, and a suitable landing place in the uterus. If sperm and egg meet in the *fallopian tube* (the conduit from the ovary down to the uterus), join together to form a fertilized egg, and then float down to a uterus with a lining that's exactly the right thickness to facilitate implantation, then pregnancy occurs. If any of those factors are amiss, well, that's when things get complicated.

Producing a mature egg

Before she's even born, a woman has all the eggs she'll ever have. Unlike sperm, no new eggs are produced over time; the original eggs just mature, usually one at a time. Mature eggs are produced from immature ones (called *oocytes*), located in the ovaries, through a complex interaction of three hormones during the menstrual cycle. Those hormones — *estradiol* (a form of estrogen), *follicle stimulating hormone* (FSH), and *luteinizing hormone* (LH) — work like this:

1. Day 1 of the menstrual cycle begins when your partner's period starts. FSH stimulates the ovaries, which produce estrogen.

2. Estradiol production starts to mature a number of egg-containing *follicles*, small, cyst like structures that contain the immature eggs.

3. One follicle, called a *lead follicle,* continues to develop while the rest atrophy.

4. Around day 14 of the menstrual cycle, LH kicks in to mature the egg and move it to the center of the follicle so it can release. Ovulation occurs 14 days before the last day of your partner's cycle, so day 14 is based on an average 28-day cycle. If her cycles are longer or shorter than 14 days, she'll ovulate earlier or later.

5. The egg releases from the follicle and begins to float down the fallopian tube. This is where you and your sperm come in.

TIP

If you're interested in really getting into the nitty-gritty of how the menstrual cycle works, check out *Getting Pregnant For Dummies* by Lisa A. Rinehart *et al* (John Wiley & Sons).

Figure 2-1 shows the events of a menstrual cycle when pregnancy does not occur.

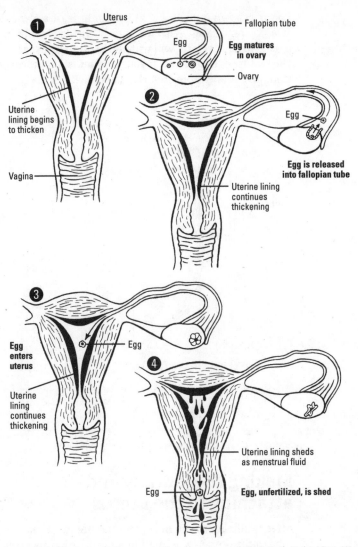

Illustration by Kathryn Born, MA

FIGURE 2-1: Every event in the menstrual cycle has a purpose.

Sending in some good sperm

Sperm can only fertilize an egg that's mature, so you need to either have sperm waiting in the tube when the egg is released or get some there within 12 to 24 hours after ovulation, because that's how long the egg can live.

Sperm (shown in Figure 2-2) live for at least a few days — up to five, in some cases — so having sex the day before ovulation, or even two days before, will usually result in live sperm waiting for the mature egg to arrive. If your partner is monitoring her ovulation, give it one more shot the day of ovulation.

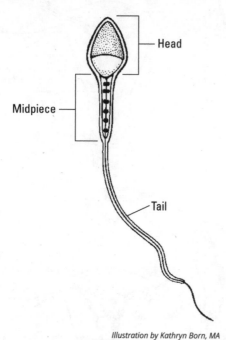

Head

Midpiece

Tail

Illustration by Kathryn Born, MA

FIGURE 2-2: Sperm are compact swimming machines.

Making the journey and attaching to the uterus

After fertilization, the new potential life must make it down the tube to the uterus, where it implants. The journey from fallopian tube to uterus takes five to seven days, on average, and implantation normally occurs seven to ten days after conception. The fallopian tube is normally a fairly straight tube, but if it's twisted or dilated because of previous infection or pelvic inflammatory disease, the embryo may wander around in the crevasses and never get to the uterus.

WHY SO MANY SPERM?

Women produce one egg a month, most of the time, and men produce millions of sperm. Why the huge disparity? Because one sperm isn't enough to get the job done — it needs lots of friends to help. Although only one victorious sperm makes it into the egg, breaking down the coating that surrounds the egg takes many sperm. And although eggs get to drift downward from the ovary to the fallopian tube, sperm have to swim upstream. Needless to say, some fall by the wayside, either because they tire or because they take a wrong turn somewhere.

Sperm are also produced in large quantities because many are abnormal, having two tails, no tails, round tails, small heads, large heads, or abnormally shaped heads. Abnormal tails make navigation difficult, and abnormal heads often indicate chromosomal abnormalities.

Only 50 to 60 percent of sperm need good *motility,* or movement, for a sperm sample to be considered normal, so lots of sperm don't make the grade, creating a need for higher numbers.

Even worse, the embryo may implant in the fallopian tube, a situation known as an *ectopic pregnancy.* The tube has no room for a developing fetus, so an ectopic pregnancy is doomed from the start and can cause serious, life-threatening bleeding if the tube ruptures. Ectopic pregnancies occur in around 2 percent of all pregnancies.

Even after the embryo reaches the uterus, it's not always clear sailing. The uterine lining has to be just right for implantation. Estrogen thickens the lining before ovulation, and progesterone released from the *corpus luteum* (the leftover shell of the follicle that contained the egg) prepares the lining after ovulation. If either of these hormone levels is low, the lining may not be able to support a pregnancy. *Note:* Your partner's medical practitioner can assess the uterine lining by ultrasound and prescribe extra progesterone if needed to achieve and maintain pregnancy.

After the embryo reaches the uterus and implants, the implanted embryo begins to produce *human chorionic gonadotropin,* or hCG, the hormone that pregnancy tests measure. hCG levels aren't detectable until the embryo implants, or around the time of the first missed period.

CONCEPTION STATISTICS

If you don't get pregnant the first month you try, the wheels in your head may start turning as you obsess over why this is taking so long. But pregnancy is by no means a sure thing, even when you do everything right and have no major fertility issues. Statistics say that

- Out of 100 couples under age 35 trying to get pregnant over a three month period, 50 achieve their goal, but 20 percent miscarry.
- If your partner is in her late 30s, you have a 10 percent chance of pregnancy each month but a 34 percent chance of miscarriage.
- If she's older than 40, you have only a 5 percent chance of pregnancy each month and more than a 50 percent chance of miscarriage.

The good news is that 90 percent of 30-year-olds trying to get pregnant become pregnant within a year, and 66 percent of 35-year-olds get pregnant in a year. Around 44 percent of 40-year-olds become pregnant within a year. Over age 40, variables such as hormone levels affect pregnancy rates, and generalizations are hard to make. Timing intercourse to ovulation can increase the chance of getting pregnant to 76 percent in the first try, for those under 30.

Answering FAQs about getting pregnant

Getting pregnant may seem straightforward, but what exactly does it take? Here are some answers to the most common concerns:

>> **How long does it take to get pregnant?**

On average, more than half of couples under age 35 get pregnant within the first six months of trying, and four out of five are pregnant within one year.

>> **Does having more sex increase the chances of pregnancy?**

>> No. In fact, due to the amount of time it takes for semen volume to build back up to normal levels following ejaculation, overdoing it around ovulation time by having sex

several times a day can deplete your sperm count, which probably won't be a problem if you have a normal sperm count but can be if your count is low.

» **Should we only have sex with my partner on her back and me on top?**

It's a myth that this standard position is the best way to get pregnant. Although it may help the semen stay in better, no scientific proof exists that the sexual position you choose has any effect on conception rates. Feel free to experiment, especially if it makes having sex less like a chore and more like something you do for fun — you know, like the good old days.

» **Does my partner's past use of the birth control pill mean getting pregnant will take longer?**

It varies from person to person. One woman can miss a single pill and end up pregnant; others may take a little longer to return to their regular ovulation pattern.

REMEMBER

The chances of getting pregnant the first month are small, but the average couple is pregnant within a year, regardless of past birth-control usage.

» **Is it okay to drink and smoke when trying to conceive?**

If you're ready to start a family, you should both give up smoking immediately. Occasionally having a drink or two when you're trying to become a mom or dad won't likely produce a negative outcome, but the general rule of thumb is to live as though your partner is pregnant from the moment you begin trying to conceive. Check out the section "Assessing lifestyle choices that affect eggs and sperm," later in this chapter, for more tips on getting healthy to improve the odds of conception.

Tracking the Journey: Using Fertility Apps and Monitors

If you need one more reason to play with your smartphone, or if you're the type that lives to organize data, using a fertility app can make getting pregnant more fun and sometimes a bit easier. Yes, you could do much the same with a diary or written calendar, but if you have an app on your phone, you'll always be able to find it. A few even have a place for dad-to-be data, to help spot possible issues.

Fertility apps, which can range in price from free to up to $100 a year, can make the baby journey easier by tracking

>> Your partner's normal cycle schedule

>> When ovulation is most likely to occur, based on her cycles

>> Symptoms that indicate ovulation is imminent

>> Premenstrual symptoms, including mood changes

Some apps go a lot further — and cost a whole lot more — by synching the app data with monitors they sell to track your temperature, saliva, or cervical mucus. These can get quite pricy.

If you want to determine when ovulation occurs in a less techy way, you can use ovulation prediction kits, which measure the amount of LH in your partner's urine to determine when ovulation is about to occur. These tests can work well if your partner has regular cycles and a good idea of when she usually ovulates, but may not work at all for women with PCOS, who often have abnormally high LH levels. (For more on this, see "Polycystic ovary syndrome," later in this chapter.) They can also get pretty expensive if your partner has irregular cycles and no idea when she's going to ovulate. You can go through a lot of expensive strips in this case.

Evaluating Health to Get Ready for Parenthood

Some health issues and bad habits can make it harder to get pregnant. A few months before trying to get pregnant, take an inventory of your behaviors and health issues and get yourselves into the best shape possible, not only so that you can get pregnant without difficulty but also so you'll be healthy new parents.

TIP

Checking out your physical health before trying to get pregnant isn't difficult. See your doctor, let him know you're trying to get pregnant, change any medications that may affect fertility, and run some blood tests.

Discovering female health issues that affect conception

Many female health problems can cause fertility difficulties. Some affect egg production and the menstrual cycle; others affect egg transport and implantation. The good news is that you can improve many of these problems after you identify them.

Sexually transmitted infections

Among the biggest fertility busters in the age of sexual freedom are *sexually transmitted infections (STIs)*, formerly known as sexually transmitted diseases (STDs). The following STIs can affect female fertility in these ways:

>> Chlamydia, if not treated promptly, increases the risk of pelvic inflammatory disease (PID) by 40 percent. PID damages the fallopian tubes. Women with PID are seven to ten times more likely to have an ectopic pregnancy. Eighty percent of women who've had chlamydia three or more times are infertile.

>> Gonorrhea also increases the risk of PID and ectopic pregnancy.

>> Human immunodeficiency virus (HIV), if untreated, can affect male and female fertility and increase the risk of pregnancy loss. Antiretroviral treatment before trying to get pregnant can significantly reduce the risks. An undetectable viral load can reduce the risk of transmission to your child during pregnancy to less than 1 percent.

>> Human papillomavirus (HPV), also called genital warts, may increase the risk of early miscarriage, and could affect sperm motility in some cases. To be safe, have treatment before trying to get pregnant.

>> Syphilis can cause miscarriage, stillbirth, developmental delays, and blindness in your unborn child.

REMEMBER

STIs need to be treated early with antibiotics before damage is done to the fallopian tubes. Having a *hysterosalpingogram* (HSG), a dye test to assess the patency of the tubes, is a good idea if your partner has any concerns about whether her tubes have been damaged in the past.

Endometriosis

Endometriosis, which is growth of the tissue that lines the inside of the uterus, called the endometrium, in places it doesn't belong, is common; 5.5 million women in the United States suffer from it, and 40 percent of women with endometriosis have fertility issues.

Endometriosis tissue bleeds at the time of the menstrual period and leads to scarring and pain. Endometrial implants can be removed in some cases, but they tend to recur. Most endometriosis is found in the pelvis, near the uterus, but it can turn up in some odd places, like the lungs. In vitro fertilization (IVF) can increase the chances of pregnancy in women with endometriosis.

Polycystic ovary syndrome

Polycystic ovary syndrome, or PCOS, affects between 5 to 10 percent of women of childbearing age and can cause *anovulation,* or failure to produce a mature egg. PCOS is associated with an abnormal rise in male hormones, called *androgens;* all women have some male hormones, but women with PCOS have more than normal. They're often overweight and have excess body and facial hair, thinning head hair (just like some men), and acne.

Women with PCOS also have a higher rate of type 2 diabetes, heart disease, high cholesterol, and high blood pressure. They may need fertility medications to get pregnant because you can't get pregnant unless you ovulate.

Thyroid problems

Thyroid problems are common in women of childbearing age and can cause anovulation. A simple blood test checks for thyroid function. Low thyroid levels can raise prolactin levels, which can also interfere with ovulation.

Fibroids

Fibroids are common uterine growths (rarely cancerous, lest you add another worry to your list) that occur in up to 75 percent of women and often cause no problems with conception. However, fibroids can grow big enough to interfere with embryo implantation or cause preterm labor in some women.

Fibroids like the ones shown in Figure 2-3 are easily seen with a pelvic ultrasound and can be removed surgically if they appear to be interfering with a woman's ability to get pregnant or carry a pregnancy.

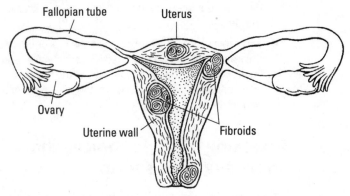

Illustration by Kathryn Born, MA

FIGURE 2-3: Fibroids (uterine growths) occasionally interfere with pregnancy.

Recognizing issues that cause fertility problems in men

Sperm take a long time to make. Sperm you ejaculate today have been three months in the making, so if you're working on health problems or making lifestyle changes, give them enough time to take effect.

Although male health issues may seem less important to a quick conception, your health problems can interfere with conception. Here are a few examples of potentially problematic issues:

>> Diabetic men often have problems with erection and ejaculation. If you have a problem with erection, you're probably well aware of it, but ejaculatory issues may not be quite as obvious. *Retrograde ejaculation,* where sperm get pushed into the bladder rather than out through the urethra, can affect diabetic men.

>> Men who take high-blood-pressure medications called *calcium channel blockers* may have sperm that don't penetrate eggs well; other blood pressure medications may cause retrograde ejaculation.

>> Toxins common to the workplace — such as lead, X-rays, inhaled anesthetics in the operating room, and a host of other environmentally damaging substances — can also damage your internal plumbing if you work with them frequently.

>> STIs can also take their toll on the male reproductive system. Chlamydia and gonorrhea can cause an infection and inflammation in the *epididymis,* part of the testes where sperm develop. Syphilis can cause low sperm count and poor motility.

Assessing lifestyle choices that affect eggs and sperm

You can improve your chances of pregnancy by adopting a healthy lifestyle. Yes, giving up bad habits is painful, but failing to get pregnant month after month can be painful, too. Take the step of cutting the following bad habits out of your life *before* you start trying to get pregnant.

Smoking

WARNING

Smoking can affect sperm and eggs and increase miscarriage rates. Nearly one in four adults smoke in America. If either of you is a smoker, quit for at least a few months before trying to get pregnant.

Compared to nonsmokers, smokers

>> Have sperm that are less *motile* (capable of moving spontaneously). Sperm have a long way to go to reach the egg, so they need all the motility they can get.

>> Have lower sperm counts and more abnormally shaped sperm, which are chromosomally abnormal.

>> Have more eggs that are chromosomally abnormal.

>> Have a 50 percent higher rate of miscarriage.

>> Are two to four times more likely to have an ectopic pregnancy.

Drinking alcohol

Alcohol has far-reaching consequences for the fetus long past the moment of conception, so cutting out alcohol before trying to get pregnant and avoiding it like the plague after getting pregnant are essential for your partner. It won't hurt you, either. Heavy drinking, defined as three or more drinks a day for a guy, can decrease sperm quantity and quality. And a drink doesn't have to be hard liquor; one beer is a drink.

Using drugs

Two commonly used drugs can affect male fertility:

>> Marijuana lowers testosterone levels in males, which isn't good in the baby-making biz because testosterone is the male hormone responsible for male sexual functioning and sperm production. Sperm counts are lower and sperm are less motile in men who use marijuana regularly.

>> Anabolic steroids suppress testosterone production and can cause irreversible damage to the sperm production line. Avoid them at all costs.

Maintaining an (un)healthy weight

Being overweight is a huge problem — one that's getting bigger all the time. Around 20 percent of women of childbearing age in the United States are obese. Overweight women may not ovulate, and if they don't ovulate, they can't get pregnant. One Australian study showed that obese women were only half as likely to get pregnant as normal-weight women.

However, being underweight can also interfere with ovulation. Overall, 12 percent of infertility issues are related to being over- or underweight. Fortunately, either losing or gaining weight in these cases results in pregnancy 70 percent of the time.

Issues that may never have crossed your mind

Sometimes, behaviors you may never have considered can negatively affect your chances of pregnancy. Here are a few:

>> **Douching:** Washing or cleaning out the vagina using water or an over-the-counter solution is referred to as *douching*.

Although between one-third to one-half of childbearing age women do it, it's not only unnecessary but also potentially harmful. Women who douche are 73 percent more likely to have pelvic inflammatory disease, which can seriously damage the fallopian tubes and increases the chance of ectopic pregnancy by about the same percentage.

WARNING

Because you want your partner around for a long time, remind her of this statistic: Women who douche are 80 percent more likely to develop cervical cancer.

>> **Not sitting on the couch enough:** No, not really — some exercise is definitely good for you. But some sports, like bicycling, may cause testicular damage from the pressure of the bike seat. Women who exercise too heavily may stop having periods (called *amenorrhea*), and good luck getting pregnant without them.

>> **Spending time in hot tubs and other heat sources:** Hot tubs, tight underwear, saunas, steam rooms, and anything else that raises the temperature of the testicles is bad for the boys. Hot tubs may also damage eggs and increase miscarriage rates, so neither of you should be lolling in the hot tub.

Keeping Sex from Becoming a Chore

As unfathomable as it seems, sex while trying to conceive isn't always fun. Couples often begin to feel a sense of duty and pressure when they segue from spontaneity to planning exactly when to have sex to increase chances of conception. Monitoring rises in body temperature, charting mucus, and even lying down afterward to give the semen time to do its job are just a few of the unromantic actions that can take your sex life from crackin' to clinical.

Pleasure may take a back seat to the goal of having a baby, and nothing takes the "sexy" out of sex faster than making it feel like work. In fact, if the sex becomes solely about trying to conceive, you may begin to feel a bit like a sperm-producing machine that's only needed during ovulation, and performance issues can arise (no pun intended).

TIP

If for some reason conception takes a while, this feeling will only increase as you both grow impatient. If you begin to suffer these feelings, share them with your partner immediately. Plan "sex dates" that don't revolve around her ovulation time and discuss ways to create a more relaxing and less stressful romantic environment.

Choosing the best time for conception

When we talk about the best time for conception, we're not talking about the phase of the moon or the alignment of the stars; we're talking about planning to have sex at certain times to increase the odds that you'll hit the day when an egg is present and ready to be fertilized. Why do you have to plan? Well, not all women have 28-day menstrual cycles — the average menstrual cycle is 38 to 35 days — and ovulation doesn't always occur on day 14 of the cycle.

Ovulation does, however, always occur 14 days before the next period is due, or, to be more accurate, your partner's period starts 14 days after ovulation occurs. You can figure out the best timing for your conception efforts in several ways, which we explore in the following sections.

TIP

The countless apps available for both iOS and Android devices that allow women to track their cycles, predict ovulation days, and help determine when they're most fertile can simplify matters. Better still, the more info your partner enters into the app, the smarter it gets about exactly when she should put down that phone and hop into bed with you. Tracking cycles with an app is a lot more sophisticated than tracking them with a boring old calendar, and it could be more fun and effective to boot.

Monitoring ovulation with a kit

Predicting ovulation doesn't take mind-reading abilities. Simple observation and a few ovulation predictor kits (OPKs) from the pharmacy are all you need to pinpoint the big day. OPKs determine the rise in luteinizing hormone (LH) that occurs just before egg release. Your partner urinates into a cup, dips the test stick into the urine, and reads the results.

WARNING

The only drawback to OPKs is that women who have high levels of LH normally, like women in or near menopause and women with PCOS, may not get accurate results.

Watching for physical signs of ovulation

Your partner may also be able to tell when ovulation occurs by these signs:

» Cervical mucus becomes more copious, thinner, and more slippery and stretchy as ovulation approaches.

» She may have *mittelschmerz,* a pain on the left or right side as the egg releases from the ovary.

» Her temperature drops slightly right before ovulation and rises afterward.

You can track ovulation by keeping a monthly temperature chart, but doing so can be a real pain because your partner has to take her temperature first thing in the morning, before she gets out of bed, and when she uses the bathroom or has a cup of coffee.

Catching ovulation with a regular visit

If you don't want to closely monitor ovulation, you can take the easy way and simply have sex on a frequent, regular schedule. Medical practitioners seem to have differing opinions on how much sex is enough when you're trying to get pregnant. Some say every other day helps build up a good supply of sperm; some say every day is okay starting a few days before ovulation and continuing (if you're not dead yet) until the day after ovulation. Masturbation has the same effect on your sperm supply as having sex, so put that on the shelf for now and save the sperm for baby-making.

TIP

The most sensible schedule suggests having sex every other day, all month if you're up for it, starting right after her period ends. Because sperm live for up to five days, having sex the day before or the day of ovulation gives you a good shot at fertilization, and if you're aiming for every other day, you're bound to hit one or the other.

Scheduling sex: The do's and don'ts

Just because you've written sex down on your calendar doesn't mean it's just another obligation that eats up your time and lacks excitement. After all, this appointment has a far bigger upside than the average visit to the dentist.

TIP

Because you have only a few ideal times each month to conceive, you need to make time for sex on those days, which requires planning. Follow these dos and don'ts to make sure your sex life doesn't suffer for the sake of conception.

>> ***Do* put sex on your calendar.** Believe it or not, looking forward to intercourse all week can be very exciting. Verbal foreplay leading up to intercourse only increases the excitement.

>> ***Do* plan a date that night if possible to make it a full-fledged romantic evening.** Making it just about the sex increases your pressure to perform.

>> ***Do* engage in foreplay.** On TV and in movies, you often see the ovulating woman demand sex the minute her body temperature leads her to believe it's the best time. Make sure to keep it romantic and intimate. Some light massage, touching, and kissing should do the trick.

>> ***Do* mix it up.** Remember that although some positions are supposed to be better when you're trying to conceive, that doesn't mean you have to stay in the same one the whole time.

>> ***Do* keep it spontaneous.** Knowing the exact date you're going to have sex doesn't mean the setting has to stay the same. Play music, light candles, take a warm bath (not too hot — remember, you don't want to overheat the boys!), or even play out a fantasy if your partner is onboard.

>> ***Do* help make the aftermath enjoyable.** Your partner may want to elevate her legs and stay in bed for a while after intercourse to give the semen the best chance to stay put. Help her elevate her legs, and then put on her favorite show or read to her from a book. Don't just get up and leave her alone.

>> ***Do* have unscheduled sex.** Letting nature run its course every once in a while is okay, even when your road to conception is more like driving in bumper-to-bumper traffic than the autobahn. After ejaculation, sperm can live in a woman's reproductive tract for up to five days.

>> ***Don't* try too hard.** Sex carries its own set of complex, anxiety-inducing expectations, but now that the expectations include creating a baby, the pressure can become downright overwhelming. If you experience performance issues, either

mental or physical, due to the stress of the moment, talk it out with your partner. You won't do anyone a favor by having sex as if you're taking the SAT.

>> *Don't* **talk about the baby.** Unless talking about getting her pregnant is a turn-on to your partner, keep the baby discussion out of the sex equation. Although trying to have a baby does indeed require sex, talking about getting her pregnant while engaging in intercourse likely won't set your bedroom on fire.

>> *Don't* **drink before you have sex.** Alcohol can cause performance issues, and the last thing you want to do is let your partner down because you had one too many beers.

>> *Don't* **assume your partner isn't interested in both pleasure and conception.** In fact, studies show that women who orgasm have a greater chance of conceiving than those who don't.

>> *Don't* **make her laugh afterward.** Keeping a sense of humor during sex is always a good thing, but keep the comedy to a minimum after you ejaculate. Laughing tenses muscles that cause the semen to come out, reducing the chance of conception.

Taking a Brief yet Important Look at Infertility

Infertility is an issue that affects more than 7 million people in the United States, but not getting pregnant within a month or two doesn't necessarily mean you're infertile. Couples under the age of 35 are diagnosed with infertility following 12 months of attempted reproduction without achieving a pregnancy.

Knowing the facts about infertility

Imagine 100 average couples under the age of 35 trying to get pregnant. The following outcomes are expected:

>> 75 couples are pregnant within a year.

>> 10 couples are pregnant after two years of trying without medical intervention.

>> 10 couples need treatment from an infertility specialist in order to conceive.

Causes of infertility can be complex and often hard to diagnose. Some are related to the health and lifestyle issues we cover in the earlier "Evaluating Health to Get Ready for Parenthood" section. Despite treatments and diagnostic practices that primarily focus on women, the statistics paint a different picture:

>> One-third of infertility is diagnosed as female-factor.

>> One-third of infertility is diagnosed as male-factor.

>> Between 10 and 15 percent of infertility cases are diagnosed as a combination of male- and female-factor.

>> About 20 percent of infertility cases are unexplained following diagnostic testing.

For women, the main causes of infertility are

>> **Ovulatory disorders:** No ovulation or ovulation on an irregular schedule.

>> **Tubal disorders:** Fallopian tubes are blocked or have an infection that interferes with ovulation or sperm travel.

>> **Uterine issues:** Fibroids and polyps (growths that can cause blockages) or an abnormally shaped uterus.

For men, the main causes of infertility are

>> **Low sperm count:** Not enough guys to get the job done.

>> **Decreased sperm motility:** The sperm has trouble moving forward into the fallopian tubes.

>> **Abnormally shaped sperm:** Abnormal shapes usually indicate chromosomal abnormalities.

>> **No sperm present in the ejaculate:** A blockage somewhere in the reproductive tract or hormonal disorders can cause an absence of sperm.

Checking on potential problems when nothing's happening

For many couples, the first step toward fixing infertility is admitting that you're having a problem. It's not an easy revelation to make because it means that at some basic level, your bodies are failing you. Fertility problems aren't fair, they're not fun, and they can be cause for a wide array of emotions, frustrations, and outright anger.

The good news is that this is an age in which getting pregnant doesn't have to be a simple matter of the birds and the bees. Throw in a doctor or two, and you may be well on your way to conceiving in no time flat.

If you're not getting pregnant after a few months, especially if your partner is older than 35, it's time to check things out — for both of you. For her, this may involve the following tests:

>> **Blood tests:** These check hormone levels, including follicle stimulating hormone, or FSH. FSH levels are normally below 9 mIU/ml on day two or three of the menstrual cycle; higher levels indicate decreased ovarian reserve and the possible need for medical intervention.

>> **Hysterosalpingogram (HSG):** This test injects dye into the uterus through a catheter placed through the cervix. The dye outlines the shape of the uterus and fallopian tubes. HSG can identify blockages in or dilation of the fallopian tubes that interferes with embryo transport, and it also shows fibroids and polyps in the uterus, which may interfere with implantation.

>> **Hysteroscopy:** This test uses a hysteroscope, a sort of mini-telescope, to evaluate the uterus for fibroids or polyps. Small fibroids and polyps can also be removed at the time of the test.

For you, it's a quick trip to the urologist for a full physical, blood work, and a semen analysis. This is the only way you can find out your sperm count and the quality and motility of your sperm.

Semen collection at a medical center is just as uncomfortable as it sounds, but it must be done. Just keep your expectations to a minimum and forget all those movie scenes showing posh rooms, dirty magazines, and absolute privacy. If you have to produce in the doctor's office or a hospital lab, you may very well find your-self in a bathroom, unable to escape the distractions of screaming children and the witty banter of the nursing staff outside the door.

Some offices allow specimens to be collected in the privacy of your home and then delivered to the lab within an hour. Ask your doctor about this alternative, as well as any special instructions for collection and transportation.

Working through it when your partner needs treatment

Some female fertility issues are easily dealt with by simply taking a pill that induces ovulation. But female infertility can also lead to daily injections of fertility medications, uncomfortable vaginal ultrasounds to assess egg development, painful surgeries to remove fibroids or repair damaged fallopian tubes, and frequent blood tests.

Fixing female fertility issues can be a drawn-out affair that combines inconvenient and uncomfortable procedures with medications that manipulate hormones, a difficult combination if there ever was one. And if your partner suddenly views childbearing as a woman's most important prerogative, her seeming inability to accomplish it and subsequent emotions can make fertility treatment a tough time for both of you.

Even though you may have your own stresses when dealing with fertility issues, remember that at least you aren't dealing with a barrage of excess hormones, and keep your cool if conversations get complicated.

Exploring solutions when your sperm don't stack up

A count of less than 20 million is considered a low sperm count. Although that may sound like a large number, due to the number of abnormal sperm in the normal sample and the distance required to reach the egg, it takes a lot of good sperm to achieve conception.

Sperm is produced on a cycle, so the semen you produce now actually was created three months ago. If your sperm count is low, start thinking back to what was going on three months prior. An illness, medications, or a hot-tub vacation may be the culprit.

Learning the components

What exactly makes a semen specimen normal? The following guidelines from the World Health Organization (WHO) are deemed the ideal for baby making:

» **Volume:** About 1.5 to 5 milliliters of semen should be present in a single ejaculate, equaling about a teaspoon.

» **Concentration:** Strength in numbers is key. You need at least 20 million sperm per milliliter of ejaculate to hit the normal range.

» **Motility:** For every man, an average ejaculate contains dead, slow, and immobile sperm. However, at least 40 percent of your sperm in a single sample should be moving.

» **Morphology:** Shape is also important to reproduction, and the lab technician examining your sample takes a close look at how many of your swimmers are normally shaped. A normal amount of normally shaped sperm is considered to be anything above 30 percent.

» **Trajectory:** Graded on a 4-point scale, this test determines how many of your sperm are moving forward. A normal score is 2+.

» **White blood cells:** Too many white blood cells can indicate an infection in your groin. A passing grade is no more than 0 to 5 per power field.

» **Hyperviscosity:** Your semen sample should liquefy within 30 minutes after ejaculation. If it takes longer, it reduces the chances for sperm to swim before being expelled from the vagina.

» **pH:** Like an AA battery, your semen needs to be alkaline to avoid making the vagina too acidic and, ultimately, killing the sperm.

A semen analysis also evaluates the following:

» **Head quality:** The head of the sperm contains all the genetic material, so if the head is misshapen, it won't be capable of fertilizing an egg.

» **Midsection malaise:** Believe it or not, this part of your sperm contains fructose, which gives your sperm energy to swim. If the levels are low, it can account for slow swimmers.

>> **Tail troubles:** Much like a fish, a good tail is required for the sperm to swim forward. If too many of your sperm have no tail, multiple tails, or tails that are coiled or kinked, they won't reach their destination.

A low sperm count may have you feeling, well, downright low. Feeling embarrassed is completely natural but also completely unnecessary. Infertility has no correlation to a man's masculinity, nor does it have anything to do with the size of his penis. Having a low sperm count is no different from having asthma — it's a medical condition that requires treatment.

Because sperm counts are created months out, you need to have a follow-up semen analysis to see whether the issue is corrected by lifestyle changes. Although you won't be in a rush to do it all again anytime soon, whether your results are good or bad, schedule a follow-up analysis four to six weeks after the first one to get a better, more complete picture.

Identifying and treating the causes

The most common cause of a low sperm count is a *varicocele*, an abnormality in the vein in your scrotum that drains the testicles. Varicoceles can cause decreased fertility in the following ways:

>> Increasing temperature in the testes

>> Decreasing blood flow around the testicles

>> Slowing sperm production and motility

Varicoceles are treatable in the following ways:

>> **Surgery:** An outpatient procedure during which an incision is made just above the groin and the swollen vein is "tied off." Recovery takes seven to ten days and requires minimal activity and no heavy lifting. Risks are minimal and include infection, nerve injury, and the collection of fluid around the testicles.

>> **Radiographic embolization:** Also an outpatient procedure, this requires the insertion of a catheter through the femoral vein in the groin. Dye is injected to show where the problem is located and, when isolated, it's blocked so blood flow to that vein stops.

Other less common male–fertility issues include the following:

>> **Hormone imbalances:** Medications to adjust hormone levels may improve sperm quantity.

>> **Chromosomal abnormalities:** One such problem is sperm that lack part of the Y chromosome, which is the male chromosome. *In vitro fertilization* (IVF) and *intracytoplasmic sperm injection* (ICSI), where the best-looking sperm are injected directly into your partner's egg in the lab, can help overcome abnormal sperm issues. (See the following section for more info.)

>> **History of cancer:** Having treatment for cancer, including lymphoma and testicular cancer, can kill or damage sperm. Many men freeze sperm before undergoing cancer treatment for this reason.

>> **Various diseases:** Diabetes, sickle cell disease, and kidney and liver diseases can cause problems. Treatment depends on your individual issues.

Even if your ejaculate has no sperm at all, a procedure called a *sperm aspiration* in conjunction with an IVF cycle may be able to remove sperm directly from the testicles.

Examining new developments in infertility treatments

Researchers are always looking for the next big thing in treating infertility. Many of the most recent research has centered around eggs, namely freezing them and producing them.

Putting eggs on ice

Freezing sperm is old hat in the infertility world. Embryos can also be quite successfully frozen and thawed years later. Eggs, however, have had less success in the freezing department because they contain more water than embryos or sperm. Enter *vitrification*, a kind of "flash freezing" technique many fertility clinics now use to preserve eggs for later use.

Although egg freezing doesn't have a lot of application for most couples, it can be a valuable technique if your partner has to undergo treatments that could seriously damage her ovaries or if a disease such as endometriosis is destroying her ovaries.

If you're not quite ready for parenthood but your partner is feeling the effects of the ever-advancing biological clock, egg freezing can buy you the time you need to travel the world, advance your careers, or climb Mt. Everest before settling down to parenthood.

WARNING

Even though some fertility clinics claim high success rates freezing eggs, the proof is in the pudding, so to speak. You won't necessarily know whether it worked until you actually try to use frozen eggs, perhaps years later, when it's too late to go back for more. In most cases, fertilizing the eggs and freezing them as embryos has a better chance of success down the road.

Circumventing early menopause

Research that's still in preliminary stages may find a way to make ovaries produce eggs in women who are in *premature ovarian failure* (POF), a condition where menopause that occurs early (before age 40) results in a shutdown of egg production.

Researchers have removed the ovaries in women experiencing POF, cut the ovary into sections, and then treated them with drugs to block a protein that prevents egg follicles from growing normally. The ovary fragments are transplanted back near their original site, where the egg follicles then begin to grow. This technique could eventually help women whose reproductive days are cut abnormally short.

Deciding how far to go to get pregnant

Deciding what steps you're willing to take to get pregnant is easier after you have a better understanding of the infertility issues you and your partner face. Most infertility treatments can be quite expensive, so check with your insurance company to see what it covers.

TIP

Making decisions on infertility treatments based on finances seems heartless, but if your insurance doesn't cover a treatment or medicines, you could be looking at bills in the thousands of dollars.

The most common procedures to aid in pregnancy are the following:

>> **Intrauterine insemination (IUI):** A lab tech takes your sperm sample, pulls out the best of the best, and adds it to a saline

solution, which is then inserted past your partner's cervix. This gives the sperm a far shorter distance to travel and a greater chance for success.

>> **In vitro fertilization (IVF):** Sperm meets egg in a lab, and then the fertilized embryo is placed into the womb. Fertilization can take place by either placing a concentrated semen sample in a dish with the egg or via *intracytoplasmic sperm injection,* or ICSI. In ICSI, a single sperm is injected directly into a mature egg. Even with ICSI, fertilization may not occur, because the egg or sperm may be chromosomally abnormal, which in some cases isn't evident just by looking at them.

TIP

Try not to make too many long-term decisions about how far you're willing to go because undergoing fertility treatments is like riding a roller coaster — after you're on, it's harder to get off. Especially when it feels like your baby could be just around the next corner. Make decisions month to month and procedure to procedure to avoid stress and allow for an open, ever-changing dialogue with your partner.

Sharing Your Decision to Have a Baby

Deciding to try to have a baby is a very big, very exciting step for most couples, and increasingly it's something many people choose to share with a select group of friends and family members. News of an expanding family is usually met with joy, cheers, and even a few inappropriate jokes about your sex life. But although sharing good news is fun, you also need to be prepared for people in the know to ask nosy questions and offer unwanted advice — all of which becomes less fun if it takes longer than expected to conceive.

Considering the pros and cons of spilling the beans

REMEMBER

Sharing the news means you're turning your quest to have a baby into a mini-reality show that your loved ones are going to closely follow. Having a well of support during this time can be great, but having your mom and dad hinting for info every time you talk on the phone can also feel intrusive.

If getting pregnant takes longer than expected, you're also setting yourself up to have to deal with the inevitable questions about the delay. On the plus side, if you and your partner must deal with infertility, you need all the support you can muster.

Just make sure you're both ready to continue sharing information and dealing with questions from the people you tell. Trust us when we say that after their curiosity is piqued and their excitement sparked, there's no turning back, especially for a first-time grandmother-to-be.

Handling unsolicited advice about reproduction

You may think you have a handle on lovemaking, but after you announce to the world that you're trying to have a baby, it may seem like all the folks in your life suddenly morph into Dr. Phil.

Now that reproduction is fodder for morning news programs and countless blogs and Internet sites, more people have more sound bites and nuggets of wisdom to offer you and your partner than ever before. If your mother tells your partner she shouldn't be eating that grilled hamburger because the *Today* show said so, or if she tells you that you really should be wearing boxers rather than briefs, you may find yourself at wit's end before you even make it to the bedroom.

TIP

If your loved ones start interfering or offering advice that you don't want, thank them for their excitement and interest, but reassure them that you have the situation under control. Remind them that people have been having babies forever and let them know that being bombarded with all this information — be it from them, the TV, or the newspaper — stresses out you and your partner, and that can decrease your chances of conception.

Not all unsolicited advice is about the act of having sex. Some people may think you're too young or too old to have kids. Your parents may chime in about how expensive kids are, implying that you're not financially ready to have a baby. Perhaps your stressed-out brother (and father of three) tells you to enjoy your freedom while you still can.

REMEMBER

Whether somebody thinks you're too immature to be a father because you still play video games or that your wife's job is too demanding for her to be a mother, remember that the only voices that matter are yours and your partner's.

Chapter **3**

Non-Traditional Dadhood

N ot all dads are part of a mom, dad and baby makes three scenario.Maybe you don't have a partner. Or maybe you do — but you're both guys. In today's world of reproductive science, you can become a dad even if you're short a few eggs. There's always a way.

That's not to say becoming a dad under these circumstances is necessarily easy, and it's often not cheap. And you'll certainly be faced with more decisions to make than the traditional Mom, Dad, and Baby household. But in this chapter, we help by walking you through the decisions you'll have to make about egg donors, carriers, and who gets to know the details.

On the other hand, you might be part of a traditional family— most of the time. But, for whatever reason — maybe you work on an oil rig, are in the military, or have decided to take a year off and live in a commune to find yourself — you can't be home for all or part of the pregnancy and birth. Although we can't magically whisk you home for all the exciting parts, in this chapter we can show you how to stay involved and help your partner feel your support even if you're half a world away.

Becoming a Two Dad or Dad Alone Family

If you're a guy, you can supply half your baby's DNA, but you still need someone to supply the other half. This is true whether you're a single guy alone or if you have a partner who's also a guy. In either case, your first order of business will be to find someone who can donate an egg to you. Unfortunately, donating eggs isn't nearly as simple as donating sperm, so finding a friend or someone altruistic enough to donate to you might be difficult. In that case, many fertility clinics have egg-donor programs in which carefully screened women of childbearing age go through the donation process in exchange for a monetary fee.

The legality of this gets tricky from one state to the other, so make sure you know what your state's regulations on egg donation are before going too far into the process.

If just finding the right egg were all you needed to do, this process wouldn't be so difficult. But, you also need someone to carry the baby for nine months and give birth to them. You also want to make very sure — as sure as is humanly possible — that the person you choose will want to give your baby to you at the end of nine months. States have regulations on surrogacy as well, but this is the kind of sticky mess you want to do everything in your power to avoid.

Who's supplying the egg? The sperm? The womb?

There are more than a few moving parts to coordinate in this type of baby-making scenario. If you're a couple, you and your partner need to decide whose sperm is going to be used. You also need to determine whether your egg donor and your gestational (pregnancy) baby carrier are going to be the same person. This is a complicated question that deserves some really hard thinking on your part.

If you're using a relative as egg donor, you may feel fairly comfortable using her as the carrier also. After all, you probably have a reasonably good relationship and you know where she lives if there are any problems. If your relative or friend feels funny giving you her eggs, you could use an anonymous egg donor and someone you know as gestational carrier. Or the other way around. You can see why this takes some serious thought.

It's a little trickier still if you don't know your egg donor or gestational carrier. In this case, choosing a separate egg donor an a gestational carrier can be a prudent decision. The carrier won't have a biological tie to your baby, which could prevent legal issues if something goes wrong.

Giving up a few good sperm

If you're a single guy alone, identifying the person responsible for supplying the sperm is pretty straightforward — that would be you. If you have a male partner, this question becomes a bit more complicated. Does one of you already have children? Does one of you have better sperm than the other? Is one of you more invested in the whole idea of having kids? Talking through these issues to make a decision can take time, so don't rush it. You can also mix your sperm together and let nature make the decision.

Sperm donation is simple and not very time consuming. Some centers let you donate ahead and have sperm on ice waiting for the day it's needed. Others let you collect the sperm at home, as long as you can bring it to the center within a reasonable time frame. The center will concentrate the sperm and optimize it for fertilization.

Understanding the egg-donation process

Egg donation is not a simple process, at leasy not compared to sperm donation. The egg donor has to take powerful ovary stimulating medications, usually by injection, for 10 days or so, sometimes longer, depending on the clinic's protocol. The egg donor must undergo a number of ultrasounds, and her blood word must be monitored frequently to make sure she's producing the right number of eggs — not too many and not too few. The ins and outs of in vitro fertilization are beyond the scope of this book; check out "Pregnancy for Dummies" if you want to know exactly what egg donation involves.

Some fertility clinics have an egg-donor program and can match you up with a donor. As with a sperm donor, you can choose someone who has characteristics similar to yours — or exactly the opposite, if that's what you're looking for. There are also businesses that will match you with an egg donor, if your clinic doesn't have a donor program. Anonymous egg donors and the companies that find them for you both need to be paid, usually in amounts in excess of $10,000. If you're using a known donor, you might have to pay for her medical expenses, if she isn't covered for fertility treatment.

Looking at the legalities of surrogacy

The term *surrogate* usually refers to a woman who is genetically related to the child — that is, her eggs are used — who also carries the pregnancy. Whether you're asking a family member or looking for someone you don't know to act as a surrogate, it's vital to know your state's surrogacy laws before getting too far into the process. Being a surrogate involves a nine month commitment that can include taking medication to assure a healthy pregnancy, coordination of her menstrual cycle with that of the egg donor, frequent monitoring, and dealing with an anxious parent-to-be (you).Some states don't allow surrogacy or offer no legal protection if a legal battle ensues down the road. The following states are, in 2022, not surrogacy-friendly:

>> Michigan

>> New York

The following states allow compenstated surrogacy and are generally considered surrogacy-friendly:

>> California

>> Connecticut

>> Delaware

>> District of Columbia

>> Maine

>> New Hampshire

>> Nevada

>> Oregon

>> Rhode Island

>> Washington

The rest of the states have more complicated regulations, some of which may be favorable in some aspects of surrogacy and some not so favorable. In any case, a lawyer well-versed in reproductive law is essential to this road of parenthood. They'll be up on the most recent changes and can advise you accordingly.

The American Academy of Adoption and Assisted Reproductive Technology Attorneys (AAARTA) maintains a list, found at www.aaarta.org.

Involving a family member in egg donation or carrying the baby

Having one side of the family more involved than the other in your baby-making project can have consequences down the road. Keeping boundaries in place in such an emotional situation can also lead to problems, sometimes for years to come. Families, unlike friends or acquaintances, are generally around for the long haul, and your child will likely be involved with them for most of their lives. However, families can and do make this work, and it can be the best of all possible worlds if the stars align and your relatives are all solidly behind you.

If you're a gay couple, both of your family's genetics can be in the mix if one of you has a sister willing to donate the egg. (Obviously, the guy whose sister donates the egg doesn't donate the sperm.) This would be the best-case scenario — everyone has a genetic claim — but altruistic sisters may be in short supply in your families. Or the whole idea might just not sit right with one of you.

Monetary issues can also complicate the issue of using a family member; do you offer them a financial stipend or will your relative or friend simply want to do this out of the goodness of their heart? How "legal" do you need to be in terms of a contract? It's always advisable to draw up a legal document to protect all parties down the road, no matter how unnecessary it seems at the time or how close you are to your family member. Life circumstances change, the question of whether or not to disclose all the details to your future child or other people can suddenly become important, or the donor who thought she'd have no problem giving away her eggs discovers after the baby is born with her eyes and nose that it matters way more than she thought it would.

Both egg-donation and surrogacy programs generally require physicals and possibly genetic testing. Some also require a mental health consultation. Unexpected issues can be uncovered during testing, which could eliminate your potential family member or friend as a donor or carrier.

Finding a friend who's willing to donate or carry

Asking a friend to go through egg donation or even to be your gestational carrier is another possible option, whether you're single or partnered. The plusses include having a known entity to work with over the next nine-plus months — although this can be a good thing or a bad thing — and having more access to the pregnant person than you will likely have with a paid surrogate. Having a friend rather than a family member might also add a useful extra layer of emotional distance between you and the surrogate if things start to get complicated. After all, it's much easier for a friend to keep their emotional distance than it is for a family member, who's at hand for every major holiday and birthday.

If you're involving a friend — even a really good friend — in your future child's creation, it's very important to make sure all your legal Ps and Qs are in order. Friends break up more often than families do, and keeping this part of your friendship as more business than sentiment is essential.

Acting as a gestational carrier requires a huge time commitment, as well as a possible loss of income for a time period. Asking someone you know to be a carrier is asking a lot, but even so, a friend or relative who loves being pregnant — it's really best if your carrier has already had a child — may jump at the chance.

Working with an agency

If you want to have a paid egg donor or gestational carrier, that is, someone that you don't know, you'll need to find an agency to work with. In some cases, this could be a local fertility clinic. Additionally, some agencies are devoted strictly to matching egg donors with recipients, or finding gestatonal carriers or surrogates. Lawyers who specialize in reproductive law may also work with certain agencies to find intended parents the right match. You can also look into agencies that work in other countries with women who donate eggs, act as gestational carriers, or serve as surrogates. Although this may be cheaper than working with an agency at home, a greater number of risks may be involved. In such cases, doing your research and having a solid legal plan in place is essential.

Drawing up a contract

The agency you choose to work with may already have a lawyer that handles all their legal paperwork. Although that makes things simpler, it doesn't mean you can't also have your own lawyer look over the contracts. Some issues that the contract should cover include, among others:

>> Monetary compensation

>> Insurance coverage, yours and the carrier's

>> Contact information, including whether you'll be able to be present at doctor's appointments, the delivery, or other times during the pregnancy, in the case of a carrier or surrogate.

>> Creation of an escrow agent to handle money transfers between you.

>> What will happen if the baby has any health issues discovered during the pregnancy

>> Plans for the baby if your relationship dissolves for any reason, or if you die (yes, grim but essential)

>> Nutrition, travel, and lifestyle guidelines for your carrier, including how much say you'll have in any or all of these things

You'll also need to file a court order that establishes your child's parentage so that your name can be placed on the birth certificate. This is called a *pre-birth order*. If you don't have this done, you may need to adopt your own child after she's born.

Deciding how involved you'll be in the pregnancy

How involved you'll be during the pregnancy should be spelled out in your legal documents. However, things can change during the pregnancy: You and your carrier may really hit it off and find yourselves going out to dinner once a week and calling each other on a regular basis. Or you may find that you're not crazy about each other and keep contact to the bare minimum. If you're dealing with a family member, you probably already have established routines for how often you see each other. In either case, realize that awkwardness wll probably be part of this new relationship.

Becoming comfortable with a stranger

It's always a little strained when you're getting to know someone new. It's especially awkward when that person is carrying your child. This is something you really have to feel your way through; a legal document only covers so much. As the pregnancy goes on, you may feel more comfortable with each other and find that talking about constipation, swollen feet, and sex is more natural than you thought it would be. Or not.

It's important to let your carrier take the lead on this, though. If she's not comfortable letting you in on all the details of her personal life, you'll have to accept that. If she wants to overshare and you're really not that into knowing all the details of what she did last night, you may have to grin and bear it in order to maintain a good relationship. Don't expect to be best friends right out of the gate. And don't push for too much when you're still basically strangers. Hopefully, over the next nine months, you'll work out a comfortable balance between friendship and business relationship.

Maintaining boundaries with a friend or family member

Friends or family members can present a different sort of problem. With friends and family, you most likely have already set some boundaries in place in your lives, even though you might not think of it that way. When that person is carrying your baby, the rules may shift, sometimes to the point that one or the other of you isn't comfortable with it. For example, your partner's sister might not want both of you — or either of you — at her doctor's appointments. Your best friend might not want to share all the details of her sex life with you now that she's pregnant with your baby — even if she always did before.

Boundary setting won't just involve your carrier. Your parents, other siblings and other friends may want to put their oars in the water and tell you how you should be handling things or what they think about the situation. Parents, in particular, often can't seem to help but share their opinions about what's going on in your life, especially when a new grandchild is in the offing. Think this through ahead of time, considering what you already know about your family or friends, and set limits, at least in your mind, on how much interference couched as advice will be acceptable.

Being Involved When You're Not Able to Be Around

Sometimes, even in traditional mom-dad-and-baby families, you aren't able to be around during a pregnancy. Your job might take you to another part of the country, or out of the country altogether. Dads today expect to play a much bigger role as a support person and active participant during pregnancy than they did a generation ago. Being unable to be as involved as you want can make for a difficult pregnancy, for both of you.

Fortunately, it's never been easier to stay involved when you can't be there physically, in most cases. No, it's not the same as actually being there, but it's better than it was 20 years ago, when today's stay-in-touch technology was just a gleam in someone's eye. With a little work, you can stay in the loop and involved during a long-distance pregnancy.

Keeping up to date when you're out of town — or country

No doubt you already have the basics covered — setting up accounts on Facetime, Skype, Whatsapp, or Zoom, if you can. If you're a servicemember, video chats are difficult, if not impossible. The timing can be off, especially if you're on the other side of the world. You're also presumably away to do a job, a job that may not be very flexible as far as sitting in the front of the phone or laptop goes. Getting your schedules synched can take some doing, especially if your partner is also still working on the other side of the world at a job without a lot of flexibility. And for some assignments, particularly in the military, you may be completely out of touch for weeks at a time.

The best thing to do in this type of situation is for your baby to be born at a time when you're not fathoms under the sea and completely out of contact. But babies don't always come when we plan them, which, if this is your situation, you're undoubtedly all too aware.

One of the best things you can do in this type of situation is to make sure your partner has a lot of support at home; in some cases, this might mean having her stay with her family or having family members stay with her while you're gone. She gets to make the decisions as to what kind of help she wants and for how long. Even if you and her mom are at constant odds at the best of times, this is the time where you just have to deal with having her mom, sister or best friend knowing more about what's going on at home than you do.

After you've helped line up a support team, take care of as many of the household tasks ahead of time. Replace things that might need replacing before you leave, create an up-to-date list of repair people, get the car's routine maintenance out of the way, and generally take everything you can off your partner's shoulders before you leave.

It's also important for you to keep up with what goes on during different months of pregnancy. This book gives you a lot of info on what happens during each stage of pregnancy, and you can find other books that go into greater month-by-month detail, such as *Pregnancy For Dummies* by Joanne Stone and Keith Eddleman (John Wiley & Sons). Knowing what's going on at different stages allows you to ask relevant questions and to empathize with what your partner's experiencing at different points of pregnancy.

Dealing with the frustrations of long-distance pregnancy

Being separated during such an important time will be hard on both of you, but your partner is the one dealing with hormonal changes that can make going through pregnancy alone really difficult. Although you're probably feeling the strain of not being there as well, remember that she's dealing with much, much more. Some guys don't want to hear the details of her pregnancy, baby shower, doctor's appointments, and so on because it reminds them of everything they're missing. If you're one of those guys, try really hard to overcome it. And although it's okay to mention how hard it is to be away at such a special time — your partner will probably be upset if it doesn't upset you, honestly — remember not to make it all about you.

The complex emotions of a far-away dad can be hard for a mom-to-be to understand, since she feels just as lonely and sad that you're apart at such an important time — and she's the one dealing with taking care of the house and herself, not to mention heartburn, swollen feet, and the inability to bend over.

Staying involved is more than just sitting in front of the camera while you talk. Although you don't need to write out a script before every video chat, keep a list of things that you want to ask about or talk to your partner about. It's easy to get caught up in the moment when you're chatting — and also hard to keep yourself present and ignoring everything that's going on around you — and you may end the chat without ever touching on all the things you really wanted to ask about. So, keep a list.

As hard as it can be at times, it's also important to stay present during your calls. Whether you're talking to each other every day or once a month, make sure you're totally there during your conversations. Obviously, no playing games on your phone while you're talking! And no talking with other people in the background, if you can manage it. Having other people around can hinder both of you from saying what you really want to say.

Last but not least, remember that this too will pass. Yes, it's a time you'll never be able to get back, and it's hard, but you're going to have years to spend with your new baby, and plenty of time to make it up to them — and to your partner, too.

2

The Final Countdown: Nine Months (or Less!) to Baby

Become an educated dad-to-be by reading about your baby's physical development throughout pregnancy so you can dazzle your partner with how much you know.

Participate in the fun parts of pregnancy — putting together a baby shower wish list, readying the nursery, and picking out a name.

Feel prepared in case things don't go according to expectations. Although the odds are certainly in your favor, things can and do go wrong in pregnancy.

Handle the emotional ups and downs of the final three months as the reality that dadhood is just around the corner truly sinks in.

Find out all about birthing options — what they are, how they'll affect your role as labor coach, and how to support the choices your partner makes.

Chapter **4**

Balancing Joy, Anxiety, and Nausea: The First Trimester

F ew new fathers-to-be actually pass out when they get the big news that there's a baby in their future, despite what you see on old TV shows. That's not to say you may not feel a bit blown away by the news, though. Whether you've been trying for ten years or just met your partner last month, hearing that you're about to be a dad is life-changing.

Early pregnancy is not without its physical, mental, and emotional challenges, and although mom bears the brunt of it, you can expect to experience a few symptoms, too. In this chapter, we tell you what happens in the first few months and help you adjust to one of the biggest events in your life.

Baby on Board: It's Official!

Nothing is more momentous than hearing the words, "It's positive! I'm pregnant!" If you've been trying to get pregnant for a while, these words are your cue to breathe a sigh of relief — your boys can swim! In fact, you may feel more relief than excitement at first. Trying to get pregnant can be quite stressful, as we discuss in Chapter 2, and the news that your worst fears can be put aside is reason for relief.

On the other hand, if this was a big "oops" on your part — and many pregnancies are, even in this day and age — your first reaction may be more like, "Oh . . . *heck*," or worse. Don't feel guilty if your first reaction is negative; most of the world's babies were an "Oh, heck" at one time. In many cases, pregnancy takes time to get used to.

THE LATEST IN PREGNANCY TESTS

Pregnancy tests have come a long way from your mom's day, when she had to carry a jug of urine into the doctor's office to have a pregnancy test done or offer up her arm for a blood test. Home pregnancy tests have been around for a few decades now, but they've gotten more sophisticated than ever in the last few years.

Although many still break the news with just a big plus or "thumbs up" sign (no, not really), others go a step further and estimate how many weeks pregnant you are. This isn't all that accurate because a woman's human chorionic gonadotropin (hCG) growth levels — the hormone pregnancy tests measure — go up at quite different rates. Twins or other multiples can also confound the issue because a multiple pregnancy usually results in higher-than-normal hCG levels. Sure, this type of test is fun, but the information it adds is limited, unless your partner has wildly irregular menstrual cycles. In any case, her first step is still to make an appointment with her OB/GYN, who can pin things down much more accurately with an ultrasound.

Reacting when your partner breaks the news

When your partner tells you the big news, try to mirror her reaction, at least outwardly. If her reaction is, "Oh . . . *heck*," you can go along in that vein also, at least for a minute or two. Remember, though, that she's gauging your reaction to the news, and if you act like having a baby is a huge imposition in your life, she'll be really upset, even if it *is* going to be a huge imposition and even if she just said the same thing five minutes before. Try to throw in a few encouraging statements about how you wanted kids eventually, how having a baby will be fun in the winter when there's nothing else to do, or whatever encouraging babble you can come up with at a stressful time.

Some women get very creative with their announcements, from filling the living room with balloons to baking a cake with a pair of booties inside. Just try not to choke on one, literally or figuratively. If she's gone all out to break the news, you can safely bet that she's really excited, so make sure to be as supportive as possible.

REMEMBER

Even if you've been trying to conceive forever, an initial reaction of fear isn't uncommon. Remember that your partner may also be feeling some sudden doubts and fears, and allow her to express them. Under no circumstances is "We spent $20,000 for fertility treatments and now you're not sure this is the right time?!" the right response to her concerns.

Making the announcement to friends and family

Deciding when to tell family and friends is tricky. On one hand, telling them on the first day of the missed period makes the pregnancy seem about 15 months long, and telling early means you'll need to go through the grief of telling everyone if a miscarriage occurs, which happens in around 20 percent of pregnancies.

On the other hand, you may have told people you're trying, and they, like you, may be obsessively counting the minutes until your partner can take a pregnancy test. If that's the case, saying, "Gee, we don't know yet; we forgot to do the test" is going to come across as a big insult, and "We've decided not to tell anyone" will probably get you thrown out of the will. If you've been going through fertility treatment, you may feel the need to tell your

WHEN YOU HAVE A HUNCH . . . AND SHE DOESN'T SEEM TO HAVE A CLUE

Moms-to-be aren't the only ones who can have premonitions about pregnancy. Sometimes the male partner — that's you, the one with the undeserved reputation for being obtuse at times about all things female — may suspect that your partner is pregnant before she does. Early pregnancy can have a host of symptoms, from extreme tiredness to forgetfulness, and if you notice these things before your partner does, don't be afraid to speak up. Also, if you haven't noticed the usual habits that go along with her period, you just may be on to something.

Don't ignore your gut instinct or the evidence, but do tread lightly. Inquire about the last time your partner had her period. Saying something as simple as, "Hey, I know this may sound kind of weird, and I'm sure I just missed it, but it seems like you haven't had your period in a long time." If your partner is very open-minded, just ask outright. Gauge the situation and your partner — just be honest and open about your suspicions because the last thing you want to say is, "I knew it!" if she does find out she's pregnant and you remained silent.

fertility friends right away, because they know exactly when your embryo transfer and pregnancy test took place.

If you've already had to deal with a miscarriage, you may be understandably more reluctant to tell people in the first trimester. Nearly all miscarriages occur in the first 12 weeks of pregnancy, and most of those occur before 8 weeks, so waiting until you're pretty sure the pregnancy is going well may be prudent.

Whenever and whoever you decide to tell, realize that keeping news this big to yourself is hard. Even if you and your partner make a solemn pact not to tell a soul until after the first ultrasound, don't be shocked and disappointed to find out she's already told her best friend, mother, and entire online support group. In fact, she may have told them before she told *you*. Be understanding and sheepishly admit you secretly told your parents, the guys at the gym, and half your coworkers, too.

WHEN TO TELL WORK

For you, letting your work know that you're a father-to-be may not be such a big deal because many workplaces still don't have any sort of daddy maternity plan. If yours does, though, let your boss know after the first three months, when you're reasonably sure things will go well with the pregnancy.

Overcoming your fears of being a father

You have a lot of time to get used to the idea of being a dad, so don't worry if you have a lot of fears at first. Even if you aren't sure you're ready to become a father, you'll be surprised how quickly you come around to the idea. Besides, the baby will be here before you know it, ready or not.

REMEMBER

It's important, however, to use this time to confront your fears about parenting. Spend time with the male role models from your past (and present) and use them as learning tools. Ask them what they did right, what they would change, and what advice they have for you when raising your own child. You may feel like you're the first father ever, but you don't need to reinvent the wheel when it comes to parenting. If you admire other people's skills, monitor and mimic their behaviors.

Working on overcoming your fatherhood fears is doubly important if the father in your life wasn't the best role model for the type of dad you want to be to your son or daughter. To attempt to come to terms with any wrongdoings your father may have committed, talk with a counselor or therapist, or even a trusted friend, about your relationship with your father and try to identify the mistakes you don't want to repeat. Talking about your experience with your own father can also help heal some of the emotional wounds. Being a father is hard work, and you don't want to wait until after the baby arrives to start overcoming your fears or past traumas.

Early Prenatal Care: Kicking Off a Nine-Month-Long Relationship

Finding the right practitioner to help birth your baby isn't as easy a decision as it once was. Even if your partner already has a gynecologist, she may not want her as a pregnancy practitioner, for whatever reason. Or her current doctor may not deliver at the facility where you want to deliver — especially if that facility is your own home or a birthing center. Or, possibly, she may worry that you won't care for her current doctor. Maybe he's incredibly good looking or brilliantly witty and charming.

Whatever the reason, your partner may find herself shopping for a new medical practitioner. Even if she doesn't, you'll find yourself in the sometimes uncomfortable position of getting to know her practitioner — and learning what it's like to sit in a room full of pregnant women, only one of whom you actually know. Not to mention the experience of going with her to the somewhat embarrassing vaginal ultrasound. Pregnancy brings lots of new experiences, so take these early ones in stride — more will come later.

Finding a medical practitioner who works for both of you

When we talk about finding the right medical practitioner, we're not talking personality, although that's important, too. Finding the right pregnancy "partner" primarily means finding someone whose basic philosophies on pregnancy and birth are similar to yours, so that you aren't debating every single pregnancy and birthing decision with your partner's practitioner.

Medical practitioners' views can vary tremendously on every facet of pregnancy, from medication in labor to the vitamins your partner should take, so make sure you're all in agreement on the biggies before signing up for nine months of visits.

Finding a medical practitioner whom both of you like and trust isn't as easy as looking in the phone book for the first obstetrician listed under A. For one thing, many women already see a gynecologist for routine care. However, not all gynecologists deliver babies; as they age, they often choose to stop doing the middle-of-the-night phone calls and races in to the hospital and just do gynecology.

The situation can get sticky if your partner's gynecologist doesn't do OB (obstetrics) but the other practitioners in his medical group do, and your partner isn't crazy about the gynecologist's fellow practitioners. Or you're thinking about a hospital birth, but you find out her gynecologist has the highest Cesarean section rate in the city. Or, in some cases, you and your partner may opt for a low-tech birth and want to use a midwife for the pregnancy and delivery. If your partner has been seeing her current gynecologist since she was 13, she may be concerned about hurting his feelings by seeing someone else during her pregnancy.

Your partner and you, if you go to the appointments, will be seeing a lot of the person who's going to deliver your baby over the next many months, so being comfortable with each other is essential. Chapter 8 contains a list of interrogations — um, *questions* — you want to ask your prospective medical practitioner before planning on spending the most important occasion of your life with him. In addition, keep the following tips in mind:

>> **Ask who covers when your practitioner is off.** Even the best doctors and midwives take vacation and get sick, and getting the partner you really dislike for your delivery can make the birth a bit stressful (although in the end you'll have the same baby you were going to end up with anyway, no matter who delivers her).

>> **Discuss birthing options right upfront.** Although this conversation may seem premature, the day your partner's water breaks is no time to find out that bed rest–labor induction–epidural and a 50-percent rate of C-sections is your practitioner's standard labor plan. Asking about a doctor's rate of Cesarean, for example, can give you insight into his practices. Throwing out a few questions about water birth or unmedicated delivery also allows you to gauge his feelings by his response.

>> **Find out where your practitioner delivers.** Next to how much you like your practitioner, how much you like the birthing facility is the most important thing.

>> **Remember that doctor shopping is not a sin.** Your insurance company may refuse to pay for visits to several

medical practitioners, but if you can afford it, you may want to see a few to better decide which works best for you. The office mood, the length of time you wait, and the answers you get to your pointed questions can give you a much better idea of whom to choose than just going with a friend's recommendation or the information you find on the Internet.

If you want a midwife delivery, you may be extremely limited in choices if you don't live near a large city. Some hospitals have midwives who run clinics but don't do private practice, which may not be what you want. If you can't find a midwife, look for an obstetrician who treats childbirth more like a natural event than a medical condition.

Although you want to be involved, this isn't your show. Let your partner ask the questions and remember that she makes the final decision on the medical provider she feels most comfortable spending the next nine months with.

Attending the first (and longest) prenatal visit

Many dads now attend prenatal visits, in stark contrast to the dark ages before 1970 when fathers never went near the obstetricians — or the labor room, either.

This is what you can expect during the first prenatal appointment:

>> **Blood tests:** Your partner's blood will be drawn to determine her blood type and check for certain diseases, such as HIV and syphilis, which can affect the baby. A complete blood count, or CBC, to check for anemia will also be done. Her practitioner will likely check her blood type and run a test to see whether she's immune to rubella, a viral infection that can cause birth defects. She'll also probably test for hepatitis B.

>> **Hormone levels:** Blood may be drawn for exact levels of human chorionic gonadotropin (hCG), the hormone pregnancy tests check for, or for progesterone, if your partner has had trouble carrying a pregnancy in the past.

>> **Time to talk:** Your practitioner or the ancillary staff will go over the prenatal schedule, prescribe vitamins, and discuss your specific concerns. Because obstetricians, like other

doctors, often seem to have one foot out the door even in the middle of important discussions, make sure you pipe up and ask about what's important to you. Writing your list of questions down ahead of time keeps you from leaving anything out.

>> **A vaginal exam:** Many guys aren't comfortable watching their partner undergo a vaginal exam. Discuss this with your partner before you go because it will definitely happen.

The first prenatal appointment is the longest one and is probably the most important one for you to attend, so if you're going to have trouble getting to a lot of appointments, make sure you're at this one if at all possible. The later appointments are often so short you may wonder why she has to go at all, but rest assured that periodic visits, even short ones, can help prevent big-time problems.

Going to the first ultrasound

Your partner's practitioner may decide to do an ultrasound in the first few weeks, often as part of the first OB appointment, especially if your partner has any vaginal bleeding, the time of conception hasn't been determined, or your partner did fertility treatments. Ultrasounds are done at the doctor's office, hospital, or radiology office. Even though you won't see much, seeing that "something" is in there is still a thrill! If you can get to this appointment, go. You may even get to see the tiny heartbeat flicker if your partner is six-plus weeks pregnant.

Baby's Development during the First Trimester

When the embryo first implants in the uterus, about a week before a menstrual period is missed, it's too small to be seen without a microscope. Within a week, though, you can see the first signs of pregnancy via vaginal ultrasound. Although the embryo still isn't discernible, the gestational sac that surrounds the embryo shows up as a small black dot. From this point on, fetal growth is an astounding miracle.

He may not look like much now, but . . .

In six weeks, your baby embryo grows from a ball of cells to a recognizable creature, although the exact species is difficult to define. Following are the changes that occur in the first six weeks of pregnancy, which include the first four weeks, the time from the last menstrual period to the first missed period.

>> **Week 2:** Egg and sperm meet, usually in the middle of the fallopian tube. The zygote formed by the union of egg and sperm drifts down to the uterus over several days.

>> **Week 3:** Implantation occurs 7 to 12 days after fertilization. There may be a small amount of *implantation bleeding* as the embryo burrows into the uterine lining.

>> **Week 4:** Your partner misses her menstrual period. A pregnancy test, which detects minute amounts of *human chorionic gonadotropin,* or hCG, may be positive as early as week 4. The embryonic cells divide into two sections during this week, one that will become the embryo and one that will become the placenta.

>> **Week 5:** The yolk sac, which nourishes the embryo before the placenta forms, may be visible next to the gestational sac on ultrasound. The embryo now consists of three layers that will develop into different areas of the body. On ultrasound, a small dark spot, the gestational sac, may be seen.

>> **Week 6:** During this week, the embryo looks like a bent-over bean with a slight curve at the end. The heart is still a primitive tube, but you can see a flickering heartbeat on ultrasound as blood begins to circulate. Arm and leg buds are sprouting, and the eyes, ears, and mouth begin to form, although they're still a long way from a finished product at this point.

Amazing changes in weeks 7 to 12

Although few people would say "Yes, sir, that's my baby" by week 6, between weeks 7 and 12, the embryo really starts to look human (see for yourself in Figure 4-1).

>> **Week 7:** In week 7, the baby is huge — around the size of a blueberry! At least he's something you can see with your own two eyes, and it's a 10,000-times increase over his original size. The brain and the internal organs are all growing, and the arms and legs have primitive hands and feet.

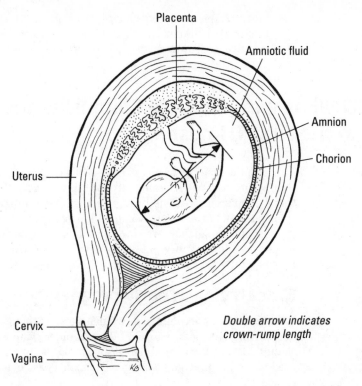

Placenta

Amniotic fluid

Amnion

Chorion

Uterus

Cervix

Vagina

Double arrow indicates crown-rump length

Illustration by Kathryn Born, MA

FIGURE 4-1: By the end of 12 weeks, the fetus actually looks like someone who just may be related to you.

>> **Week 8:** Fingers and toes start to form, and the nervous system starts to branch out. Those new limbs are moving, although it'll be weeks before your partner can feel movement, even if she swears she's feeling it already.

>> **Week 9:** The baby's heartbeat may be audible via ultrasound or a Doppler, which amplifies sound. You'll never forget the first time you hear that rapid beat and realize that a real human is attached to it.

>> **Week 10:** The kid doesn't even have knees yet, and he's already forming teeth in his gums! He does have elbows, though, and knees aren't far behind.

>> **Week 11:** Your 2-inch bundle of joy is beginning to look like a real miniature person, one who has brand-new fingernails and an admittedly large head.

> **Week 12:** The internal organs are growing so much that they protrude into the umbilical cord (they'll start moving back into the abdominal cavity shortly), and the baby is making urine.

Dealing with Possible Complications in the First Trimester

Although the majority of pregnancies really do go like clockwork, things can and do go wrong. In early pregnancy, the biggest threat is miscarriage. One in four women has a miscarriage at some point in her reproductive life. Another, less common threat is an ectopic pregnancy. We cover both miscarriages and ectopic pregnancies in the following sections; we also provide some tips for coping if you experience either of these complications.

Miscarrying in early pregnancy

Miscarriage is more common as women age, and though you may not consider your partner "old" if she's older than 40, Mother Nature does, at least for childbearing purposes. In fact, doctors used to refer to pregnant women older than 35 as "elderly."

The reason that miscarriage increases with age is that her eggs, which have been hanging around since before she was born, have aged, and you can't put face cream on eggs and have them look younger. The good eggs get used up first, so the ones left are more likely to be chromosomally abnormal. Miscarriage rates by age break down like this:

> **Under age 35:** 15 percent

> **36 to 40:** 17 percent

> **41 to 45:** 34 percent

> **Older than 45:** 53 percent

REMEMBER

Keep in mind that these miscarriage rates are averages and that a woman's actual risk depends on many other health factors. These numbers describe the potential risk *after* a pregnancy is diagnosed. Before the first missed period, many pregnancies are lost when they start to implant but then stop growing, usually because they're chromosomally abnormal.

The symptoms of miscarriage are bright red bleeding that becomes heavier over time, passing clots, and abdominal cramping. If your partner is newly pregnant, she may just have what seems like an unusually heavy period around the time of her period or shortly afterward. Pregnancies that end this early are often called *chemical pregnancies.*

Some women have spotty bleeding that isn't continuous, sometimes called a *threatened abortion.* (*Abortion* is the medical term for a miscarriage.) Some medical personnel still prescribe bed rest for women with spotting, although studies show it really doesn't change the risk of miscarriage.

REMEMBER

Chromosomally abnormal embryos cause an overwhelming number of miscarriages. You and your partner didn't cause the miscarriage, and neither of you could have prevented it. But although miscarriage is a natural event, it's still an emotional loss (to varying degrees for different people), and talking about how you feel is an important part of coping. Allow yourself and your partner to mourn the loss of the baby, no matter how early in the pregnancy it occurs.

REMEMBER

Having one or two miscarriages doesn't increase the risk of it happening again, but women with three or more miscarriages should see a fertility specialist to determine the cause, if possible. Following are some of the possible causes of *recurrent miscarriage* (defined as three or more losses):

>> **Chromosomal abnormalities:** You or your partner may carry genes that are causing recurrent miscarriage. Genetic testing can help determine the cause.

>> **Immune system problems:** Women who have autoimmune disease can have recurrent miscarriages. Treatment with medication may reduce pregnancy loss.

>> **Incompetent cervix:** An incompetent cervix dilates prematurely because it's been weakened by trauma, congenital deformities, or a previous surgical procedure. Women whose moms took DES to help prevent miscarriage may have incompetent cervixes. Miscarriage usually occurs after 12 weeks. Incompetent cervixes cause around 5 percent of recurrent miscarriages and can be treated by placing a stitch in the cervix to hold it closed.

>> **Low progesterone levels:** Sometimes progesterone levels are too low to sustain a pregnancy. In these cases, supplementation helps.

>> **Uterine abnormalities:** Fibroids, polyps, scar tissue, or congenital uterine malformations can prevent the pregnancy from implanting properly in 15 to 20 percent of recurrent miscarriage cases. Surgical correction of the abnormality may help.

After a miscarriage, many women pass all the tissue and need no further medical care. Others need tissue surgically removed so it doesn't cause infection or continued bleeding. This procedure, called a *dilatation and curettage,* or D&C for short, is done as an outpatient procedure.

REMEMBER

If your partner passes tissue, be sure to save it and take it to your medical practitioner so she can see that everything's been passed and possibly test to figure out what happened. When cramping intensifies, keep a clean container with a lid in the bathroom so you can collect any tissue as it passes. Take the tissue to your practitioner's office as soon as possible; keep the container in the refrigerator or follow your practitioner's instructions on where to take it if a miscarriage occurs during the weekend.

The miscarriage may be diagnosed afterward as a *blighted ovum,* a pregnancy where the embryo stops developing and only the placenta grows. Blighted ovum is the most common type of chromosomally abnormal pregnancy. It can't be predicted or prevented; a certain percentage of embryos are chromosomally abnormal, and one blighted ovum doesn't mean the problem will recur in the next pregnancy.

Understanding ectopic pregnancy

Sometimes a pregnancy implants in the fallopian tube, or rarely, in another location, such as the ovary, abdominal cavity, or cervix. A pregnancy that implants outside the uterus is called an *ectopic pregnancy.* Ectopic pregnancies are more common in women who have damaged fallopian tubes and occur in 1 in 100 pregnancies.

An ectopic pregnancy usually seems to be developing normally up until around seven weeks. An early pregnancy test is positive, but if an ultrasound is done, nothing shows up in the uterus. If the embryo is in the fallopian tube, the tube may appear distended.

If an ectopic is diagnosed early enough, you can take medication to stop the pregnancy from growing, which saves the tube or other implantation sites from being removed. The products of conception are absorbed naturally and don't need to be surgically removed if you take the drugs early enough and they're effective.

When an ectopic pregnancy gets too far along, bleeding starts, and the tube is in danger of rupture. At this point, removal of the fallopian tube is the only way to prevent serious blood loss that may threaten the mother's life. An ectopic pregnancy can't be removed and replanted elsewhere, so the embryo will be lost.

WARNING

Signs of ectopic pregnancy in danger of rupture include slight bleeding, abdominal pain on one side, lightheadedness, shoulder pain, or passing out. Ectopic pregnancy is a life-threatening emergency. Call your medical practitioner and get to the hospital immediately!

Coping with pregnancy loss

Losing any pregnancy can be devastating. Many people you tell won't make coping with the loss any easier with comments suggesting it was "for the best" or that "you'll have another one," either. Many people don't really see early pregnancy loss as something to grieve over and may not understand why it's hitting you or your partner so hard.

In fact, one of you may not understand why the other is taking it so hard. Whether you're on the same page or not, be respectful of each other's feelings and give yourselves time to grieve. It can be gut-wrenching to attend christenings, family gatherings with lots of kids running around, or children's birthday parties during this time.

REMEMBER

Don't try to handle what you're really not up for. If your partner doesn't want to go see your sister's new baby right now, run interference for her. Hopefully your sister will understand that this is a temporary situation, not a permanent rejection of her and your new niece or nephew.

Reducing Early Developmental Risks

The first three months of pregnancy are the time of organ development, so it's also the time when your partner needs to be most careful about what she eats, drinks, and ingests. Let her know — nicely — that you're willing to do whatever you can to help her quit any bad habits or to stay as healthy as possible during these critical months.

Around 15 percent of women of childbearing age smoke, and around 65 percent drink at least occasionally. A lesser but still significant percentage — around 15 percent — of women over age 18 used illegal recreational drugs during the past year. It's no secret that all these habits have the potential to harm your developing baby, so, at least for the duration of the pregnancy, all three should be off both of your bad-habits lists.

Smoking and development problems

Cigarette smoking exposes your partner and your baby to nicotine, carbon monoxide, and tar. All these potentially noxious and harmful substances reduce the amount of oxygen that reaches your baby through the placenta. Additionally, babies born to smokers are often smaller than normal. A 2014 report from the U.S. Surgeon General also warned that smokers have a 30 to 50 percent higher risk of having a baby born with a cleft lip or palate.

Smoking also increases the risk of stillbirth and *placental abruption,* where the placenta prematurely dislodges from the uterus and cuts off your baby's oxygen supply. After birth, babies whose moms smoke have a greater risk of dying from sudden infant death syndrome (SIDS).

Do whatever it takes to help your partner quit, preferably before you even start on the pregnancy journey but at the very least with the first positive pregnancy test. And consider quitting yourself; inhaling secondhand smoke can be as damaging as smoking yourself. If you do continue smoking, never smoke in the house, around your partner, or, later, around the baby.

WARNING

Don't suggest or let your partner think that she can swap her regular cigarettes for e-cigarettes. Sure, at first thought, switching to e-cigarettes, which often contain nicotine but no tars or carbon monoxide risk, may seem like a good idea. But the jury is still out on the safety of e-cigarettes, and many do still contain nicotine. They can also contain other toxins, such as cancer-causing chemicals nitrosamines and formaldehyde. Because they're not regulated like drugs, you can't be sure exactly what you're getting when you vape.

Nicotine causes blood vessels to constrict, which reduces oxygen delivery to your baby — never a good thing. Ultimately, it's safer for both of you to quit all nicotine products during pregnancy.

Drinking during pregnancy

The risks of alcohol use during pregnancy are well documented. Fetal alcohol syndrome can cause learning disabilities, physical abnormalities, and brain alterations that affect mood — for life. Because no one knows exactly how much alcohol is "safe," it's better not to drink any at all during pregnancy.

So what does that mean for you? That's really up to you and your partner. If she was never much for alcohol or can easily live without it, she may not have a problem if you still have a drink or two in her presence. For some couples, women prefer that men don't drink because if the pregnant woman can't, why should her partner? It may sound extreme, but think about it like you would someone who is dieting. Would you eat a huge piece of cake around someone trying to lose 50 pounds? Regardless of how you and your partner feel about the situation, always drink in moderation; you never know when you may need to be lucid enough to drive to the hospital.

OTC and prescription drugs and their health risks

Over-the-counter drugs may seem like they must be safe or they wouldn't be so available, but that's not always the case. Non-steroidal anti-inflammatory pain relievers such as aspirin and ibuprofen and Naproxen can affect nearly every system of your baby's developing body and are best known for their potential effects on heart development.

Your partner's medical practitioner will undoubtedly discuss any medications she's taking at her first visit. She'll probably supply a list of acceptable over-the-counter medications and review any prescription medications your partner currently takes.

If your partner takes certain classes of medications, such as antihypertensive drugs or antidepressants, her practitioner will weigh the risks and benefits of different medications and may change your partner to one with fewer known fetal side effects. If her practitioner doesn't bring this up, make sure you do or your partner does so she doesn't worry unnecessarily about medications she's taking or, worse, stop taking them out of fear.

The bottom line during pregnancy is not to take anything not prescribed by a medical practitioner who knows your partner is pregnant. That includes health food supplements, herbs, and commonly used cold, allergy, and flu medications. If you or your partner ever has any questions over whether a medication or supplement is safe to take during pregnancy, just pick up the phone and call her medical practitioner. It's always better to ask, for peace of mind if nothing else.

Autism spectrum risks and prevention

The increase in mental disorders on the autism spectrum has been staggering over the last few decades. As a result, you may be understandably anxious to do anything you can during pregnancy to reduce the risk that your child will have an autism spectrum disorder. Sadly, there's no one sure way to prevent autism, which may have a genetic component in up to 90 percent of cases.

Taking folic acid — the B-complex vitamin that also helps prevent neural tube defects such as spina bifida — before getting pregnant and early in pregnancy may help reduce the risk of autism, according to one Norwegian study. Ultimately, though, avoiding any known toxins, eating well, and steering clear of unnecessary medications gives your baby the best shot at dodging the autism diagnosis.

Common First Trimester Discomforts — Yours and Hers

Early pregnancy can be uncomfortable — for both of you. Though your partner bears the brunt of it, the first three months of pregnancy may bring some unwelcome changes into your life as well. Hang in there, though — it'll all be worth it in the end!

Helping your partner cope with early symptoms

Early pregnancy brings extreme fatigue, the overwhelming desire to take a nap, food cravings, food aversions, nausea, vomiting, and a constant need to urinate — not to mention hormonal changes that cause pendulum-like mood swings, from crying to euphoria almost before you can ask what's wrong.

TIP

Knowing the symptoms ahead of time helps you keep your cool when all around you seems to be falling to pieces. Following are more things you can do to help your partner through these first topsy-turvy months of pregnancy:

» **Accept her limitations.** Maybe you went out to eat several times a week and now the sight of restaurants makes her sick. Hang in there. By the middle (2nd) trimester she'll be eating everything in sight, and the Szechuan restaurant will still be there.

» **Don't take emotional outbursts seriously.** Not letting her outbursts get to you is hard when they're pointed at you and all your shortcomings, but listen to what she says, accept what may actually be true, and disregard the rest. Don't forget to fix any shortcomings you can, though.

» **Help her.** Shoulder some of her chores for now, especially the ones that make her nauseated, such as cooking, garbage patrol, dishing out the dog food, and cleaning toilets. Remember that handling cat litter is strictly verboten for pregnant women, so that's your job, too.

» **Let her rest.** Although sitting at home all weekend watching her take two naps a day may not seem like a whole lot of fun, use this time to get projects done around the house or catch up on your parenthood reading.

» **Plan pit stops.** If you're the type of driver who doesn't stop the car unless the road abruptly ends before you reach your destination, realize that pregnant women really do have to pee every five minutes; she's not making up an excuse to go in to the gas station shop for a frozen custard. Also, because blood volume increases during pregnancy, blood clots can develop if she doesn't move her legs regularly. Let the woman get out of the car every few hours!

» **Satisfy her cravings.** Not that many pregnant women really want pickles and ice cream, but if your partner does, get some for her. Try not to gag as you watch her eat them; you may have to leave the room yourself.

Getting used to strange new maternal habits

At times, you may look at your partner and wonder who this woman actually is. The sweet-tempered woman you once knew may have been replaced by someone whose head appears to be rotating at times, and the woman who used to party all night long barely makes it into the living room to collapse on the couch after work. You knew having a baby was going to change your life, but you probably didn't expect things to change this much so early in the game.

Take heart: These are temporary changes. After her body adjusts to the new hormone levels, many of the symptoms will decrease, and your original partner will start to emerge again.

In the meantime, some of her new habits may be affecting you in a big way, and you may need to find ways to cope with them. The following sections help you deal with a few of your least favorite early pregnancy things.

Vomiting

Although she's the one vomiting, sometimes you may not be far behind. Many people have a hard time dealing with vomit, whether it's their own or someone else's. If you have a sensitive stomach, hearing her heave may inspire the same reflex in you. Staying supportive while holding on to your own cookies can be difficult. You may want to try the following tips if the sight, sounds, and smell of vomiting are getting to you:

>> **Avoid trigger foods.** If certain things really get to her, make sure they don't enter your house, no matter how much you crave them.

>> **Dab something under your nose that smells good to you.** This really helps. Peppermint oil can get you through some tough moments. Nose plugs may also work, if your partner doesn't take offense at them. She probably doesn't want you to start vomiting too, so she may be okay with them.

>> **Stay cool.** People are less likely to vomit when cool air is blowing on them, so turn the fan all the way up and get a small fan that can blow right on you. This may help keep your partner from vomiting, too.

Gaining weight

Although weight gain isn't such a problem during the vomiting weeks, when the nausea ends, your partner may start eating like food is going to be taken off the market next week. This can be bad for her waistline, sure, but it can also be not so good for yours, because you may find yourself overeating just to keep up with her and matching her weight gain pound for pound. The woman who never let a chocolate-covered donut in the house may now be eating them by the cartload.

For both of your sakes, try to put a stop to the madness. You don't have to remind her how hard this weight is going to be to lose later. Just talk about your own weight gain and how you're afraid you're not going to be able to play Frisbee on the beach with the kid if you keep eating like this. Don't turn into the food police; no one responds well to being told what they should and shouldn't eat.

Even if your pleas for healthier food choices don't get her out of the junk food aisle and back into the vegetable section, force yourself to cut back on the unhealthy foods. She's eating for two, but you aren't, although you may look like you are about halfway through the pregnancy. And, all kidding aside, that extra weight will interfere with your ball-playing and horsey-back-ride abilities down the road.

Coping with your cravings

If an active sex life was part of your semiweekly (or more) agenda, you may be in for a rough few weeks. Sex may be the last thing on your partner's mind in the first trimester. And some types of sex may trigger her gag reflex, which is the last thing you want to associate with a previously enjoyable activity! Although turning into a monk may not be on your list of fun things, you can cope with the words "Not tonight, honey" by doing the following:

>> **Be flexible:** Some women are ready for sex sooner than others, and for some, when the sex drive returns, it's strong. It may come and go throughout the day. Be ready to perform when your partner is ready because the window of opportunity can be slammed shut before you've had a chance to look outside.

» **Experiment with touching:** Depending on how open your partner is to experimentation, you can do a lot to pleasure each other that doesn't involve intercourse. In fact, this may be a great time to start understanding your partner sexually more than ever before. Find out what she's up for by taking it slow, working together to find comfortable positions and techniques, and being supportive if at any moment she needs to stop.

» **Practice self-release:** Masturbation isn't something most adults like to talk about, but if you have a voracious sexual appetite, and both you and your partner are okay with the idea, there's no shame in taking the matter into your own hands, so to speak.

» **Watch her patterns:** If morning sex used to be your thing but her new thing is promptly vomiting every time she wakes up, shake things up. Try to engage in sexual activity at times of the day when she's generally not tired, nauseated, or weepy.

REMEMBER

A desire to have sex is normal, and becoming frustrated during the time she isn't up for it doesn't make you a pig. Don't push the issue or make your partner feel bad about the lack of sex, but do let her know that you miss being with her and look forward to when she's up for having sex again. In the meantime, work off that extra steam with a nice run or a game of tennis.

Taking on your emerging support role

Don't think of yourself either as your partner's personal assistant or as the pregnancy police. She may become a diva in her pregnancy, but it's not your responsibility to do it all. And try to avoid becoming overprotective of your partner's physical capabilities, especially early in the pregnancy. If everything goes well with the pregnancy, she won't have many restrictions on her activities. But that doesn't mean she's going to be up for taking care of everything she's always managed.

For the first several months — and for the last few — your partner may be too tired/nauseated/hot/and so on to make dinner, walk the dog, or perform many of the household chores you used to split. Pick up the slack until she feels good enough to contribute again. When she's back in the swing of things, she can move around and help again. After all, physical activity is beneficial for both mom and baby.

One of your main roles is ensuring that she eats healthfully and exercises if and when possible, but the way to do this is by example, not with a whip and chain in hand and bathroom scales placed in front of the refrigerator. Ask her to take walks with you and help by preparing meals that settle her stomach and feed baby's growing systems.

REMEMBER

Pregnancy doesn't turn your partner into a child, even though she's carrying one around with her. She still gets to make her own choices about what she eats and when, or if, she exercises, and you may have to bite your lip if she starts exceeding the weight limit for your delicate Queen Anne chairs.

In addition to supporting your partner physically, you need to support her emotionally. She'll likely be weepier and more sensitive than normal. If you're not the kind of guy who likes to talk about feelings, we suggest you become that guy for a month or so.

As hormones surge and wane, roll with the punches. Let the little things go without a struggle because your partner won't always be able to control her reactions the way she used to. Let her dictate what's for dinner, and if her stomach turns when you plate the exact dinner she asked for, don't take it personally.

REMEMBER

Being a rubber wall isn't easy, but the more you can let things bounce off you, the easier this time is for everyone. Supporting your partner throughout pregnancy is a constant game of choosing your battles and helping her make healthy decisions for her and the baby. Don't tell her what she should do — lead by example. It's good practice for when you have a kid in the house.

Chapter **5**

Growing into the Second Trimester

Welcome to the best three months of pregnancy, for both you and your partner. The second trimester is universally regarded as the "golden era" or "honeymoon" of pregnancy — she's big enough to look pregnant and not just pudgy, morning sickness is left in the dust, and the aches and pains of late pregnancy are still in the distant future. Enjoy these three months because the next three will bring much more upheaval into your partner's life — and consequently into yours!

In this chapter, we walk you through the garden of the second trimester, covering the development of both baby and your partner over those three months, the tests your partner will need to undergo, and more.

Tracking Baby's Development during the Second Trimester

By the end of the first trimester, your baby's vital parts are all in place and beginning to perform the functions they'll carry out for the next 80 or so years. By the end of the second trimester, the baby's lungs, one of the slowest organs to mature, are almost capable of supporting life with assistance if he's born very prematurely (23 to 24 weeks is considered the earliest that a fetus can survive if born early). But the lungs aren't the only area experiencing change; every body system is becoming more refined with each passing day.

Growing and changing in months four and five

Even though baby's basic structures are in place, they undergo further refinement in months four and five:

>> **Week 14:** The baby's eyes close for several months while they develop on the inside.

>> **Week 15:** Some women may start to feel flutters when the baby moves; many women, especially those in their first pregnancy, don't feel movement for several more weeks.

>> **Week 16:** Hair (including eyebrows) begins to grow.

>> **Weeks 17–18:** Air sacs start to form in the lungs, but the lungs aren't able to support life for another six weeks or so. If you're having a girl, her future eggs are developing. Your baby can hear and respond to sound. Her fully formed fingers include unique fingerprints.

>> **Week 19:** The permanent teeth form in the gums. The baby can swallow.

>> **Week 20:** By this week, the midpoint of pregnancy, the fetus is around 6.5 inches long and weighs around 10 ounces.

>> **Weeks 21–22:** The fetus now has a functioning tongue! A baby girl's ovaries contain all the eggs she'll ever have in life, around 6 million.

>> **Week 23:** The baby can now hear, but more important, if born now, she has around a 15 percent chance of survival.

Figure 5-1 gives you an idea of what these changes look like.

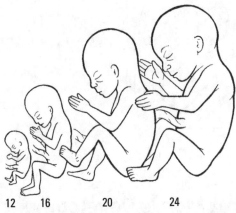

12   16   20   24

Illustration by Kathryn Born, MA

FIGURE 5-1: Months four and five of pregnancy.

Refining touches in the sixth month

The sixth month continues the refining process; all the major components are in place, and all the baby has to do is grow and mature.

>> **Week 24:** Your baby has around a 50 percent chance of survival if born at this point. She now weighs around 1.3 pounds.

>> **Weeks 25–26:** The spinal cord and lungs are forming more completely, and the eyes reopen at last!

>> **Week 27:** At the end of the second trimester, your baby approaches 2 pounds and 14.4 inches. The lungs, spine, and eyes continue their refinement process. Every week increases the odds of survival if born early.

Check out Figure 5-2 to see how much baby has developed by the end of the sixth month.

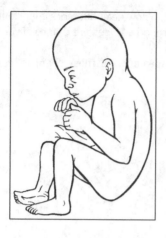

Illustration by Kathryn Born, MA

FIGURE 5-2: By the end of the sixth month, the fetus is likely to survive if born early.

Checking Out Mom's Development in the Second Trimester

The middle trimester of pregnancy may be the best time of your partner's life: She feels good, looks "cutely" pregnant, and usually enjoys these three months, which means you get to enjoy them, too! It's also the time when her sex drive may return, and the urge to begin getting the home ready for baby kicks in.

REMEMBER

During this time, make the most of your waning days as a twosome. Later in the pregnancy, your partner may not be up for doing as much, and after baby arrives, all bets are off. So get out now! Go on dates, take a vacation, or just indulge in all the things that you and your partner enjoy doing one-on-one.

Now is also the time when your partner's body goes through a lot of changes, so your support is more important than ever. Giving up her body for a baby isn't easy, and the more you help her deal with the ups and downs of pregnancy, the easier it will be for everyone.

Gaining weight the right way

One of the most overwhelming concerns for many pregnant women is weight gain: They're afraid they're gaining too much, aren't sure how much they should gain each month, and are desperately afraid that extra weight will be with them for a lifetime.

It's not unusual for dads-to-be to begin packing on the pounds, too. Perhaps you also indulged in your partner's first-trimester cravings. Maybe she wasn't feeling up for those long walks you used to take after dinner so you skipped them, too. If you're gaining weight right along with her, you may have some concerns in this area, too. The following info may help you help her (and yourself) with weight gain issues:

>> After the first trimester, a weight gain of around a half a pound a week is considered normal. Weight gain should be based on partner's BMI at start of pregnancy

>> Total weight gain, on average, should be between 25 to 35 pounds, with underweight women gaining a little more (28 to 40 pounds) and overweight women less (15 to 25 pounds).

>> Pregnant women need only an extra 100 to 300 calories a day.

>> The baby contributes around 8 pounds to the total weight; amniotic fluid, placenta, breast tissue, and an increase in uterine muscle each add another 2 to 3 pounds. The rest is stored fat and increased blood, each adding around 4 pounds.

REMEMBER

Keeping the emphasis on eating well during pregnancy helps you and your partner ensure that the baby grows well — and that your partner doesn't end up with 40 extra pounds after the pregnancy. Rather than worry about daily weigh-in numbers, focus on eating plenty of fresh fruits, vegetables, and healthy protein sources and limiting junk food. Pregnancy isn't the time to keep an obsessive weight chart; even if you fear that your partner will never get back to her normal weight, rest assured that she most likely will.

Pregnancy is also not a time to lose weight or avoid gaining it, unless she's very overweight and is working with a medical practitioner. If she's really cutting down on food intake, she may need some help dealing with her fear of weight gain. Talk to her medical practitioner about how to handle the issue because it's a pretty sure bet she'll take her practitioner's advice over yours when talking about weight gain.

And remember, leading by example is always the best option. The healthier you both are during this time, the more likely you are to continue those healthy eating habits after baby comes. Don't wait until baby arrives to start living healthy because it won't happen. Soon enough, it will be your responsibility to teach your child how to eat as well as you.

Looking pregnant at last!

One annoying aspect of early pregnancy is looking not quite pregnant enough and worrying that you look pudgy rather than pregnant. Thankfully, by the end of the second trimester, most women definitely look pregnant, although if your partner is overweight, it may still be difficult to tell, something that may frustrate her to no end.

The days of voluminous maternity wear are, for the most part, long gone, although most women invest in a few pairs of maternity pants with an elastic tummy and a few shirts either in a larger size than they normally wear or made of a stretchy fabric. Women who have to dress well for work will probably break down and buy actual maternity clothes so they don't look sloppy if their clothes are just overall too big for them or to avoid the skin-tight "Hey, I'm pregnant, look at my belly!" look that may be considered out of place in an office.

Many pregnant women today do accentuate their bellies with tight T-shirts, hip-hugger pants, and two-piece bikinis (not on the streets of Manhattan, hopefully, although stranger things have happened). If you're extremely conservative, the let-it-all-hang-out look may bother you.

WARNING

Approach your partner carefully with any suggestions as to how she should dress in pregnancy. Pregnancy hormones may be under control in this trimester, but they make an immediate reappearance under duress. There's really no nice way to say, "I hate the way you're dressed," so you may just need to keep your opinions to yourself.

TIP

You can try buying her a few articles of clothing that fit your image of what a well-dressed pregnant woman should wear. She may just wear them, if for no other reason than that she doesn't want to hurt your feelings!

Figure 5-3 shows where the uterus is during the fourth, fifth, and sixth months of pregnancy and where you can expect it to go throughout the rest of the pregnancy. You can see why pregnancy gets really uncomfortable in the third trimester.

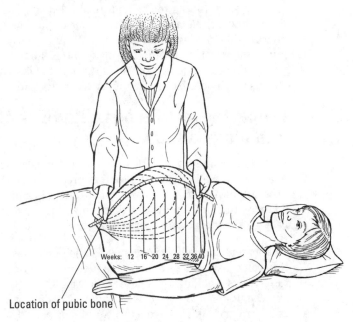

Weeks: 12 16 20 24 28 32 36 40

Location of pubic bone

Illustration by Kathryn Born, MA

FIGURE 5-3: Uterine height changes during pregnancy.

Testing in the Second Trimester

The second trimester is often the time for blood tests and ultrasounds that show that the baby's development is on target and no major problems exist. Blood tests to assess the risk of genetic defects are usually done between weeks 11 to 13 or 15 to 20, depending on the tests being done. Screening ultrasounds, which look at the baby's major organs for anomalies and can often determine the baby's sex, are done around week 20.

REMEMBER

Some babies are extremely reluctant to show their private parts on ultrasound, so not all parents learn their baby's sex at the first ultrasound, and insurance may not pay for a second without good medical cause. If you can't find out your child's sex, don't stress about it. Buying gender-neutral clothing and nursery décor is easier than ever. Greens and yellows work for boys and girls, and you'll always have time to add touches of traditional gendered colors, if you want to, after baby comes home.

And, if you're willing to shell out the bucks, you can always opt for an informal "fetal portrait" from one of the commercial sites offering these nonessential but fun looks into the womb. Keep in mind, though, that having too many ultrasounds in pregnancy poses some theoretical risks. Resist the urge to take weekly snapshots, even if your bank account can afford the hit.

Preparing for the possible risks of tests and ultrasounds

Having screening blood work and an ultrasound done brings risks of a kind, as well as benefits. Neither procedure carries any significant physical risk to either mom or baby, but the procedures do carry a risk of finding out that something is wrong with the baby — knowledge some parents would rather not have.

Most parents prefer to know whether their baby has problems so they can consider their options and prepare for potential difficulties. Others wouldn't consider terminating the pregnancy under any conditions and prefer not to know. This is a personal issue that every parent has to consider for him or herself.

If you opt not to undergo testing, make sure your partner's OB/GYN is supportive of that decision. Be upfront about your preferences so you don't feel pressured by your medical provider down the road. Most midwives allow you to make special considerations so long as those decisions pose no risk to the baby or mother.

Understanding blood tests and amniocentesis

Although some prenatal screening tests are for your partner's overall well-being and check for potentially harmful medical conditions, second-trimester quadruple-screen blood tests are aimed at determining the risk of genetic anomalies in the fetus. Some of these tests are generally used for high-risk moms-to-be and may not be offered to your partner. Talk to your medical practitioner if you have questions about why — or why not — these tests are offered in your case.

Also used in conjunction with second-trimester ultrasound, quadruple screens help predict the risk that the fetus has Down syndrome, trisomy 18, or neural tube defects such as spina bifida or *anencephaly*, where part of the brain is missing.

Quadruple screens test the blood for four things:

>> **Alpha feto-protein, produced by the fetus:** High levels of AFP may indicate neural tube defects, abdominal wall defects, or a multiple pregnancy.

>> **Estriol, a form of estrogen made by the placenta and liver of the fetus:** Estriol levels are low in Down syndrome pregnancies.

>> **hCG, produced by the placenta:** hCG levels may be higher than normal in Down syndrome pregnancies.

>> **Inhibin A, produced by the placenta:** Inhibin A levels are elevated in cases of Down syndrome.

Newer blood tests that extract DNA from mom's blood rather than from the placenta or from amniotic fluid — both procedures that carry considerably more risk — can assess your risk for having a baby with trisomy 13, 18, or 21 and can also test for baby's sex. These tests are expensive and not routinely offered; insurance may cover the cost if your partner has risk factors, such as being over 35 or having a previously affected child. Talk to your medical practitioner about the benefits of these blood tests, which can be done as early as the 11th week of pregnancy. They're more than (99 percent accuracy) 90 percent successful in detecting these chromosomal abnormalities but also have about a 5 percent false positive rate.

In the second trimester, amniocentesis may be done between weeks 15 and 20, when amniotic fluid is easily accessible. A thin needle is inserted into the fluid through the abdominal wall, and the fetal cells in the fluid are analyzed.

Amniocentesis comes with a slightly increased risk of miscarriage afterward, so most medical practitioners don't recommend doing an amniocentesis routinely. Women older than 35, who have a higher risk of having a child with chromosomal abnormalities, and those with a family history of genetic problems may consider doing amniocentesis, which can determine whether chromosomal defects such as Down syndrome, hemophilia, cystic fibrosis, and other genetic disorders are present.

Following up on the test results

REMEMBER

Remember that second-trimester blood tests are screening tests only. They don't diagnose congenital defects; they merely indicate the odds that a congenital defect exists. The risk also varies with maternal age: The older your partner is, the more likely you are to have a child with a genetic defect, although the risk is still low.

If your partner's screening test comes back abnormal, the most important thing to do is stay calm. An abnormal result indicates nothing but a need for further testing. Try hard to keep both of you thinking positive until you have a clear answer on what, if anything, is wrong.

REMEMBER

The March of Dimes reports that 5 percent of screening tests are abnormal, but only 4 to 5 percent of fetuses with abnormal test results actually have Down syndrome. This is a very small percentage, so stay optimistic; the odds are highly in your favor for a good outcome.

Scrutinizing ultrasounds

As excited as you both are for your second-trimester ultrasound, the actual event can sometimes be a bit of a letdown. Reading ultrasounds is an art, and unless the ultrasonographer is really patient about pointing things out, you may be unsure of whether you're viewing the baby's head or his tush.

Much depends on the direction the baby's facing. You may get a somewhat frightening straight-on face shot, which looks far more like the creature from *Alien* than any relative of yours, or you may get a front-on foot view that looks like nothing more than five round balls. You may be happy to know the baby has five toes on each foot, but that's usually not the main information parents-to-be want. The next sections describe what the ultrasonographer is trained to look for.

Measuring growth

First and foremost, your medical practitioner wants to know that the baby is growing as he should. Some of the measurements taken to check for normal growth include

>> The length of the longest leg bone, called the *femur*

>> The head circumference

>> The head diameter, called the *biparietal diameter*

>> The abdominal circumference

Comparing these measurements to standards assures your practitioner, and you, that the fetus is growing as he should.

Checking for genetic markers

Genetic markers indicate an increased risk of congenital problems, but as with the blood tests described earlier in this chapter, genetic markers merely indicate the risk potential; they don't diagnose the disease. Some ultrasound markers are known as *soft* markers because they're often misinterpreted and not as diagnostic as other signs. Soft markers may also be transient and no longer seen in later ultrasounds. Following are genetic markers, including soft markers:

>> **Bowel abnormalities:** Around 12 percent of Down syndrome babies have gastrointestinal defects that may be spotted on ultrasound.

>> **Cardiac defects:** Around 50 percent of Down syndrome babies have cardiac defects, which may be visible via ultrasound.

>> **Kidney abnormalities:** Dilated kidneys, missing or small kidneys, and other anomalies may indicate genetic disorders.

>> **Missing nasal bone:** Failure to see the nasal bone or a shortened nasal bone on ultrasound may indicate Down syndrome.

>> **Polyhydramnios:** An increased amount of amniotic fluid may be associated with congenital defects.

>> **Shortened arm and leg bones:** Children with congenital abnormalities often have arms and legs that are shorter than normal.

>> **Thickness of the skin on the back of the neck:** Called *nuchal translucency,* thicker-than-normal neck skin indicates an increased risk of Down syndrome.

Determining the sex on ultrasound . . . or not

Whereas the ultrasonographer's priority is looking for information that shows the baby is growing properly, your consuming interest during the second-trimester ultrasound may be the baby's sex. Ultrasonographers who do prenatal ultrasounds are well versed in not blurting out the baby's sex and usually ask whether you want to know. Most generically use *he* or *she* to avoid calling the baby *it* if you don't want to know, so don't assume anything by the choice of words if you've requested that you not be told. You can feel legitimately concerned if the ultrasonographer starts using the term *they*, though!

REMEMBER

Ultrasounds generally aren't done just to satisfy parental curiosity but rather to catch any potential problems early on. If the baby's sex can't be determined in the first ultrasound and you absolutely must know in advance, your insurance will likely require you to pay out-of-pocket for another ultrasound.

If you had your heart set on a girl and it's as plain as the nose on your face, even to your untrained eyes, that a little boy is on the way (or vice versa), remember that feeling a twinge of disappointment is normal and okay. Try to keep it to yourself and concentrate on what you're probably seeing — a healthy, normally developing child.

TIP

If one of you really wants to know the baby's sex and the other doesn't, strategize before the appointment so you don't argue in front of the ultrasonographer. One method of keeping the news to just one person is to have the ultrasonographer write down the sex and put it in an envelope. That way, one of you can look and find out, and the other person doesn't have to. This tactic also works if neither of you wants to know at the moment, but you're concerned that your curiosity may get the better of you later. If you have the answer, you can look at it any time, but you don't have to.

Obtaining 3D or 5D ultrasounds

Newer 3D and 5D ultrasounds can pick up far more detail than 2D images. In some cases, newer ultrasound techniques allow practitioners to filter out extraneous detail and add color and shadows to images for a far more realistic look at your baby's features and activities.

Early in pregnancy, if your partner has an ultrasound, it will often be a 2D ultrasound, because honestly, there's not a whole lot to see at 6 weeks of pregnancy. After 13 weeks or so, the ultrasound you have done may be a 3 or 4D version, which will show much greater detail of your baby's face and features. If you want a 3 or 4D picture later in pregnancy and your practitioner doesn't offer it, you can still take advantage of improving ultrasound technology by going to the nearest commercial facility offering non-medical ultrasounds for a photo shoot. Just keep in mind that the people running and working at these centers may not be medically trained professionals.

Ask for credentials so you know that the person doing your ultrasound actually knows what he's looking at. Also, talk to your medical practitioner about any concerns she may have about this type of ultrasound before signing up.

Having Sex in the Second Trimester

For many women, the libido is back on the ascent during the second trimester, which is a big sigh of relief for any guy who has patiently waited through nausea, exhaustion, discomfort, and a lack of sexual energy for some long-awaited sex. In fact, some women become very sexual during this time because they're flush with hormones and feeling in touch with their bodies.

Maintaining a healthy sex life during pregnancy

Forget what you may have heard — sex during pregnancy is safe as long as your partner is having a normal pregnancy. Her desire to have sex may change by the day because of fluctuating hormones, tiredness, or body aches. She also may struggle with being a sexual being as she transitions into the role of mother.

The most important thing to do is to keep talking about sex. As you get back into the swing of things, be open and honest about what you both need. Explore ways to satisfy each other's romantic and physical needs, even if your partner isn't up for sex.

Don't be surprised if your partner needs to take it slowly in the beginning. Stop at any signs of discomfort. As the baby bump continues to expand, you'll likely find yourselves exploring new positions that offer support for your partner's stomach. Many women are most comfortable on their sides or even up on their knees and can use pillows for stomach support.

Spotting and cramping that can last up to 24 hours can occur after sex. If you or your partner has any questions or concerns about either, call her medical practitioner.

WARNING

If your partner desires oral sex, it's absolutely safe. Just make sure not to blow air into the vagina because, in very rare cases, this can cause an embolism, which can be fatal for the baby and the mother-to-be.

Addressing common myths and concerns

We'll just get the myths out of the way right now: Your penis isn't long enough to hit or poke the baby during sex. The baby can't see your penis when you're having sex, and she isn't afraid of your penis during sex. Your semen won't get all over the baby upon completion of sex.

REMEMBER

Sex is perfectly healthy during pregnancy. Your baby is protected by an amniotic sac and the cervix, which is sealed tightly by a thick mucus plug, which keeps out foreign and unwanted intruders. In a few instances, however, sex during pregnancy isn't recommended. Talk with your partner's doctor or midwife prior to having sex if your partner has dealt with any of the following issues:

>> **Bleeding:** Sometimes vaginal bleeding ranging from normal to potentially life-threatening can occur during the early months of pregnancy. Sex can cause the cervix to bleed, which can be alarming if you're already worried about bleeding.

>> **Leaking amniotic fluid:** Any time amniotic fluid is leaking, the sterile barrier between the baby and the outside world is broken, and infection can enter into the uterus and infect the baby. No sex after her water breaks!

>> **Miscarriage:** If your partner has ever had one or if a medical professional has said that she is at risk for having one, check before having sex.

>> **Multiple pregnancy:** Because multiples often deliver early, you need to avoid anything that can upset the delicate balance between no children and two — or more — children, sex included. Semen contains substances that may bring on labor if the tendency for preterm delivery exists. Besides, your partner probably has enough going on in there already.

>> **Placenta previa:** With the placenta close to or overlying the cervix in placenta previa, having sex can cause life-threatening bleeding.

>> **Preterm labor:** If your partner gave birth to a previous child prematurely, get clearance to make sure having sex is safe.

>> **Weakened cervix:** Sometimes called an *incompetent cervix,* this condition can lead to the cervix dilating before the baby is full term, which can lead to miscarriage. A stitch is often placed into the cervix to keep it closed. Sex can cause uterine contractions that disrupt the stitch.

REMEMBER

A female orgasm during low-risk pregnancy won't cause your partner to go into labor prematurely. Contractions of the uterus associated with sex aren't the same as those experienced during labor (and your partner is *very* thankful for this!). However, orgasm achieved by any method can start contractions that can lead to preterm labor in high-risk pregnancy, so put the vibrator away for the duration as well.

Some medical practitioners recommend avoiding sex during the final weeks of pregnancy because of the *prostaglandins* in semen, which are hormones that can stimulate contractions. On the flip side, if your partner is overdue, you may get a "prescription" for sex to jump-start the contractions.

Exploring Different Options for Childbirth Classes

Yes, you're expected to attend childbirth classes if your partner wants to go. The good news is that today's market offers a variety of choices that are welcoming to both mother and father. And they aren't just about learning how to breathe! These classes are an opportunity to ask questions, build confidence, and connect with other couples going through the same experiences you are at the exact same time. You may actually enjoy it.

Regardless of the type of class you sign up for, you'll be taught the basics in the following areas:

>> Techniques for coping with labor and delivery pain

>> Your role in assisting your partner

>> What labor feels like/signs of labor

>> When to call your doctor/midwife/doula

>> Choosing the birthing option that's right for you and your partner

REMEMBER

Selecting the class that's right for you has a lot to do with the kind of childbirth experience you and your partner want to have. Whatever class option you select, make sure to meet with the instructor prior to signing up (and paying the fee) to make sure he's the right teacher for your needs. Ask what's covered in the class, how many couples are in the class, where the class is held, and how many weeks the class runs.

Following are the most popular types of classes offered:

>> **The Alexander Technique:** These classes focus on utilizing techniques that reduce tension in the body and offer the mother-to-be freedom of movement during childbirth.

>> **BirthWorks:** The philosophy of this program is that women instinctively know how to give birth and that they can be empowered to understand their bodies and respond accordingly to their own labor experience.

>> **The Bradley Method:** Also focusing on medication-free, natural childbirth, these classes cover breathing techniques and the roles that diet and exercise play in childbirth. They generally include a heavy emphasis on the father's role.

>> **HypnoBirthing:** Sometimes called the *Mongan Method,* this class teaches couples how to use relaxation and visualization — self-hypnosis — to have a natural, intervention-free childbirth when possible.

>> **International Childbirth Education Association (ICEA) classes:** Although they don't adhere to a particular philosophy, these classes offer certified instructors. Check with the teacher to find out what to expect.

>> **Lamaze:** Developed in the 1940s by a French obstetrician, Lamaze focuses on empowering women to be confident in their abilities to birth children. Its teachings are rooted in natural childbirth options, and it follows the philosophy that women shouldn't be required to have routine medical intervention in childbirth.

If you've decided to use a doula (see Chapter 9 for more information on doulas), she may also offer childbirth classes.

Dealing with Insurance (or a Lack Thereof)

The better you understand your insurance coverage, the less likely you are to receive an unexpected (and unexpectedly large) hospital bill upon your return home. The second trimester is a perfect time to dive into your insurance benefits so you can make sure you have a crystal-clear picture of what's covered and what's not prior to delivering your bundle of joy.

Understanding your insurance

Although navigating your insurance plan may sound as impossible as understanding your income taxes, it's an important pre-delivery step for couples. Talk with someone from your human resources department at work, as well as with your insurance company to fully understand your coverage.

REMEMBER

Unites States law says that pregnancy can't be deemed a preexisting condition by insurance companies, so if you or your partner switched jobs or insurance plans in the middle of pregnancy, you're probably still covered. However, the law is limited to group policies, not individual policies, and it has multiple loopholes, so be sure to carefully research your coverage. Also, if you've recently changed insurance plans or signed up for coverage through the Affordable Care Act, understanding what your plan covers is of utmost importance and ultimately spells out how much you'll owe when all is said and done.

Your personal insurance plan dictates the following factors:

>> **Elective procedures:** Whether it's a scheduled Cesarean or a circumcision, not all insurance companies cover procedures that can be deemed as elective.

>> **Length of stay in the hospital:** The Newborns' and Mothers' Health Protection Act is a U.S. federal law that requires all insurance companies to cover the hospital stay for 48 hours after a standard delivery and 96 hours after a Cesarean. It does not, however, require that insurance companies cover any or all of the birth itself.

>> **Percentage of total cost:** 80 percent coverage may seem like an awesome deal, until you realize your entire stay cost $10,000, and you're now on the hook for two grand. Knowing what to expect allows you to save ahead so that when the bills start arriving, you don't have to scramble.

>> **What drugs are covered:** It may seem like your insurance is obligated to fully cover any drug or medicine your doctor provides your partner, but that's not always the case. Find out how much of the total cost of an epidural is covered because they're quite expensive, and you may need to plan ahead for the costs you may incur.

>> **Where you can give birth:** Unless you want to get stuck footing a huge portion of the bill, make sure the hospital or birthing center of your choice is on your insurance company's list of approved facilities. You've hopefully done this well before the third trimester, but it never hurts to double-check and make sure your policy hasn't changed.

>> **Who can attend your birth:** Not all medical practitioners are covered by your insurance, so make sure yours is early in pregnancy, and recheck with your insurance company as the date approaches. If you're opting for a midwife, investigate the coverage your insurance provides and make sure your midwife is willing to work with your insurance company. In rare cases, some insurance plans cover part of a doula's fees.

TIP

Midwives are generally less expensive to employ than a doctor, and if your insurance covers the cost of a midwife, you'll likely save money going that route. Many midwives even deliver in hospitals and partner with a doctor to ensure emergency care when needed.

Home births are the cheapest option of all but are generally recommended only for women who fall into the low-risk pregnancy category. However, if you and your partner are opting for a home birth, check with your insurance provider to find out how it handles such situations and what's covered in case of an emergency.

In the case of multiples, the cost will increase by a great deal because there are two — or more — babies who need care, and the babies are more likely to be born early and need to stay in the neonatal intensive care unit. Again, assuming 80 percent coverage, you could be responsible for 20 percent of a bill that quickly escalates into the six figures. Also, keep in mind that after mom is discharged, the costs of travel and staying at or near the hospital while your baby/babies are in the NICU are up to you.

Here are some other important questions to ask your health insurance provider:

» Do you need to notify the provider upon admission into the hospital?

» Are childbirth classes covered by your plan?

» Will any portion of a doula's services be covered?

» Is lactation consultation covered?

» What newborn care is covered in case of emergency?

» Are any prescriptions or medications *not* covered?

» Are any procedures (circumcision, scheduled C-section) or prenatal tests (amniocentesis) *not* covered? Are there exceptions?

TIP

During open benefits season at your work, which usually occurs sometime around the end of the year, check into the labor and delivery coverage of any alternative insurance plans that your company offers and consider switching plans or providers to one that best suits your needs. Doing so may save you thousands of dollars in hospital bills.

Having a baby without insurance

Under no circumstances is living without health insurance a preferable idea, especially if you're pregnant or have children. If your employer doesn't provide it, you can purchase it in the health insurance marketplace via www.HealthCare.gov. Having a baby is expensive, so having coverage of some sort is preferable. Even if you cringe at the expense of insurance, that expense will pale in comparison to the expenses ahead of you if you choose to have a baby without coverage.

In the U.S., you may be eligible for programs such as Medicaid or Children's Health Insurance Program (CHIP), which insure your partner and baby during pregnancy and for some period of time after, if you meet certain income requirements. You can sign up for these programs at any time, not just during the traditional "open season" for insurance changes.

REMEMBER

The costs of all the tests, ultrasounds, and medical practitioner visits leading up to and following childbirth are an enormous expense, and many medical providers won't even accept you as a patient if you're paying out-of-pocket. However, others are happy to work out a payment plan, which may require a larger upfront deposit. Your provider options may be limited, but with a little legwork you can find someone.

Aside from the cost of your partner's medical practitioner, you have to make similar arrangements with the hospital for your stay and any medicines, procedures, or operations you may undergo. The same goes for the anesthesiologist, who may require that you pay the fee for an epidural upfront, which runs between $1,000 and $2,000, depending on the provider. And after baby is born, she'll need more checkups and vaccinations, and you'll have to find a pediatrician who accepts patients without insurance.

TIP

With all those expenses, an insurance plan you buy on your own will probably pay for itself. In the case of job loss, pay for COBRA coverage for as long as it's offered to your family.

Chapter **6**

Nesting, Registering, and Naming (Oh My!)

s the calendar inches closer to baby's arrival date, usually around month five of the pregnancy, many soon-to-be parents get the urge to bring order to the home. What may start as getting the nursery ready often triggers an avalanche of do-it-yourself projects and more items added to the ever-growing registry list.

To make this whole baby thing even more real, the five-month mark is also prime time to think about names. In this chapter we tell you how to get through all the planning and preparing without any major blowups.

A Guy's Guide to "Nesting"

Put down the twigs and leaves — we're not talking about that kind of nesting. The nesting we're referring to is all about making the concept of baby a real thing in your everyday life.

Nesting can give you a sense of progress in the seemingly endless pregnancy and serves as the first of many acts of giving and loving that you'll show your baby. It can also be a great motivator for finally repainting the kitchen cabinets and replacing the broken bathroom tile.

Making the house spotless — and then some

For many pregnant women, the biological need to nest can be powerful. It can also veer into the seemingly irrational as your partner donates or trashes perfectly good linens, rugs, and towels because they may have unseen germs. Some women even get the urge to grab a toothbrush and some disinfectant and literally scrub the house top-to-bottom. This is perfectly normal — if mildly aggravating at times.

TIP

Try your best to be supportive without breaking the bank on unnecessary purchases. If your towels aren't in need of replacing, suggest having them professionally cleaned instead. Sometimes, however, the best thing to do when your pregnant partner is going through a bout of nesting-induced hysteria is to just let her do it. It's a natural process, and, as with all things, this too shall pass.

However, don't just sit back and watch. She may not ask, but she definitely wants you to help with the cleaning and organizing. Even if you don't think everything she's doing is necessary, she may be unable to see why it's not as important to you as it is to her. Simply ask her how you can help or just join in with the express knowledge that this is a fleeting phase of late pregnancy.

This is also a time when your partner feels the need to launch a new set of rules regarding safety and cleanliness, such as no more shoes in the house or no more dogs allowed on the sofa. If your partner feels very strongly about something you disagree with, work together to find a compromise.

TIP

Some pregnant women are so bothered by the idea of pet hair, cat litter, and the suspect grooming habits of animals that they may start talking about re-homing the family pet. As best as you can, try to delay any decision-making regarding your pet's future until after the baby arrives. Hormones change following pregnancy, and the last thing you want is a crying partner feeling guilty about giving up Rover in the heat of the moment. Offer to take over the duties of pet maintenance for the remainder of the pregnancy and reevaluate monthly.

Pregnant women have to be a little more cautious than normal while doing work around the house. Take note of the following household projects and their do's and don'ts:

>> **Cleaning:** Using eco-friendly cleaning products is always better, so start during pregnancy. Your partner will avoid exposure to harsh chemicals, and you'll already be prepared for the day when baby is crawling around and putting everything in his mouth.

>> **Lifting:** It's a myth that lifting heavy objects lowers a baby's birth weight or causes birth defects. (Also, raising her hands over her head doesn't cause the baby to become tangled in the umbilical cord, although her mother — and yours! — may insist otherwise.) But a woman's center of gravity changes as her stomach grows, and her tendons and ligaments soften. Lifting objects heavier than 25 pounds in the last few months of pregnancy can throw off your partner's balance and result in a fall, so have her leave the heavy lifting to you.

>> **Painting:** Pregnant women should avoid the urge to paint the nursery — or anything else, for that matter — because, among other potentially harmful chemicals, latex paint may contain mercury, and old paint can contain lead, both of which can cause harm. Sanding, which can release lead from old paint, is also a no-no. As many as 75 percent of houses built before 1978 contain some lead paint. If your partner is going to be around while you coat the walls, make sure the room is well ventilated and that she consumes no food or beverages in the room where you're painting.

>> **Pet care:** According to the U.S. Centers for Disease Control and Prevention, pregnant women shouldn't clean a cat's litter box because of the risk of *toxoplasmosis,* a parasite in cat feces that can cause congenital defects in the baby. To further decrease the chance of toxoplasmosis, make sure you clean the litter box frequently, keep your cats indoors, and avoid adopting new cats during pregnancy.

Engaging in Instagram preparedness

Chances are your significant other has been collecting her favorite recipes, outfits, quotes, and home décor styles for years now. In fact, your whole future — from what next year's Thanksgiving centerpiece will look like to what kind of house you're going to live in ten years from now — very well could be planned out on social media.

Instagram is an app where users can peruse content on their favorite topics and save ideas and inspirations for things they'd like to buy, make, or do in the future. It's the perfect place to share likes, dislikes, styles, and dreams, which is why it's an ideal place to begin planning for baby's arrival.

Surprise your partner by creating a secret board that only the two of you can see, and begin searching for the things you want for your baby. Nurseries that speak to you, things for which to register, names, your favorite stroller, parenting inspirations — it's all there and more, and it will give you the chance to be an equal voice in the decision-making process.

Although Instagram isn't the most popular app for men, being able to share what you like with each other and comment on each others' ideas in a safe online space often is easier and less stressful than spending hours and hours at store after store trying to make a decision together. You'll learn a lot about each other, and knowing what your partner likes versus what you like ultimately makes compromise much simpler . . . and you may just avoid an argument or two.

Setting up the nursery

Fun *should* rule the day when it comes to setting up the nursery, but overanxious parents-to-be often try to tackle too much at once. Begin your nursery designing with a planning session. Draw a bird's-eye floor plan of the room. Then start filling in the space with all the things you need and decide on the placement of all the furniture. Before you run out and start buying, measure the allotted spaces to make sure you don't end up with an overstuffed debacle à la the Griswold family Christmas tree.

Clearing and painting the room

Unless you're starting with an empty space, the next step is to empty the room and find a home for all your displaced things. This chore is the least fun thing to do, but don't put it off. Having an organized room just for your baby makes you feel less anxious about bringing her home.

When the room is empty, painting is a cinch. Because pregnant women shouldn't paint, this is your job. If you don't have the time or desire to paint, find a friend, family member, or local painter to do it for you. Opt for odorless, VOC-free paint; it's more expensive but emits fewer harmful chemicals that you and your baby would otherwise breathe in.

After the room is painted, have the carpets and rugs deep cleaned or refinish the floors if they need it.

Buying and assembling the furniture

When the paint's dry and the floors are ready, it's all about shopping and assembly.

TIP

Budget some alone time for assembly if possible. Cribs often come with instructions that seem to be written in Swahili, and they don't just pop together. They're solidly constructed, which is good for baby's safety but bad for your frustration threshold. Take your time and plan on spending a few hours on assembly. Lay out all the parts and read through the instructions (yes, actually read through the instructions!).

Most of today's instructions offer picture-only guidance, which can be quite vague and frustrating. If you can't understand what you should do based on the company's illustrations, don't just do what you think should be done. Take the time to call. The safety of your child is at stake — and your warranty, too.

TIP

Assemble the crib in the nursery because many cribs are too wide to fit through doorways, and won't you be frustrated if you have to take it apart and do it all over again!

Some parents opt to use *co-sleepers,* which are small, three-sided cribs that butt up to your bed, keeping the baby very close at hand. This arrangement is ideal for late-night feedings but less ideal when considering the amount of your personal space you have to sacrifice.

WARNING

Putting an infant directly in bed with you isn't safe because adult bedding is soft and presents a smothering risk. Adults or other children in the bed can also smother an infant.

THE HAZARDS OF CRIB BUMPER PADS

An important crib-related item to consider doesn't even come with the crib itself, but it's downright controversial: *Bumper pads* are quilted pads that attach to the crib's inner four walls, just above the baby's mattress. Their purpose is twofold: to keep baby's arm or leg from getting stuck between the crib slats (theoretically, anyway) and to add to baby's nursery décor.

Opinions differ on bumper pads. The Canadian government discourages their use because of the chance of suffocation, and a 2007 study in the *Journal of Pediatrics* determined them to be unsafe because an infant can get stuck beneath them or have his face pressed into the bumper, causing him to smother. Babies, unlike older children, can't move themselves away from an object they get stuck up against. Some states and cities, including Chicago (coauthor Matt's hometown), have made the sale of bumpers illegal. Some medical practitioners believe that with the use of a crib positioner, which keeps baby sleeping on his back, bumper pads cause little increased risk. However, some experts think positioners themselves also pose a smothering risk.

Whether using bumper pads is worth the risk is up to you and your partner, but there *is* a risk. If you choose to use bumpers, remove them if you notice your baby creeping toward the bumper in his sleep. Another option is to use mesh bumpers, which aren't padded but do offer a breathable barrier between baby and the crib's slats.

Arranging the nursery for two or more

Not all nurseries accommodate just one little baby. Whether you're welcoming multiples or adding a second child into a pre-existing nursery, creating a space that works for more than one takes a little extra effort.

Multiples

The only real challenge in accommodating multiples is making room for them to sleep. Changing tables, dressers, and closets can easily be shared when you invest in closet-organizing systems that allow you to store more items in less space.

For twins, some people opt to use a single crib with a crib divider that literally splits the bed down the middle. It's great for space-limited parents, and research shows that twins sleep better when placed near each other as they were in utero. However, crib dividers are a short-term solution because as the babies grow, each needs more space.

If money and space allow, you have many options for twin cribs that are smaller versions of full-sized units and are generally built side by side. And if you're having more than two, you may want to look into bunked cribs, which offer an individual space for each baby. Most aren't very stylish, but if you're having more than two babies, stylish cribs are probably the least of your worries.

Separate-birth siblings

If you're going to have an older child cede space to the newborn, the situation won't be all that different from having multiples. Most of your work concerns organization and maximizing storage space with closet-organizing systems, baskets, and bins. However, investing in a co-sleeper or a portable crib can be a lifesaver when the older child and the baby aren't on the same sleep schedules. And if your older child is still a baby, this setup allows for a secure place for the older child when you're tending to the newborn.

Baby-proofing 101

You have some time before baby starts getting into things, but that doesn't mean that the nesting period isn't the perfect time to baby-proof. In fact, doing it early allows you plenty of time to adjust to the complicated life of cabinet locks, outlet covers, and doorknob locks.

To make sure your baby's safe, take the following precautions:

>> Get down on the floor, look at the room from baby's level, and clear all potential hazards.

>> Install rubber stoppers at the top of doors to keep baby's fingers from being pinched.

>> Remove rubber tips from doorstoppers at floor level because they're choking hazards.

>> Install mesh baby gates in dangerous locations.

- ❯❯ Plug in outlet covers on all outlets below waist level.

- ❯❯ Install cabinet locks.

- ❯❯ Add a toilet-lid lock.

- ❯❯ Make sure all rugs and mats have slip-proof pads underneath.

- ❯❯ Add foam coverings to the edges and sides of sharp furniture.

- ❯❯ Apply doorknob covers to keep toddlers from being able to open doors.

- ❯❯ Find an out-of-reach location for pet supplies and the cat litter box.

- ❯❯ Remove any toxic plants or chemicals that are within baby's reach.

- ❯❯ Cover the bathtub waterspout with a plastic cover to avoid head injury.

- ❯❯ Put your trash cans in an inaccessible place — to baby, not to you.

- ❯❯ Keep bags and purses off the floor.

TIP

When in doubt, move it or remove it. Get into the habit of looking for small items on the floor, closing doors, putting the toilet seat down, and putting all potential choking hazards out of baby's reach. After years of not having to think about where you throw your keys, retraining your brain takes a while, so start now.

Understanding the Art of the Baby Registry

If the mere suggestion of free stuff has you lacing up your sneakers to run out to the nearest baby goods store, slow down. Registering isn't as easy as it sounds. Babies need a lot of gear, but they don't need everything, so you have to think through your particular wants, needs, and style before you point the scanner and click.

WARNING

When you get into the store, registering can be an overwhelming, almost paralyzing experience. Some parents-to-be first realize how unprepared to care for baby they feel when forced to choose among different styles of bottles, diapers, and baby monitors.

MONITORING OPTIONS

Baby monitors have come a long way. Most parents today are interested in systems that offer smartphone apps that allow them to check on baby from the next room, the grocery store, or work. If that level of coverage doesn't suit you and you live in a larger home, you'll at least need a video monitor to check on baby from afar. It will save you a lot of late-night trips to the nursery to check on noises. Even in smaller homes, having a video- or app-based system can be useful to check whether that little noise was a minor disturbance or something requiring your immediate attention. Some high-end monitors even come with a crib pad that detects baby's heartbeat, breathing, and movement in an effort to lower a child's risk for sudden infant death syndrome.

Regardless of your choice, make sure the unit you purchase can effectively communicate at the distance between the nursery and the other rooms of your home. Most monitors today can provide whole-home coverage and, with the addition of an app, there are no boundaries.

Some couples enter panic mode and start registering for one of everything because they feel like their baby *might* need it.

You only get free stuff once, so be sure to make the most of it by getting prepared before you register. The more online research you do about the differences among various products, the more competent and confident you'll begin to feel about your parenting duties to come. Registering is the perfect opportunity to familiarize yourself with exactly what it takes to raise a baby.

Doing your homework ahead of time to get what you want

When it comes time to register, everyone who has been a parent will tell you the things that you won't be able to live without. In truth, you *have* to have very few items to raise a baby, but a lot of modern inventions can make raising a baby easier.

First, consider your space. If your nursery is too small to fit an entire bedroom set and a glider, you and your partner need to prioritize. The room's size helps dictate the size and number of items you can add to it and the style of crib, dresser, changing table, curtains, and every other accoutrement you can imagine. If a rocking chair is the one thing you must have, plan the rest of the room around that to make sure you have enough space.

REMEMBER

Register for the essentials first, and don't make your registry too long or you run the risk of not getting everything you need. Also, don't register for too many clothes because, although clothes are necessary, everyone will want to buy clothes first, and you may not get other, more vital things. People often throw in an outfit along with whatever registry gift they purchase, anyway.

TIP

Spend time thinking about how you're going to use your stroller. If you're a runner, investigate the best running strollers and try them out at the store. If you live in a city, make sure the stroller is durable enough to handle bumpy, uneven sidewalks but not too big to make you the enemy of your fellow pedestrians. If you drive a lot, make sure the stroller folds up small enough to fit in your car and still leave room for shopping bags.

TIP

Before you register for anything, check safety ratings and parent reviews online. Visit Consumer Reports' baby section (`www.consumerreports.org/cro/babies-kids/index.htm`) for recalls and safety information.

A SYSTEM FOR TRAVEL

Travel systems that offer a compatible stroller, infant car seat, and car seat base in one package are a popular option for new parents. If you're on a tight budget, a travel system is an ideal solution to get everything you need for less than $200. However, many travel systems are quite bulky, and the included strollers generally aren't top-of-the-line quality.

Travel systems come in many styles, so start by picking the car seat of your choice. Make sure it has a five-point harness system and that it's the appropriate size for your vehicle. Consider the size of the stroller, too, and make sure it fits comfortably in your trunk. Collapse the stroller in the store before you buy it to see how small (or big) it is when not in use.

Finding out what you need — and what you think you won't need but can't live without!

When you've never before had to care for a baby, knowing what you need — and how many of each thing — is nearly impossible. Use the basic checklist in this section as your guide.

Note: We don't mention certain items, such as a high chair, jumpers, and play mats, because you don't need them right away. However, if you have room to store them, pick the ones you want and register for them. Remember, though, that when you meet your baby and get to know him, your idea of what he might like may change. The play gym you picked out before you met him may not really suit him. It's kind of like signing him up for college before he's born; you may think Harvard is the best, but he may not like it.

Following are the items you absolutely must include on your registry (in our opinion, at least).

» **Clothing:**
- Eight to ten onesies
- Six pairs of socks
- Three to six newborn hats
- Four to six warm, footed pajamas
- Two to six bibs
- Six to eight burp cloths
- Hangers

» **Feeding:**
- High-quality breast pump (if breast-feeding)
- Milk storage bags (if breast-feeding)
- Nursing pads (if breast-feeding)
- Nursing support pillow
- Lanolin and/or gel nursing pads
- Bottle brush
- Bottle drying rack

- One each of six different kinds of BPA-free bottles
- Four nipples for each type of bottle

>> **Furniture:**
- Nursery seating
- Baskets/bins for closet organization

>> **Just in case:**
- Smart thermometer
- Dye-free infant acetaminophen
- Dye-free gas relief drops
- First-aid kit

>> **On-the-go goodies:**
- Infant car seat
- Stroller
- Backseat mirror
- Car window sun shades
- Diaper bag
- Portable baby wipe container
- Travel-size hand sanitizer

>> **Sleeping and changing essentials:**
- Cradle/bassinet/co-sleeper/crib
- Two to four fitted sheets
- Crib mattress
- Two to four swaddling blankets
- Nursery monitor
- Changing table or station
- Two to three changing pad covers

>> **Toiletries:**
- Diapers (As many as you have room to store!)
- Wipes
- Diaper cream
- Baby powder
- Baby shampoo

- Baby lotion
- Infant manicure set
- All-natural hand sanitizer

REMEMBER

Not all babies take to every type of bottle; you may end up trying many different brands before you find the right one. Avoid registering for too many of the same brand in case your baby refuses to use them. You can always return any unopened bottles and nipples if your baby takes to the first or second brand you try.

Navigating the online-versus-local-registry decision

Nothing is simpler than registering for your shower at an online retailer or big box store. Practically everyone has immediate access to buy and ship what you and your partner want for baby. Their sophisticated websites store your address for simple shipping and track purchases to avoid duplicate gifts arriving at your door. If you're having a baby shower in person, however, it's definitely worth supporting a local store and expanding the options for friends and family. It feels good to support your local small business owners, and these retailers make it easy to try out and explore potential options when you are registering. Nothing makes up for testing out potential gear in person. Just make sure not to use your local shop as a testing ground and then make an online registry.

Discovering five things you don't have to have but will adore

Yes, some things are luxuries, but they can become necessities if you use them every day and they save your sanity. These five items may well fit into your "don't need it, gotta have it" category:

>> **Ergonomic bouncy chair:** Not all bouncy chairs are created equal. Finding one that sits baby upright (great for gas relief) and allows her to grow with the chair saves you down the road — but not upfront. A bouncy chair is a perfect sanity-saver for the shower-starved parent and a great place for naps and playtime for baby.

>> **Hands-free baby carrier:** Whether in a sling, a front carrier, or a pouch, wearing your baby in a hands-free carrier allows

you to get work done around the house and move about more freely. Most babies love the body-to-body contact. Make sure to try them on first to make sure the carrier you're getting fits your body.

Recent recalls of baby slings have called their safety into question, so make sure you get a model that keeps the baby upright and able to breathe freely. When a baby slumps in a curled position, her airway can be compressed.

» **Snap-and-go stroller:** This stroller provides only the skeleton of a traditional stroller with no seat. Instead, it has bars for a car seat to snap into and a bottom basket. Infants aren't in the bucket-style car seat for very long, which makes the idea of having a second dedicated stroller seem a bit extravagant. But it's the smallest stroller on the market, which makes it ideal for car travel and easy use. You literally snap the car seat into the stroller and you're ready to roll.

» **Wipe warmer:** This may seem unnecessary, and in reality, it probably is. A lot of babies, however, cry less during diaper changes when the cold, wet wipe straight from the package is replaced by the warm, cozy wipe straight from the warmer. A wipe warmer also helps keep the wipes from drying out when accidentally left open.

» **Yoga ball:** All babies are gassy, and nothing helps get the gas out better than bouncing. Save your legs and back a lot of undue stress by sitting on a yoga ball and bouncing the burps right out of your baby. It's also a great alternative to a nursery chair for those with space limitations and a great late-term pregnancy chair for the woman who can't get comfortable.

Checking out five things you don't have to have and will never adore

Some baby items, luxurious or otherwise, are just downright unnecessary — especially the ones that don't actually make a new parent's life any easier. Here are five things you should consider omitting from your registry:

» **Baby bathtub:** Why exactly does your baby need a smaller version of the same device you already have in your home? Many parents opt to bathe with newborns, and most others use a clean sink in lieu of the tub. As baby grows, your existing tub will work just as well. Besides, it's not like you're going to give baby his bath-time privacy while you stream YouTube videos on the back patio.

>> **Baby DVDs/CDs:** Before your child has the ability to ask for the latest Jonas Brothers album/Baby Einstein DVD to be played ad nauseum, why on earth would you voluntarily spend your time engaging with this entertainment? Babies shouldn't be watching TV, and your child will be just as happy listening to music from your collection. Besides, we live in a streaming world, and services such as Netflix and Spotify have you covered.

>> **Car-charger bottle warmer:** If your baby is breast-fed, the milk will most likely be frozen or straight from mom, and the warmer won't help. If your child is formula-fed, you'll be making bottles as needed. Either way, how often will you need warm milk in the car? Most babies are just as happy with room-temperature milk. Unless you plan on using it for your coffee, skip this one!

>> **Crib mobile:** It only takes one time of knocking into a crib mobile while putting your sleeping baby down to realize that the thing is more of a nuisance than it's worth. Instead, opt for a soothing sound machine.

>> **Infant shoes:** If your child gestates for 18 months and comes out walking as nimbly as a newborn horse, you'll need lots of fancy footwear. Otherwise, forgo the shoes. Most babies are annoyed by socks, let alone shoes, and for the most part, babies under the age of six months spend most of their time in sleepers with attached feet.

Celebrating the Wee One's Impending Arrival: Baby Shower Basics

These days, baby showers often aren't just for the mom-to-be and the other women in your life. If you want to be involved, by all means, tell the people planning your shower that you want it to be a unisex affair. If you don't want to attend, that's okay, too, as long as your partner is fine with that decision. Deciding how much you want to be involved is up to you and your partner, but don't forget that the more involved you are on the front end, the more connected to and involved with that baby you'll be down the road.

Traditional showers are female-centric and a bit on the cheesy side. Men often don't go because they don't feel welcome. So if you don't want to spend an afternoon sniffing diapers filled with melted candy bars, let the planners know what kind of shower you and your partner desire. It can be anything from a lunch at a nice restaurant to a traditional streamers-and-balloons affair or anything in between.

TIP

If you opt to have a coed shower, make sure that everything about the event is inclusive to people of both sexes. Here are some simple ideas to make your shower welcoming to all:

>> Send invitations that aren't overly cutesy and frilly because they're addressed to both men and women.

>> Invite all the fathers you know to ensure you're not the only man at the shower.

>> Pick a fun, unique setting or theme, such as a park or a backyard barbeque.

>> Plan some separate men-only and women-only activities. For example, see which guy can chug beer from a baby bottle the fastest, if you're a drinking crowd.

>> Play a creative game, such as constructing babies out of clay or holding a diapering competition to see who can wipe, powder, and diaper a doll the fastest.

>> Have guests write down a funny story from their childhoods and then try to match the guest to the story.

>> Open gifts with your partner. It's awkward to send her up there alone and for you not to be part of the fun.

>> Set up an assembly station where you can put together the new gifts after you open them (this idea works best if you have the shower at your home).

Opting into — or out of — gender reveal parties

We've all heard the horror stories of the pink or blue fireworks that announced an expectant couple was having a girl or a boy only to cause a forest fire or some other serious accident. Gender reveal parties are designed as a way to celebrate the pivotal moment when soon-to-be parents discover the sex of their baby. For some couples, that's a significant moment. Instead of simply finding out at the doctor's office, the couple allow that information to be passed to a designated person, who plans a gathering that will culminate with a blue or pink surprise. This can be as basic as slicing into a cake to discover the hidden cake color or as over-the-top as the aforementioned fireworks spectacular. Gender reveal parties aren't for everyone though, so if you're someone who's less-than enthusiastic about celebrating your baby's sex, make sure to let your partner (and friends and family) know. Gender is a sensitive topic for some people — maybe even your partner — so if she doesn't want to fete your unborn baby's sex, respect that decision.

Throwing virtual parties

Virtual parties — whether they're gender reveal parties or baby showers — are a modern option that allow people to gather without travel, germs, or the need to wear fancy clothes. If you or your partner would rather host a virtual event, make sure to let your friends and family know before they start booking rental facilities. Not everyone will be onboard but remember — this party is for you and your partner, not your relatives.

Because virtual parties can get difficult to navigate with too many guests, consider scheduling smaller groups at different times throughout the day. Group presents for each time slot to make it easy to open the gifts from those in attendance. Also, consider planning one game for each group. This will provide a unique experience for every guest, give everyone in attendance the chance to interact and speak, and you won't have to repeat the same game — or get mired in small talk — which can be exhausting.

Also, if budget allows, send every guest a beverage and food (and perhaps a few party favors!) that you will all share together. Doing the same thing at the same time, even virtually, is a great way to come together to celebrate baby.

Naming Your Baby

When people find out you're having a baby, the first thing they ask is, "Is it a boy or a girl?" Question number two is inevitably, "Do you have names picked out?"

Choosing a name for your baby is one of the most fun and most challenging decisions you'll ever make in your entire life. Soon-to-be parents spend hours upon hours combing through books and websites, searching for the perfect name and making lists of their top choices. And with so many options, the list can easily become mind-numbingly long and a point of contention. Getting two people to agree on the same first and middle name for a baby can devolve from a congenial conversation into something resembling a congressional hearing.

This section helps you and your partner choose the perfect name for your baby with as little stress as possible.

Narrowing down your long list

Just like a to-do list at work or that never-ending list of weekend projects you've been meaning to tackle for years, a long list of baby names only distracts and overwhelms you. Keeping the list at a reasonable length makes you more likely to engage in a meaningful conversation about the names that are truly in play.

TIP

Remember that just because you really like 30 names doesn't mean you don't like some more than others — you just may not realize your preferences yet. Stop trying to choose among Evan, Graham, Dexter, and Jude all at the same time. Instead, pit two names against each other at a time and choose one. It's like filling out your March Madness bracket; you don't pick the champion without first picking the winners of the early rounds. This tactic allows you to begin crossing some names off the list while continually pitting new names against the winner of the previous round.

At this point, you and your partner shouldn't take the opinions of others into consideration. The name is your choice, and unless you're ready to justify your choices, get frustrated with other people's input, and stand up in the face of criticism, keep the contenders to yourselves until you've made a final choice.

Reconciling father/mother differences of opinion

In a perfect world, your favorite name is also your partner's top choice. The chances of that happening, however, are slim to none. When differences of opinion arise, don't get defensive. Be able to articulate why you like the name, and even do your research about the history of the name, the name's popularity, and any family history regarding the name.

If your partner still doesn't like it or you don't like a name she adores, allow each other absolute veto power. With so many names from which to choose, don't waste your time fighting a losing battle. And besides, do you really want your partner to cave in and name your child something she despises?

TIP

For more background information on baby names, check out the following resources:

>> **Social Security Administration's Popular Baby Names** (www.ssa.gov/OACT/babynames): For some people, the relative popularity of a name can have a huge impact on the decision-making process. The SSA provides a comprehensive look at the top 1,000 names from 1880 to the present year and can help you keep your kid from being one of 17 others in her kindergarten class with the same name — if that's important to you.

>> **The Baby Name Wizard** (www.babynamewizard.com): This interactive site takes the info from the SSA site, pumps it into an innovative chart, and provides site-user input about how names are perceived, an encyclopedia-like "Namipedia" entry for each name, and a "Namemapper" that charts the popularity of names by state.

>> **Baby Namer** (www.babynamer.com): This site is an encyclopedic reference of names that allows you to create a digital list as you find names and offers similar names, famous people with the same name, and possible drawbacks of using the name, including bad nicknames.

>> **Baby Names Country** (www.babynamescountry.com): This site is an exhaustive resource for unique baby names and their meanings from around the world.

Discussing choices with friends and family

If you think talking about names between the two of you is hard, just wait until your loved ones start offering their two cents' worth. No matter what name you choose — be it classic, modern, or something in between — someone you know is going to tell you she doesn't like it. You'll probably hear it from multiple people, friends and strangers alike.

Don't feel the need to defend your name choice. In fact, the more you defend it, the more likely the person is to continue to challenge you on it. Instead, focus on why you chose that name and don't be afraid to let other people know that the matter isn't up for debate. A playfully delivered "I guess it's a good thing this is my baby and not yours" can put them in their place without too many hurt feelings.

Even after the baby is born, the name will be under scrutiny. From coworkers to cashiers at the supermarket, everyone will inquire about your baby's name, and you'll be confronted with a variety of reactions. Remember that everyone has his own association with the name of your child, but at the end of the day, your only association with the perfect name you chose will be the perfect baby on whom you've bestowed that name.

Some people are reluctant to share baby names with others for fear they may get "stolen" by another friend or family member. If your partner has this concern and you don't, be very careful about sharing the name you've chosen. Though you may think it's silly, she won't take it lightly.

IN THIS CHAPTER

» Handling common maternal pregnancy problems

» Dealing with difficult ultrasound discoveries

» Knowing what to expect if baby comes early

» Managing multiples

» Resolving money matters without panicking

Chapter **7**

Preparing for What Could — But Probably Won't — Go Wrong

M ost parents-to-be expect pregnancy and childbirth to go off without a hitch, but many women experience some sort of complication. Complications may be related to your partner's health, the baby's well-being, or the pregnancy itself. Some complications are relatively minor, but others can pose a serious threat to mom or baby.

In this chapter, we explore what can go wrong in pregnancy and guide you through the process of supporting your partner while dealing with your own fears.

Managing Pregnancy-Related Medical Issues

Problems that affect your partner's health sometimes develop with frightening speed. Other times problems develop insidiously and build to a crisis point. Neither type of problem is easy to deal with, especially if you feel like you need to stay strong to support your partner during a tough time. We take a look at some of the most common maternal pregnancy problems in this section.

Hypertensive conditions in pregnancy

Hypertensive disorders — *hypertensive* means high blood pressure — are not uncommon in pregnancy. According to the American Congress of Obstetricians and Gynecologists (ACOG), hypertensive disorders include:

>> Chronic hypertension, which is present before pregnancy

>> Chronic hypertension with superimposed preeclampsia

>> Gestational hypertension, which begins after the 20th week of pregnancy

>> Preeclampsia-eclampsia, a more serious hypertensive disorder of pregnancy

Approximately 6 percent of women develop gestational hypertension, which is characterized by high blood pressure readings but no protein in the urine. Approximately 25 percent of women with gestational hypertension develop preeclampsia.

Your partner is more likely to develop preeclampsia if

>> This is her first pregnancy.

>> She's older than 35.

>> She had high blood pressure before she got pregnant.

Hypertension in pregnancy is dangerous because it reduces blood flow to the baby and also to the mom's major organs, including the liver, kidneys, and brain. In severe cases of hypertension, decreased blood flow to the baby can cause *intrauterine growth retardation*, known as IUGR, which means the baby isn't growing the way he should.

In severe cases of preeclampsia, your partner may experience the following symptoms; new onset of anything in this list requires an immediate call to your medical practitioner:

>> Abdominal pain

>> Blurred vision

>> Decreased urine output

>> Light sensitivity

>> Severe headaches

Women with gestational hypertension or preeclampsia often end up on modified or complete bed rest (see the later section "Mandatory bed rest") or may at least have to stop working or work a reduced schedule.

TIP

Resting on the body's left side increases blood flow through the placenta. In some cases, decreasing sodium intake can help lower blood pressure. However, medical practitioners no longer recommend routinely decreasing sodium intake during pregnancy, so your partner should do this only if her practitioner advises it. The practitioner may prescribe blood pressure medications if her pressure rises too high, more frequent visits, and possibly more frequent ultrasounds to check on the baby's well-being.

WARNING

Although it's rare, women with preeclampsia may need hospitalization to control the symptoms and decrease the chance of *eclampsia*, which is severe gestational hypertension/preeclampsia with seizures. Eclampsia can be life-threatening for your partner and the baby and may require immediate delivery, even if the baby is premature. Part of your job is to watch for changes in your partner's mental status, such as confusion, irritability, or disorientation, because these changes may precede a seizure.

Gestational diabetes

Gestational diabetes, high blood sugar that develops during pregnancy and disappears after delivery, affects 2 to 5 percent of pregnancies. Glucose testing for gestational diabetes is normally done in the second trimester. Women who are diagnosed may be treated with oral medications to lower blood glucose levels or may be managed by dietary modifications. A few will need insulin injections.

The problem with high blood sugar in pregnancy is that it causes the baby to also develop high blood-sugar levels. Gestational diabetes can affect the baby (and your partner) in several ways:

>> The baby may grow larger than normal, which can make for a difficult delivery and increase the chance of a Cesarean delivery.

>> Babies whose moms have gestational diabetes are more likely to be born early and can have a severe and potentially dangerous drop in blood-sugar levels after the delivery.

>> The baby may have to be monitored in the neonatal unit for a short time until her blood sugars stabilize, which is probably not the way you envisioned your time in the hospital.

WARNING

If your partner is older than 35, is overweight, or has a family history of diabetes, she's more likely to develop gestational diabetes. Studies indicate that gestational diabetes is often a sign that she may develop type 2 diabetes later in life; as many as 50 percent of women with gestational diabetes develop diabetes later in life.

The introductions of daily injections and monitoring can add a whole layer of annoyance to pregnancy, for both you and your partner. If she cooks, her cooking will probably become a whole lot healthier, which you may or may not appreciate. If you're the chef, you may be expected to devise a new repertoire of healthy yet appealing meals. The bonus is that you'll both probably be healthier by the end of pregnancy if you follow her new diet.

Pregnancy in women with previously diagnosed diabetes

Between 1 and 2 percent of American women have either Type 1 and Type 2 preexisting diabetes when they get pregnant. Both Type 1 and Type 2 diabetes can lead to an increased risk of miscarriage, stillbirth, birth defects, high blood pressure, and other health issues for both mom and baby. If your partner has known diabetes, it's essential that she sees her healthcare provider before getting pregnant and follows instructions to the letter. You play an integral part in maintaining both mom's and baby's health by supporting and encouraging her without slipping into the role of diet and exercise overseer.

As hard as it is sometimes, you need to walk the fine line between supporting and nagging, when it comes to her lifestyle choices. Making some changes in your own lifestyle may be the best way to do this, and will be good for you as well.

Placenta previa

Placenta previa is a condition in which the placenta implants too low on the uterine wall (see Figure 7-1). Usually the placenta, which transports nutrients to the baby, implants near the top of the uterus. If it implants too low, all or part of the placenta can cover the opening to the uterus, the *cervix*, and cause bleeding.

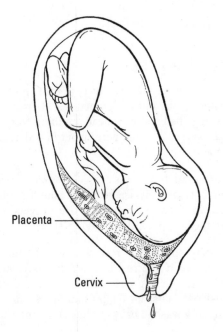

Placenta

Cervix

Illustration by Kathryn Born, MA

FIGURE 7-1: Placenta previa.

WARNING

Bleeding from placenta previa is painless, can happen without warning, and can be severe enough to require immediate delivery. A known placenta previa can necessitate bed rest and possibly a prolonged hospital stay to try to hold off delivery until the baby is less premature.

A marginal placenta previa, one that's near but not covering the cervix, may allow for a vaginal delivery, but usually a Cesarean is required. And sex is out of the question because anything that causes contractions or any cervical movement can start heavy bleeding.

Your partner is more likely to have a previa if

>> She's had a previous Cesarean delivery.

>> She's older than 35.

>> She smokes.

>> She's of Asian descent.

>> She's having more than one baby.

Mandatory bed rest

If your partner has a risk of early delivery or other problems, your medical practitioner may put her on bed rest. Depending on the condition's severity, bed rest can mean anything from not going to work and taking it easy to not getting out of bed at all, even to go to the bathroom.

REMEMBER

Having your partner on bed rest is difficult for both of you. However, if your practitioner advises bed rest, take it seriously. Bed rest brings its own risks — mostly the risk of blood clots from inactivity — so medical practitioners don't suggest it lightly.

Although you may think bed rest sounds like fun for your partner — especially if you're the one running around trying to cook, clean, take the dog out, run errands, and set up the nursery — trust us, she's not happy that she's unable to help put away the freshly washed baby clothes and hang the pictures on the wall.

Many women on prolonged bed rest get depressed, especially if they have to stay in the hospital rather than at home. Make sure to keep your partner in the loop of baby stuff; if it's okay with her medical practitioner, have friends visit regularly. You can even suggest that her baby shower be held while she's on bed rest to give her something to look forward to during those interminable days. (See the sidebar "Setting up a bed rest station" for more ideas on helping her through the restrictions of bed rest.)

SETTING UP A BED REST STATION

Your bedroom may not contain all the elements needed to entertain a sometimes bored, often dejected woman who's just itching to get up and paint the nursery. But you can turn any space into a home inside your home — or inside the hospital, if necessary. Make sure your partner's living space has all the following comforts:

- **Entertainment:** A TV, reading material, cards, games, puzzles, and a laptop, tablet, or smartphone all help pass the time.

- **Exercise ideas:** Even if she can't run around the bed, she needs to keep the blood flowing to prevent blood clots in her legs. Depending on what her medical practitioner says is okay, encourage position changes, ankle circles, and calf flexes several times a day. Discourage a cross-legged position, which decreases blood flow.

- **Extra pillows:** Spending time in bed is really hard on your back, especially when you're pregnant! Invest in extra pillows to facilitate position changes. And take the Star Wars pillowcase off, too; give her something pretty and cheerful.

- **A method of communication:** Unless your house is really small, yelling back and forth isn't the best method of communication. Cellphones work well, but walkie-talkies also work in most houses.

- **Somewhere to jot down shopping ideas and other thoughts:** She may see something on TV or think of something she'd like to try for dinner, so give her a way to write down ideas as they come to her. Though pen and paper work perfectly well, tablets and smartphones are usually on hand at all times and easier to find than scraps of paper.

- **Space to work and something to do:** No, she can't load the dishwasher from the bed, but she'd probably love to fold baby clothes.

- **A table to hold food and drink:** A drawer for snacks means she won't have to call for help every time she's hungry, and a cooler filled with drinks by the bed also gives her a little independence. Some tables fit over the bed, but a table next to the bed works fine, too.

    Venting room: In this context, *venting* has nothing to do with fresh air and everything to do with letting her get frustrations off her chest. Discourage constant negativity, but she'll need to express her aggravation, and better she vents to you than to her medical practitioner — or her mother! So be available to her, not only to keep her company but also to let her vent when she needs to.

REMEMBER

Bed rest is a vital job despite its simplicity — stay put so the baby stays put for as long as possible. Remember to make your partner feel good about the hard yet boring work she's doing. In case you've never noticed until now, women often feel guilty without a reason for feeling that way. If your partner has to worry about how all the extra work is affecting you, she won't be resting peacefully, and staying calm and relaxed is essential on bed rest.

Handling Abnormal Ultrasounds

Many couples don't really relax about a pregnancy until they see the baby on ultrasound. But some couples don't come away from the ultrasound appointment with reassuring news. Although ultrasounds aren't perfect and can miss some abnormalities, they recognize many problems.

In most pregnancies, the first ultrasound is done either between 6 and 9 weeks (to establish pregnancy) or between 18 and 20 weeks (to evaluate whether all baby's major organs are in place and growing as they should). An ultrasound may also be done at a different time if your partner is bleeding or if her medical practitioner has any concerns about the pregnancy. If your medical practitioner sees anything suspicious on ultrasound, she may schedule a level 2 ultrasound, which is done in the same way as a regular ultrasound but takes a more detailed look at the fetus.

REMEMBER

Always research your insurance company's policy on ultrasounds during pregnancy because some may not cover routine ultrasounds or repeat ultrasounds done just to find out the baby's sex. Knowing what's covered and what isn't prevents shocks to your pocketbook when an unexpected bill arrives in the mail.

Birth defects

Hearing that your baby has a problem is devastating. Even if a birth defect is minor, you or your partner may mourn the loss of your "perfect child." This reaction is normal, and neither of you should feel guilty. If a serious defect is found, you need to make decisions together about what to do.

Following are some of the most common birth defects in the United States, according to the March of Dimes:

>> **Heart defects:** 1 in 115 births

>> **Musculoskeletal defects:** 1 in 130 births

>> **Club foot:** 1 in 735 births

>> **Down syndrome:** 1 in 900 births; risk increases with the age of the mother

>> **Spina bifida (abnormal opening in the spine):** 1 in 2,000 births

>> **Anencephaly (lack of part of the brain):** 1 in 8,000 births

The most important thing to do when you get bad news is to find out exactly what you're dealing with. You may need to see a *perinatologist* — a doctor who specializes in complicated pregnancies — and possibly a genetic counselor.

REMEMBER

You and your partner may not be on the same page when it comes to making decisions about birth defects. One of you may be more optimistic about the situation and the other more pessimistic. Your feelings will be a jumble, and emotions will run high. Try to support your partner in whatever she's feeling, but don't discount your own feelings and grief, and don't feel like you can't let your feelings show. No one expects you to be emotionless at a time like this, and crying with your partner can be a bonding experience.

Expect to go through the five stages of grief: denial, anger, bargaining, depression, and acceptance. Getting to acceptance can take a long time and a lot of anger. Give yourself the time you need.

Talking to someone outside the situation who listens and doesn't tell you what to do — like a friend, religious advisor, or relative — can be a godsend. And most important of all, don't play the blame game. Congenital birth defects are rarely anyone's fault.

Fetal demise

Even more devastating than the discovery of birth defects on a routine ultrasound is the discovery of a fetal demise. The term *fetal demise* is usually used to describe the death of the fetus in utero after 20 weeks. Fetal demise occurs in 6.8 per 1,000 pregnancies overall.

Fetal demise has many potential causes, and few — if any — can be anticipated or avoided. It may be discovered because the baby doesn't seem to be moving much, bleeding starts, or amniotic fluid begins to leak, but it can also be found during a routine gynecological checkup.

Most fetuses are delivered vaginally after labor induction. Parents are encouraged to hold their baby and give him a name, but this practice won't be forced on you if you don't feel it's the right thing to do.

REMEMBER

In many cases, parents are better able to get through a fetal demise if they know exactly why it occurred, but sometimes the reason isn't obvious. Not knowing why can be very difficult, but blame has no place in the aftermath of a fetal demise.

Preparing Yourself for Preterm Labor and Delivery

More than 12 percent of all baby deliveries in the United States are *preterm*, which means they occur before 37 weeks. Of those,

>> 70 percent are born between 34 and 36 weeks.

>> 12 percent are born between 32 and 34 weeks.

>> 10 percent are born between 28 and 32 weeks.

>> 6 percent are born before 28 weeks.

The chances of delivering a very small preemie are low. Babies born between 28 weeks and term may require prolonged hospital stays, but most ultimately do well.

Recognizing the risks of preterm delivery

Many preterm deliveries occur without any known cause, but in a good percentage of cases, doctors can pinpoint the reason. The following situations all increase the risk of preterm delivery:

>> **DES exposure:** Diethylstilbestrol (DES) was a drug given to millions of women between 1938 and 1971 to prevent

miscarriage. Women whose mothers took the drug may have structural abnormalities that cause preterm delivery.

>> **Hypertension:** High blood pressure can reduce blood flow through the placenta to the baby, causing poor growth that may necessitate early induced delivery.

>> **Infections:** Urinary tract infections can start uterine contractions if not promptly treated.

>> **Multiple births:** A large percentage of twins, triplets, and other multiples deliver before 37 weeks.

>> **Structural abnormalities:** An abnormally shaped uterus or an *incompetent cervix,* one that starts to dilate from the increased uterine weight, can cause labor.

Handling feelings of guilt

Guilt is common after a preterm delivery, just as it is after any other setback in pregnancy. Don't get caught up in what you and your partner could have done to prevent the preterm delivery or whose fault it is that you went for that long walk the day before the delivery. Even if one of you did something you consider foolish, rehashing it now is pointless.

TIP

Put your energies into working with your partner to help your baby get healthy as quickly as possible. Visit often, and if support groups are available, get involved; studies show that parents involved in support groups have less anxiety, anger, and depression.

Navigating the NICU

The *neonatal intensive care unit* (NICU) is like nothing you've ever seen before. Although hospitals put more emphasis than they used to on keeping NICUs quiet, they are, by necessity, fairly noisy and busy, with alarms going off, lights on day and night so hospital personnel can see what they're doing, and at the center of it all, your little baby. She may be hooked up to just a single monitor or perhaps so laden down with medical equipment and IV lines that you can scarcely find her, as shown in Figure 7-2.

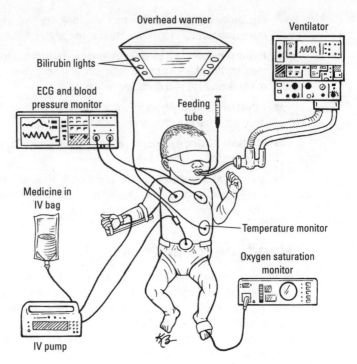

Overhead warmer

Ventilator

Bilirubin lights

ECG and blood
pressure monitor

Feeding
tube

Medicine in
IV bag

Temperature monitor

Oxygen saturation
monitor

IV pump

Illustration by Kathryn Born, MA

FIGURE 7-2: A preemie baby in the NICU.

REMEMBER

The best way to deal with the NICU is to focus on your little part of the world. Get to know your baby's nurses and stay near your baby's incubator. Asking what's wrong with other babies is really bad etiquette, and the nurses won't (or shouldn't) tell you, anyway.

Preterm babies are often moved from the hospital where they're born to a level 3 nursery with advanced technology to handle complicated preterm issues. This can make your life difficult, especially if the new hospital is some distance from your house, but your baby's care is ultimately worth it.

Some hospitals with large, regional NICUs have facilities that allow parents to stay overnight for a small charge or for free. Ronald McDonald houses are examples of facilities available near some hospitals.

TIP

If your partner is still in the hospital and can't see the baby right away, make sure you take lots of pictures — not just of the baby but also of the neonatal unit and, if possible, of the people taking care of her. That way your partner can get a real sense of where the baby is and picture her in an actual place.

Some regional NICUs provide a video feed to community hospitals so that moms who are separated from their babies can maintain a connection until they have a chance to see the baby in person.

Expect the first time you hold your baby to be extremely awkward; she may be festooned in IV lines, and you'll probably be scared to death of picking her up. Don't worry; it gets easier with time. She'll have less equipment attached, and you'll get to be a pro at dealing with dangling wires.

Knowing what to expect with a preemie

Preemies don't exactly look like the babies you've pictured in your mind, especially if they weigh less than 5 pounds. If your baby is born before 35 weeks, this is what he may look like:

>> **Big-eyed:** The lack of fat in his face gives your preemie a wide-eyed look.

>> **Boys may have underdeveloped genitalia:** Don't worry, dad — they'll grow.

>> **Hairy — except on his head:** Preemies often are still covered with *lanugo,* a fine, downy hair that helps keep them warm before they develop enough *subcutaneous* (under-the-skin) fat. Babies born before 26 weeks, on the other hand, may have no hair anywhere and may have very red, gelatinous skin.

>> **Skinny:** Babies born before 35 weeks often don't have a good layer of fat.

>> **Thin-skinned:** The blood vessels are more visible in a preemie's skin.

If you think your baby looks really odd, check with the nurses for reassurance that everything's okay — just not within your partner's earshot. No matter what the baby looks like, your partner will think he's the most beautiful person on the planet. As a new dad, you may not have that same rush of parental feelings that blind your partner to your baby's obvious — to you — shortcomings, such as no hair, a lopsided head, and limbs that seem to fly off in all different directions.

Parents often have a sixth sense or are just very observant of the little changes in their babies, and they may notice a change in their baby's condition before the staff does. Don't be afraid to speak up if you feel something's not right!

Clarifying common problems

Premature babies often have respiratory problems because their lungs aren't well developed. Artificial ventilation may be started almost immediately and is gradually decreased as the baby tolerates the reduction in extra oxygen. Some babies need special types of ventilation to overcome resistance in their lungs.

Most premature babies have feeding problems. Tiny babies, under 28 weeks, may not be fed by mouth for weeks or months because their digestive systems are too immature to handle food. Intravenous feeding is given instead, and as the baby grows, tube feeding is started. Nippling is begun very slowly because it can tire a preemie and use up her energy stores.

Many babies grow very slowly in the NICU. Infections, stress, and any number of complications can slow growth. Reading the weight chart and seeing the weight increase by a few grams can be the highlight of an NICU parent's day.

Learning the ropes — er, wires

Sometimes knowing what's what when it comes to the wires and machines attached to your baby can calm your anxiety. Your average preemie may sport the following wires and attachments.

Breathing apparatus

If the baby can't breathe on his own, he may be attached to a ventilator via a tube that goes through his mouth or nose down to his lungs, which delivers a certain number of breaths per minute, or to nasal prongs, which deliver extra oxygen to his lungs via — naturally — prongs that fit into his nose. Try very hard not to do anything that may dislodge the breathing tubes.

Monitoring equipment

Because preemies have an unfortunate habit of forgetting to breathe, often even babies who don't need breathing equipment are hooked up to a monitor that flashes a series of incomprehensible numbers, some with little flashing hearts next to them. The monitor is attached to the baby by wires that lead from the baby's chest, and possibly also from his hand or foot, or even from his umbilical cord if a line was placed there right after birth.

The machines monitor pulse (that's the flashing heart), respiration (the number of times the baby breathes each minute), and oxygenation levels. Preemie heart rates are from 110 to 160 beats per minute, on average. Respirations are 40 to 60 per minute. Oxygenation in the 90s is good. Blood pressure may also be continuously monitored in very sick babies.

The baby's temperature may also be monitored frequently, if not continuously. Because preemies have little in the way of fat stores, they get cold easily, and stress and the extra work of being sick and trying to grow can use up energy that may otherwise help keep them warm. The incubator or bed the baby's lying on also has its own thermometer to make sure it doesn't get too hot or too cold.

Intravenous lines

Most NICU babies receive intravenous medications and nourishment, at least at first. IV lines can be very precarious in preemies and need to be replaced frequently. The medications are sometimes hard on the veins, which "blow," necessitating a new IV. The NICU nurses don't do it on purpose, believe us; spending time putting a new IV in a preemie is rarely on the "fun things to do in the NICU" list.

If your baby has an umbilical line, he may not have a *peripheral line* (a line in the extremities or head), but umbilical lines can't be used for very long because they're a potential source of infection.

Preparing for preemie setbacks

Just when you think things are finally moving in the right direction, your preemie may get sick. Because preemies have a decreased ability to fight off infection, and because they're attached to invasive equipment that can serve as a portal into their little bodies, infections are very common among preemies.

Some common NICU complications include the following:

>> **Intraventricular hemorrhage (IVH):** IVH is a bleed into the brain that can range from mild (graded I) to very serious (graded IV). Around a third of babies born between 24 and 26 weeks have a bleed, but any baby born before 34 weeks can have an IVH. Bleeds may occur at the time of delivery or afterward.

>> **Necrotizing enterocolitis:** Called *NEC* by the NICU staff, this inflammation of the immature digestive system usually occurs after feedings are started. NEC can seriously damage the intestines. Feedings are temporarily stopped so the gut can heal, and IV feedings are given instead.

>> **Respiratory disease:** Long-term ventilation can save your baby's life but can also contribute to *bronchopulmonary dysplasia,* damage to the lungs that can take months or years to fully heal. This problem is more common in tiny babies known as *micropreemies.* Some babies with respiratory disease are discharged to home while still receiving oxygen, which is decreased gradually as they develop the ability to breathe better on their own.

>> **Respiratory infection:** The tubes can allow entry of germs into the lungs. Pneumonia may develop, and the baby may need antibiotic treatment.

Taking baby home

Preterm babies don't always have to stay in the hospital until they reach their original due date, and they don't always have to weigh 5 pounds before being discharged, either. NICUs generally assess the baby's condition, the parents' ability to handle possible problems, and the parents' willingness to learn the baby's care so they can do it at home.

Many parents take home babies who are still being tube-fed or who are on monitors to make sure they keep breathing. Others don't feel at all comfortable with technical equipment and would rather have their child in the hospital a little longer to be monitored. In fact, feeling completely unprepared to take home a preemie who has spent weeks or months in the NICU is very common.

TIP

If you or your partner starts to go into panic mode about coming home with your preemie baby, get involved with a preemie support group if you haven't already. Knowing that other families have done this and have survived is reassuring. And seeing a former 2-pounder tooling around the block on his bike is the best possible assurance that most preemies come through their early trauma just fine.

Seriously, going home with the inept pair of you is not the worst thing your baby will have to face in life, so just do it. Keep that NICU number on speed dial for a while, though!

Hi, Baby Baby Baby: Having Multiples

The birth rate of twins, triplets, and more has exploded with the advent of in vitro fertilization (IVF) and other advanced reproductive technology. Seventeen percent of twins and 40 percent of triplet births are results of infertility treatment. In 2019, the multiple-birth statistics in the United States broke down as follows:

>> Twin births occurred in 32 of 1,000 live births

>> Triplets or higher-order multiples (quadruplets, quintuplets, and more) occurred in approximately 88 of 100,000 live births

TIP

If you're expecting multiples, find a support group pronto. Support groups are a great source for used twin or triplet baby paraphernalia, which can be extremely expensive, and also for practical info on how to handle more than one baby.

Multiple identities: What multiples are and who has them

Although infertility treatments are the largest risk factor for multiples, you're more likely to have multiples if

>> **Your partner is black.** Black women have the highest natural twinning rate of the different racial groups; Asian women have the lowest.

>> **Your partner is older than 35.** Twins occur naturally around 3 percent of the time in women 25 to 29 and 5 percent of the time in women 35 to 39.

>> **Fraternal twins (nonidentical) run in your partner's family.** Your family history doesn't seem to have any bearing on the statistics, but if your partner is a fraternal twin, she has a 1 in 17 chance of having fraternal twins.

Twins can be either fraternal or identical. *Fraternal twins* are created from two different eggs and are no more similar than any other two siblings. *Identical twins* are the result of one embryo splitting into two at a very early stage of development. *Siamese twins,* also called *conjoined twins,* are always identical twins who didn't completely split as embryos. Conjoined twins are usually identified on ultrasound before delivery.

Obviously, boy-girl twins are always fraternal, but if you have two of the same sex, identifying whether they're identical or fraternal may be difficult at first. The majority of twins, especially twins from IVF cycles, are fraternal, although IVF also increases the risk of having identical twins. DNA testing is the only definite way to determine whether twins are identical or fraternal, although sometimes it's obvious that twins are fraternal if they look quite different.

WARNING

Many IVF parents who implant only two embryos are surprised to find themselves carrying three fetuses. If this happens to you, don't accuse the doctor of putting in an extra embryo he had lying around! What happened was that one of the embryos split into identical twins. Yes, it's possible.

Health risks for mom

All the usual pregnancy complaints are intensified during a multiple pregnancy. Annoying issues such as morning sickness, weight gain, heartburn, constipation, shortness of breath (especially on any type of exertion), urinary problems, and hemorrhoids are all likely to be magnified.

Many of the health risks of pregnancy for your partner increase with the number of fetuses she's carrying. Multiple pregnancies are often medically complicated by the following:

>> **Anemia:** This is low red blood cell count in the mother.

>> **Cesarean deliveries:** Cesarean deliveries are pretty much a given in higher-order multiple births because it's unlikely that all the babies will be head down. Additionally, high-order multiples are so small that even if they're all head down before birth, one or more are likely to flip as soon as the first baby is delivered and the rest have more room, possibly necessitating an emergency Cesarean.

>> **Gestational diabetes:** The increase in placenta size and hormone production may raise the risk of gestational diabetes in multiple pregnancies.

>> **Hemorrhage:** This is severe blood loss at the time of delivery.

>> **Placental abruption:** Women with multiples are three times more likely to have the placenta come off the uterine wall prematurely, possibly resulting in severe hemorrhage.

>> **Pregnancy-induced hypertension (PIH):** Defined as high blood pressure after 20 weeks of pregnancy, this affects one in three mothers of multiples.

For high-order multiples (triplets or more), bed rest during pregnancy is very likely.

Risks for the babies

Twins are five times more likely than single babies to have problems at birth or to die before or soon after delivery. Multiple pregnancies often deliver early because the womb has less room for all the occupants, and preterm babies are known to have more complications, so these factors account for some but not all of the risks multiples face. Statistics show that

>> Approximately 60 percent of twins deliver before 37 weeks.

>> 36 percent of triplets deliver before 32 weeks.

>> 80 percent of quads and more deliver before 32 weeks.

Twins are also more likely to have the following complications:

>> *Twin-to-twin transfusion syndrome* occurs only in identical twins who share the same placenta. One twin receives too much blood; the other, too little. Both can cause problems.

>> Birth defects such as cerebral palsy are much more common in multiples, and the risk increases with the number of fetuses.

>> Cord accidents can occur, such as knots in the cord or entanglement in a cord. Cord accidents reduce blood flow to the fetus. Identical twins, who develop in one amniotic sac, are more likely to become entangled in their own or their twin's cord.

Your medical practitioner may well suggest that you deliver at a medical center equipped for high-risk births, but if she doesn't, you should still plan to do so. Knowing that your babies have all the technological advances that may be needed in place from the moment of delivery can really reduce the stress you and your partner feel.

REMEMBER

Babies can be transported, if necessary, but doing so is stressful for the babies and for the parents. And if one baby is transported and the other isn't, you'll be trying to split your visiting time between two hospitals, which is unnecessarily stress-inducing.

Keeping Cool in Monetary Emergencies

Not all pregnancy emergencies involve medical crises: Some are all about cold, hard cash — or the lack of it. You may have taken a quick glance at your health insurance policy before you got pregnant, just to make sure you had the sterling coverage you thought you had, and you may have even checked the limits of coverage without ever dreaming that you might rack up a hospital bill of more than a million dollars for one little baby.

You may also have a new insurance provider and policy under the Affordable Care Act and don't fully understand your coverage. Worse, you may have let your policy lapse just before getting pregnant — surprise!

It's possible (probable, even, if you're normally a healthy twosome) that you have no idea what your insurance actually covers. Take time to dig through the drawers and find that policy because pregnancy illnesses and hospitalization costs can blow your socks off. Many hospitals today have counselors who help educate you on your fiscal responsibilities before they let you walk out the door, but it's nice to know your coverage ahead of time.

REMEMBER

If you find yourself without insurance or with minimal coverage, ask your healthcare provider or your local hospital about your options sooner rather than later. Community resources are likely available to help with prenatal care or baby care if you're experiencing financial hardship, and you may get the most benefit from them if you look into these resources ahead of time.

Checking out your insurance limits

Most insurance policies clearly list their limits, including a lifetime benefit amount. Insurance policies also may list your maximum obligation, or deductible, for the year. For example, you may have a cap of $5,000 on your out-of-pocket expenses for a year, meaning your insurance company pays everything else. However, you may have to pay every penny of your deductible before benefits kick in.

Covering the cost of unexpected medical expenses

Even the best insurance plans leave you footing a certain portion of the medical expenses. Over the next six months, don't be surprised to receive separate bills from every wing and department of the hospital in which you stay.

As many as 66 percent of all bankruptcies are related to unpaid medical bills. Even with insurance, using up your limits can leave you with a hefty bill. Most hospitals have a social worker or debt counselor who can work with you on unexpected costs that aren't covered by your insurance. Most have debt repayment plans, and many will reduce the bill in some circumstances.

You may be able to get some aid from the hospital's charity program or, if your child has an unusual medical condition, from a foundation involved in the disease.

REMEMBER

The main thing to do when faced with a bill that equals the national debt is not to panic. You have options, and you need to investigate them. You also need to be upfront with the hospital from the beginning about your coverage so you have time to resolve things before the hospital threatens to hold your partner or baby hostage. (Don't worry, it won't.)

TIP

Mistakes happen, and they can be difficult to find. Hospital bills generally list only the total charge and not each item individually. If at any point your bill doesn't make sense — or it seems like you're paying for the same thing twice or for something you didn't receive — ask your hospital's billing department for an itemized receipt. It's a lengthy document to comb through, but it allows you to challenge mistakes and suspect charges, and it may save you money.

Chapter **8**

Nearing the Finish Line: The Third Trimester

The last three months of pregnancy are when reality hits like a ton of bricks, and you and your partner realize, albeit still rather dimly, that a real baby is coming to live with you — a baby with her own personality, a separate person who's developing definite likes and dislikes even before birth and will be able to express them even when she can't say a word.

In the third trimester, all the major organs and appendages are in place, and all the baby has to do is grow. Mom is also doing her own growing, with an attendant list of common discomforts and complaints that you'll become well acquainted with. In this chapter, we look at baby's growth, mom's ever-expanding girth, and your role in your family's expansion.

Tracking Baby's Development during the Third Trimester

At the start of the third trimester, your baby is fully formed, although you wouldn't think so if you got a look inside the womb. The eyes are still fused, the skin is gelatinous, and the body fat is nonexistent, but everything that the baby needs to develop into a normal newborn is present and accounted for. The following sections provide the highlights of fetal development in the last three months of pregnancy.

Adding pounds and maturing in the seventh and eighth months

Week 28 starts off the final trimester of pregnancy, and don't think your partner will let you forget for one minute that she's been hauling this child around for six months already. Week 27 also marks the end of the "easy" trimester, so if you thought you heard lots of complaints in the second trimester, you ain't seen nothin' yet! And her complaints are justified. The baby grows from around 10 inches long and 1.5 pounds at week 27 to around 18 inches long and 4 to 6 pounds by week 36. That's a lot of growth in just nine weeks, and your partner will be feeling it.

In the seventh and eighth months, the baby develops in the following ways:

>> **Begins to see:** The eyes open around week 31, and the baby begins to perceive light and darkness.

>> **Fully develops the lung tissue necessary to breathe outside the womb:** By 36 weeks, most babies can breathe independently without oxygen supplementation.

>> **Jumps in response to loud noises and recognizes familiar voices:** Go ahead, talk just to him — he'll turn toward your voice after he's born if he's familiar with it, and "Honey, get me a beer" aren't the only sounds you want him to associate with you.

>> **Matures the digestive tract and kidneys:** The ability to breathe, suck, swallow, and eliminate in tandem is essential for life outside the uterus.

>> **Puts on some fat:** Your baby gains weight in these nine weeks (and so does your partner) because the baby is both growing and developing fat stores to help him regulate his temperature after birth.

Figure 8-1 shows the development of your baby in these final weeks.

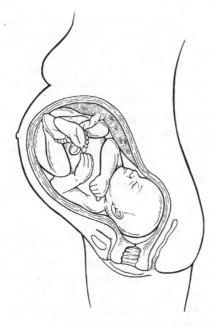

Illustration by Kathryn Born, MA

FIGURE 8-1: The fetus looks more and more like a fully developed person in the third trimester.

Getting everything in place in the ninth month

The ninth month is the home stretch. In these four weeks, the baby assumes the head-down position — the most advantageous position for delivery. After baby is head-down, she's probably that way for good. After 36 weeks, she's usually too big to go flipping around, although some babies do manage to turn themselves right-side up, which, for birthing purposes, is upside down, or *breech*. (Head to Chapter 10 for the scoop on breech deliveries.)

Your baby doesn't have much left to do in the last four weeks but grow and perfect already-in-place systems. In the last month, your baby will

>> **Be active:** Some babies are thumb suckers even before birth. They may yawn, grimace, and grab the umbilical cord in their hands. Kicking gets harder as space becomes tighter, so mom may not be able to feel the karate chops she's used to, but she should still feel some movement every day. If not, it's time to call the medical practitioner.

>> **Drop lower into the pelvis:** In anticipation of labor, the baby may drop down so that her head is pressing more directly on the cervix. This pressure helps thin and dilate the cervix and helps prevent the umbilical cord from falling below her head if your partner's water breaks, a dangerous situation known as a *cord prolapse*. (See Chapter 10 for more about cord prolapse.)

>> **Have descended testicles, if he's a boy:** Earlier in pregnancy, the testicles develop in the abdomen and descend gradually into the groin before assuming their final position outside the body. Boys whose testicles don't descend by the time of birth are evaluated periodically. Surgery may be required if they don't descend by a certain age because the increased body temperature can damage reproductive organs in males.

>> **Shed body hair and gain some head hair:** *Lanugo,* the soft downy hair that covers the fetus earlier in pregnancy, starts to disappear. Hair on the head may be abundant or nonexistent. Dark-skinned babies often have more hair at birth than future blondies.

>> **Start to develop wake-sleep patterns:** Most babies seem to be more active at night, which may give you some idea of what you're in for.

>> **Swallow amniotic fluid, urinate, and practice breathing:** Babies get ready to eat by swallowing amniotic fluid, which also gives the kidneys practice in elimination as urine is excreted into the amniotic fluid.

Finding Out What Mom Goes Through in the Third Trimester

The baby isn't the only one who changes in these final months, of course. Although your partner's changes on the outside are obvious, if somewhat unnerving at times (Can she really get any bigger than this? Won't her skin break apart?), the changes on the inside are just as dramatic, if not more so.

Getting acquainted with your "new" partner, now known as mother-to-be-with-a-vengeance, can be as complicated as getting to know the baby after he's born. Keep in mind at all times that your partner is going through physical and emotional upheavals, the likes of which you'll never be able to fathom, but you need to try.

Understanding your partner's physical changes

A pregnant woman at the end of the second trimester still looks pretty much like her normal self. Your partner may not even be wearing maternity clothes at this point, letting large shirts (probably yours) and pants a size or two larger than normal cover her cute little belly. All that changes in the third trimester for most women, although some lucky women never look all that pregnant, even when delivering 8-pound babies.

Between the seventh and ninth months, expect these changes in your partner's physique and physical condition:

>> **Backaches** are common because of the strain from the additional weight in front.

>> **Breasts may start leaking** a few drops of *colostrum,* the first fluids produced after birth. They may also look humongous because they contain around 2 pounds of extra weight — each!

>> **Constipation and hemorrhoids** can occur due to sluggish, compressed bowels. Pain and rectal bleeding can accompany hemorrhoids. Stool softeners and lots of roughage, along with physical activity, can help.

>> **Feet and ankles often swell,** especially if you're having a summer baby. Encourage her to rest with her feet up as much as possible.

>> **Heartburn** becomes more severe, but despite old wives' tales, it's in no way related to the amount of hair the baby will have.

>> **Her center of gravity shifts,** making falls more likely. Hide her high heels and, if she'll let you, take her arm when walking, like a proper gentleman.

>> **Interest in sex** may be at either extreme; it may be the last thing she's interested in or one of the things that interests her most. Hormones are funny that way. (See Chapter 5 for more about sex during pregnancy.)

>> **Itchy skin** is a huge problem for some pregnant women in the third trimester. Creams help keep the skin moisturized and decrease itching.

>> **Leg cramps** occur because of nerve compression by the growing uterus.

>> **She may have trouble sleeping,** even though she's always tired. Try tying a 6-pound, baby-shaped weight to your abdomen, and you'll quickly understand why.

>> **Shortness of breath comes with exertion** because the baby is pressing on her lungs. When the baby drops, she may feel relief, but the tradeoff is increased frequency of urination.

>> **Urination** becomes almost a full-time job. She may need to get up in the night to urinate, possibly more than once.

>> **The uterus can be felt** a few inches above her belly button at the start of the third trimester and up under her ribs by the end.

>> **Vaginal discharge increases,** so expect the reappearance of sanitary pads in the linen closet.

>> **Varicose veins** may pop out on her legs; they may itch or ache. *Spider veins,* small broken capillaries, may also occur on her face, neck, and arms.

Contractions may also begin to occur on and off, starting first with Braxton Hicks contractions, which don't change the cervix and are felt mostly in the front of the abdomen rather than in the back.

As the due date approaches, more contractions may come and go, usually with just enough frequency to have you leaping for the suitcase and putting it in the car before they peter out. Don't worry; the real thing will start soon enough!

Heeding warning signs

WARNING

Though many complaints of late pregnancy are normal and expected, some are not. Make sure your partner contacts her medical provider if she experiences any of the following symptoms:

>> **Leaking fluid:** This symptom usually indicates the bag of waters has broken. This is normal at the end of pregnancy but not in the seventh or eighth month. Always call if she notices more discharge than normal or is leaking fluid. After the water breaks, the baby is more susceptible to infection because his protective sac is breached. If labor doesn't begin within 24 hours, her medical practitioner may consider inducing labor.

>> **Severe abdominal pain:** This can be a sign of placental abruption, which can be life-threatening for mother and baby.

>> **A sudden, severe headache:** Strong headaches can be a sign of preeclampsia. (For details on the risks of preeclampsia, refer to Chapter 7.)

>> **Swelling of her face, hands, and feet:** Some swelling at the end of pregnancy is normal, but facial swelling can also be a sign of preeclampsia, especially if accompanied by sudden weight gain, headache, or a rise in blood pressure.

>> **Vaginal bleeding:** In the last few weeks of the pregnancy, your partner should tell her medical practitioner about any type or amount of bright red vaginal bleeding, with the exception of *bloody show* (blood-tinged mucus). Bleeding can indicate the premature separation of the placenta from the uterine wall, called a *placental abruption,* or a low-lying placenta, known as *placenta previa.* (See Chapter 7 for more about both conditions.)

PREGNANT DAD SYMPTOMS: COUVADE SYNDROME

In the past few years, some attention and study has been given to the idea that expectant dads may develop symptoms similar to those of their partners. This phenomenon, known as *couvade syndrome,* may affect as many as 90 percent of dads-to-be. Dads may experience nausea, backache, and other pregnancy symptoms as a psychological or physical reaction to their own weight gain, which may be due to eating more from stress or just from keeping up with their partner. Whatever the reason, rest assured in the third trimester that if you have "pregnancy pains," they too will soon be coming to an end.

Bracing for your partner's emotional changes

Hormone levels are very high in the last few months of pregnancy, and, for many women, with hormones come mood swings. Be prepared for the following emotional changes in the last trimester:

>> **Irritability:** When you don't feel your best physically, everything irritates you. Try not to be one of the "everythings" that drives your partner crazy.

>> **Self-image issues:** Pregnancy changes a woman's body image, sometimes for the better, sometimes not. Some women resent the loss of the perfect figure, whereas others are happy that pregnancy provides an excuse for the extra weight that's always bugged them. Expect to hear your partner make negative comments, and don't respond to them in kind. The answer to "Do I look fat?" is never "Yes."

>> **Weepiness:** Women find many reasons to cry in the last few months of pregnancy. They cry because they're happy, or sad, or frustrated, or angry. They cry for reasons they can't even express to you, which can, of course, be frustrating to you, but you'll get over it.

Some degree of moodiness, sadness, or depression is normal in late pregnancy. These mood changes should be fleeting, but as many as 10 percent of women become clinically depressed during pregnancy and need medical intervention. Additionally, up to 20 percent develop some depressive symptoms that may also need medical treatment.

Symptoms of clinical depression include sadness that doesn't lift, feelings of hopelessness or guilt, difficulty sleeping, constant fatigue, or behavior not typical for your partner. Don't ignore depression that seems extreme or that doesn't lift after a few days.

Antidepressant medications can be given in pregnancy if your medical practitioner feels that the benefits outweigh the risks. Some studies — but not all — have shown that certain antidepressants known as *selective serotonin reuptake inhibitors* can possibly increase the risk of a rare heart and lung condition known as *persistent pulmonary hypertension of the newborn,* or PPHN. The Food and Drug Administration in 2011 stated that reaching any conclusions about the risk of PPHN in newborns was premature given the conflicting study results.

It's important that your partner doesn't stop taking antidepressants on her own. Some drugs need to be tapered to avoid an increased risk of side effects. Staying on an antidepressant may decrease her risk of developing postpartum depression after birth. Talk to your medical practitioner about the pros and cons of antidepressants.

Sympathizing with her desire to have this over, already

Around the seventh month, many women start expressing a strong desire to have this pregnancy over and done with. Before you jump in with long-winded explanations of how the baby isn't fully developed yet, it's too early, or other pompous statements about why being pregnant for just two more months is a good idea, realize that your partner doesn't really want to have the baby early (well, maybe she does, a little); she's just tired and frustrated with being pregnant.

The last few months of pregnancy are no picnic, and unfortunately, you can't truly understand what she's going through. When she starts talking about getting this baby out by hook or crook the minute she hits 37 weeks, take it with a grain of salt. She's every bit as concerned about the welfare of this baby as you are, and she's not going to do anything rash.

Let her vent without giving her a lecture, and in five minutes, she'll probably be telling her mom how pregnancy has been the best time of her life. That's how hormones go sometimes.

Dealing with tears, panic, and doubts . . . even your own

Doing anything for the first time can be stressful, overwhelming, and scary. Facing labor, delivery, and motherhood for the first time certainly qualifies. Yes, you're also facing fatherhood for the first time — dealing with the prospect of labor, seeing your partner in pain, and a host of doubts and fears — but her concerns are fueled by hormones and the knowledge that some form of delivery, be it labor or surgery, is the only way to emerge with a baby after nine months of pregnancy. The inevitability of the end of pregnancy can be overwhelming at times.

Your partner won't be the first woman to ever express the feeling that she can't do this, that having a baby was a mistake, or that she's changed her mind about the whole thing and wants to call it off. These feelings will intensify when she's in labor, so if you deal with them rationally now, you'll be better prepared for them then.

TIP

All new parents fear they won't be good at their new role. The two of you can approach this fear together by taking the following practical steps:

>> **Read baby books and online pediatric sites.** You'll still go to pieces during the first colic episode, but if you know what to expect, it's a little easier to handle.

>> **Take a class.** Most hospitals offer pregnancy classes that touch on at least the basics of breast-feeding and newborn care.

>> **Talk it out.** Experience may change your mind about a number of parenting issues, but you'll feel more prepared if the two of you try to set out some basic ideas about how you want to raise the baby. Doing so helps avoid drama-filled discussions when one of you wants to put the baby in your bed at 3 a.m. and the other doesn't. Discussing things also gives you the sense of having some grasp of what parenthood is all about. Expect your ideas to change frequently in the first actual weeks of parenthood, though.

>> **Talk to your mom and dad — or a therapist.** Although time dims the memories of parenting, your own parents may be able to vaguely recall their early parenting days and give you some advice based on their own experiences. After all, you turned out okay, didn't you? (If you didn't, don't ask them.) Never underestimate the power of a third-party voice, too, especially when emotions are at an all-time high. Reach out to a therapist or marriage/couples counselor if the issues become too big to handle on your own.

>> **Visit friends with babies.** If you have friends or relatives with infants, hang out with them and pick their brains if you trust their judgment. Otherwise, just enjoy getting used to being around a little person.

REMEMBER

Allow your partner to vent and express doubts and concerns, but never fail to reassure her that you know she'll be a great mom, that she was born to do this, and that you'll be helping her every step of the way. Feel free to express your own fears and doubts about being a really good parent, but never in a "Can you top this" way.

WARNING

Many women at the end of pregnancy have vivid dreams about the baby or develop fears that something may be wrong with him. You can't do much about these fears except let her talk them out and reassure her that no matter what happens, you're there for her and the baby. However, if your partner becomes fixated on thoughts that she may harm the baby or that something is wrong with the baby, she may be experiencing a severe depressive disorder. Make sure she sees her medical practitioner promptly.

FACING YOUR OWN FEARS ABOUT FATHERHOOD

Old sitcom fans are well aware that it wasn't long ago that dads trotted off to work and mom stayed home (in pearls, no less) and kept the home fires burning. Dad talked to his kids for about two minutes each day to give them profound pieces of wisdom that they were extremely grateful to hear. Yesterday's dads — including yours, likely — were far more remote and less involved with their children than today's dads. Because today's new dads may not have had involved fathers as role models as they were growing up, they may face uncertainty about exactly how to approach the fatherhood thing. The idea that dad should be as involved in child rearing as mom is a fairly new one, and you may feel uncertain about what your role is.

Because no two families are alike, you and your partner will design your own family model. You set your own standards here, so don't worry about what a "good" dad does or how other people approach fatherhood. You're going to be a "good" dad, so however you decide to embrace the parenting role is the right approach for you and your partner. Being present and involved is all it takes.

Guaranteeing a Smooth Admissions Process

Think back to the last time you arrived at a crowded shopping mall with a parking lot packed to the gills with cars and you ended up walking ten minutes just to get to your store of choice. Now imagine that you drive right in and, miracle of miracles, the parking spot closest to the door is waiting for you.

If you want that experience upon arriving at the hospital when your partner is in labor — and believe us, you do — you need to make sure you fill out all the preadmissions paperwork at your hospital or birthing center. Doing so keeps you from having to fill out forms and answer an endless array of questions when you should be focused on the woman in pain.

A good time to make sure everything is in order is during your prenatal visit to the birthing center. The visit is not only a chance to get to know a few of the faces you may be seeing but also the perfect firsthand opportunity to make sure your partner is in the system.

Also, you want to make sure you contact your delivery doctor or midwife prior to going to the hospital. Some want a call as soon as labor begins; others just want a 30- to 60-minute heads-up before you head to the hospital. Many practitioners request that you call when your contractions are regularly occurring every 5 to 6 minutes and lasting 60 seconds for at least an hour, but follow your own practitioner's instructions. And because many labors begin (and end!) in the middle of the night, you want to give your doctor or midwife ample time to wake up before heading out the door.

At some point during the admissions process, you may be asked to leave the room so the nurse can talk to your partner alone. Although it may seem off-putting at first, this procedure is very important. Unfortunately, domestic violence is far too common, and one of the nurse's duties is to ensure that the woman in labor and the baby she's bringing into the world are in a safe environment during labor and delivery. Don't take it personally.

Picking a Pediatrician

Choosing a pediatrician before the baby arrives may seem unnecessary, but with so much going on in the weeks before and after delivery, you want to get it checked off the list in the third trimester. Finding someone who agrees with your stances on breast-feeding, vaccinations, and the necessity of certain in-hospital procedures may take more time than you think.

Also, a pediatrician needs to clear your baby for checkout from the hospital, and the sooner you start working with the doctor of your choice, the better. Building a relationship between a pediatrician and your baby increases the likelihood that your child will get the care she needs.

TIP

Get a list of approved pediatricians from your insurance company and start your research. Talk to other parents in your neighborhood and friends who live close by. As best you can, choose a pediatrician who's close to home because you'll be making the trip many times during the first year. Research feedback the doctor has received online, too. Considering the sheer number of hateful things people are willing to post online, take nasty reviews with a grain of salt, but do take note if a doctor has an overwhelming amount of negative feedback.

Next, schedule an interview with two or three doctors of your choosing. Here's a list of questions that you should ask any potential pediatrician to ensure you get the care you want for your baby, both during your hospital stay and beyond:

» How long have you been a pediatrician?

» How many doctors are part of your practice?

» What are your hours on the evenings and weekends?

» Is there an on-call doctor at all times? Is there a charge for after-hours calls/services?

» Are you a family practice doctor or solely practicing pediatrics?

New parents may find it easier for the whole family to be treated by the same doctor. If you and your partner have strong feelings about this, make sure to ask whether the doctor can see you too.

» Do you offer same-day appointments for illness?

» Are you often double-booked?

» How long is the average wait?

» Will I always see you at each visit or will my baby be seen by other doctors, nurses, or junior staff members?

» What's your stance on formula feeding? How long should our baby be breast-fed? What formulas do you recommend?

Whatever decisions you and your partner make about feeding your child, having a pediatrician who supports your choices is vital.

>> Are you flexible with immunization schedules?

Some parents choose to delay vaccinations or use alternate schedules. Make sure your pediatrician is onboard with your immunization wishes.

>> When do you recommend beginning to feed solid foods?

Depending on the doctor, you may be told to start feeding your child solid foods beginning at four months or as late as six months. Research varies on what's best, so get educated and make sure your pediatrician supports your feeding schedule.

>> Do you require breast-fed babies to take vitamin D supplements?

Breast-fed babies are often prescribed a supplement for vitamin D, but not all pediatricians and parents agree that it's necessary. Do your research on what feels right to you and make sure your pediatrician agrees with your decision.

>> Do you employ a lactation consultant or offer lactation support?

>> What's your stance on the use of antibiotics in children?

>> How often are the play facilities in your office cleaned?

>> Do you have a separate waiting area for sick children or for infants younger than a certain age, such as six months?

Also, feel free to show your potential pediatrician your birth plan. Her reaction to your decisions — such as whether to give the baby a vitamin K shot right after birth or whether a baby needs erythromycin on his eyes — may help guide your decision. (See Chapter 9 for more on the choices detailed in a birth plan.)

REMEMBER

Choose a doctor who most closely aligns with your wants and desires for your baby. You don't want to have to start the search all over again just because a pediatrician doesn't agree with your decision to delay vaccinations or give your child formula.

TIP

Chat up the other parents in the waiting room to find out the real dish on how long they have to wait at each visit, how often they actually see the doctor, and what their overall impressions are of her caregiving style. Parents are brutally honest and your best source of information.

If you have a long-time family physician with whom you have a personal relationship and you don't plan to have him be your child's pediatrician, let him know before the baby arrives. Doing so is respectful and helps you avoid the awkwardness of having both your family doctor and your pediatrician show up at the hospital.

Whose Baby Is This, Anyway? Dealing with Overbearing Family Members

From the time you share the news of your coming baby, you'll be inundated with advice and visitors. Nobody will want to be more hands-on than your family, and it may grow tiresome and become a source of angst very quickly the closer to labor and delivery your partner gets, and especially when you get home from the hospital and crave some family time.

Mothers, grandfathers, aunts-to-be — they all get nervous, too. Unfortunately, their offers of assistance and their constant presence can keep you and your partner from some much-needed quiet bonding time before baby arrives. Your lives are about to change forever, for the better (baby, baby, baby!) and for the worse (goodbye sleep and frequent sex!), and you need time to enjoy the waning bits of childlessness you have left.

REMEMBER

Your families love you, and their well-meaning, obtrusive advice, visits, and purchases are the only way they know how to show you just how excited they are to meet the new little person you're bringing into the family. However, if members of your family are becoming too involved or over-the-top for your tastes, be sure to thank them for their love and support and simply let them know that you and your partner need to take some time for yourselves before the baby comes.

TIP

Depending on how big and how emotionally connected your family is, consider starting a phone tree to share news earlier in your pregnancy to save you from having to call every single relative in your contacts list every time you go in for an ultrasound (see Chapter 9 for details on creating a phone/text tree). Telling the same story over and over to 13 aunts, cousins, and neighbors may take the fun right out of your fun news.

Social media is a common way for folks to share pregnancy news and ultrasound pictures, but it's a double-edged sword. Yes, social media updates are the easiest way to share information with large groups of people, but it's also difficult to filter the info to only the people you want involved. And just like with anything, too many cooks in the kitchen can bring about a lot of unwanted advice and intrusion from people you don't want involved in the process. Use social media at your discretion; only you and your partner will know how much social sharing you're comfortable engaging in.

That said, don't cut off communication altogether. Make sure to call the most important people in your life as frequently as you see fit. It's an exciting time for everyone, and you don't want to tarnish a loved one's joy by letting him get all the news secondhand.

Chapter 9

The Copilot's Guide to Birthing Options

abor is nothing like it used to be. From the au naturel days, when biting down on a bullet was the "medication," to the 1950s, when every woman was sedated up to her eyeballs while dad spent the night at the bar, labor has evolved into a family event that involves medications that really take the pain out of labor, sleepovers for dad, and champagne and steak dinners the night before discharge.

One thing about having a baby is certain: There's no one right way to do it. For every person who wants to deliver at home on her grandma's favorite quilt, another person feels that *epidural on demand* is the best phrase in the English language. Whatever you and your partner dream up as the ideal labor experience, rest assured it probably won't be the weirdest idea your birthing practitioner has ever heard.

You have more childbirth options today than ever before. Natural deliveries, home deliveries, and give-me-everything-you've-got deliveries are all possible. And the good thing is, no one will hold your partner to the ideas you both thought sounded good before labor started. If she decides she wants an epidural after all, all she has to do is scream — er, say so.

However, even though the number of options is much larger than in previous years, some of these options may not be feasible in your situation. For instance, if your partner has certain medical conditions, such as preeclampsia, or if the baby has congenital birth defects, they really need to be under a doctor's care in a hospital, even if your partner had her heart set on a home delivery. Be sure to talk to the doctor early in the pregnancy about your plans so she can advise you on their feasibility and safety and let you know if circumstances change.

In this chapter, we review the birthing options available and help you decide what may work best for you and your partner. We also provide tips on crafting a birth plan and deciding who's allowed in the delivery room.

Choosing Where to Deliver

A century ago, nearly everyone delivered at home. Fifty years ago, nearly everyone delivered in the hospital. Today, parents can choose among three options: home, hospital, or a special birthing center designed to mimic the comforts of home while providing cutting-edge medical treatment if needed.

Delivering at a hospital

Hospitals today love to stress how much like home they are while still having all the most up-to-date equipment at their fingertips. And though hospitals have come a long way in improving the overall birthing experience, they're still not home. Some, however, are better than others at creating a welcoming, open-door policy for families.

Check out the local possibilities, keeping in mind that your doctor can only practice where he has privileges and that, in the long run, a doctor you trust is far more important than lavender quilts and a pullout sleeper chair. Here's what to look for when you visit different hospitals:

>> **Is it secure?** Most hospitals have beefed up security, especially around the maternal and child health area. Hospital bracelets are embedded with alarm triggers, codes have to be activated to enter certain areas, and the staff all dresses in one color so you know who belongs there.

Walking on to a maternity floor without a pass should *not* be possible. You want security to be tight, even if it's a pain in the neck for you and your family and friends. The alternative is someone walking off with your precious bundle of joy.

» **What are the visiting policies?** What you're looking for depends on your preferences. Do you want your entire family and a three-piece band present or are you hoping to have just the two of you at the delivery and in the mother-baby unit afterward? Keeping family out is much easier if you can quote "hospital rules." During the Covid-19 pandemic, hospitals modified visiting policies from time to time, so double check on the hospital's most current policies before labor starts.

» **How much access does dad have?** Many places allow 24-hour visiting privileges, but some don't. Find out the rules ahead of time so security isn't called to remove you.

» **Is the staff helpful?** You can tell a lot by the staff's attitude, even on a short visit. Do they smile and say "hello" or do they run over your foot with a gurney without even an "excuse me"? You're going to spend way more time with the nurses than with your doctor in labor — in fact, the doctor is often in and out so fast you may not be quite sure he was there at all — so your experience will be more pleasant if the nurses are good. Although you may still draw Nurse Ratched for your labor nurse, it's less likely at a hospital with a mission statement and policies that promote a positive, family-centered mother-baby unit.

If you're planning to use a midwife or a doula, find out how the staff will work with her.

» **Is anesthesia in-house all night?** Surprising as it may be, some small hospitals don't have an anesthesiologist in the hospital all night. The anesthesiologist may have to be called in from home if your partner wants an epidural during the night. And if the hospital has only one on staff, she may be doing an appendectomy just as your partner starts getting really uncomfortable. Know ahead of time so you can ask for an epidural early, if need be.

» **How's the décor?** Consider the appearance of the hospital room, but only after you take everything else into consideration. Pretty surroundings are nice, but you'll be too busy to notice them. And ultimately that pretty quilt will be removed from the bed because the staff doesn't want anyone bleeding — or worse — all over it.

>> **What type of neonatal intensive care unit do you have?** Though no one anticipates problems, they can and do occur suddenly in labor sometimes. Having your baby transferred to another hospital because the original hospital can't handle his issues is traumatic for you. A level III unit is the best for caring for very sick infants; most level II units can handle many types of sick or premature newborns.

After you make your decision, visit the hospital again. Knowing exactly what your room will look like and even recognizing some familiar faces removes a layer of stress as you get ready for delivery. Most hospitals and birthing centers offer tours, but you can call and schedule a private tour of the facility as well.

While you're there, take note of the eating options, parking guidelines, and prenatal and postpartum classes that the hospital or birthing center offers. This allows you to plan ahead and give your well-wishers the information they need, as well as make full use of the facility's offerings.

TIP

Many hospitals hold prenatal lactation classes that are taught by the on-staff lactation consultant who visits your room after delivery. The classes are usually free and not terribly long or taxing to attend. Encourage your partner to attend a class to find out the basics of breast-feeding and to initiate a face-to-face relationship prior to the consultant's postpartum visit. Your partner will be much more comfortable asking questions and discussing any issues she and baby are having if she has met the consultant previously.

Delivering at home with a midwife

The idea of having your baby at home may appeal to you and your partner. Home delivery may be an option for you if you meet all the following strongly suggested guidelines:

>> You've found a midwife who's willing to deliver at your home. Most, but not all, certified nurse-midwives (CNM) deliver in hospitals, so a CNM willing to come to your home may be difficult to find.

>> You live fairly close to a medical facility in case of emergencies.

>> You're not delivering in Montana in January or any other area where roads are impassable during the month in which you're due.

>> You're both calm, sensible people who are really committed to the idea of home birth.

WARNING

The trouble with labor is that though 99 out of 100 times everything goes perfectly, you need to be prepared for that one time when things go bad so quickly you can't believe your eyes. Having nearby medical help is essential, unless your midwife can do a Cesarean in less than 30 minutes in an emergency.

Make sure your midwife has a backup plan to cover contingencies such as sudden illness or other problems that would prevent her from getting to you for the delivery. Does she have a partner or someone who covers for her? Discuss circumstances that may cause you to change your mind about home delivery, from ominous weather to last-minute cold feet.

If you plan to use a midwife at home, be sure to get good answers to the following questions (in addition to the questions listed in the later "Working with a midwife" section):

>> **What type of equipment will you bring with you?** You can be sure a ventilator and fully equipped operating room won't appear out of her black bag, but oxygen and basic medications such as intravenous fluids and oxytocin (to prevent heavy bleeding after delivery), plus equipment like a bag-valve mask to breathe for the baby in case of problems after birth, should be in every midwife's bag.

>> **How long do you stay?** "As long as you need me" is a good answer. She should stay at least an hour or two to make sure your partner and the baby are behaving normally and to get nursing started. On the other hand, you may not want her moving in with you — that's your mother-in-law's role. She should also visit for the next few days to recheck both mother and baby in case of any late-developing problems.

Delivering at a birthing center

Birthing centers are sort of a hybrid compromise between home and hospital delivery. In most cases, they're staffed by certified nurse-midwives or licensed midwives (see the section "Working with a midwife" later in this chapter for the difference) and have an association with a nearby hospital. If your partner's labor becomes complicated, she can easily be transferred to the hospital.

You generally can't get an epidural at a birthing center, although conscious sedation is usually available. Units range from free-standing outpatient buildings that resemble a medical facility to homes that have been converted into birthing areas.

Some birthing centers are really little more than homey labor-and-delivery units located away from the rest of the hospital, while others are truly women-oriented places that work to give you and your partner a more natural birth. Do your research when you choose your practitioner because you'll likely need a practitioner who works at the birthing center to deliver there.

Making Sure Your Birth Practitioner Is a Good Fit

Discussing your plans with your current birth practitioner as soon as you figure out what they are is important. For one thing, he may not be interested in participating if you're planning something out of his comfort zone, and you may need time to find someone who thinks childbirth in the backyard sounds like fun. If your midwife balks at assisting you during a delivery that features a medically unnecessary planned Cesarean, you need to find a medical practitioner who doesn't.

REMEMBER

Though many doctors are more flexible about childbirth options than they used to be, most doctors still have a fairly narrow comfort range, one that likely includes fetal monitoring, intravenous infusions, and limited time in the hot tub. The practices that midwives use, on the other hand, have become more mainstream in many areas, and a certified nurse-midwife may practice only slightly differently from an obstetrician. Lay midwives — although not legal in all parts of the country — are more likely to support non-traditional birthing options.

Screening potential practitioners

Whichever birth practitioner you choose, the best way to know whether you're in the right place is to ask. Accompany your partner to her visit when discussing options because if the practitioner isn't onboard with your partner's plan, she may think she can just wait and talk some sense into the absent parent — that would be you. Presenting a united front, especially on nonnegotiable items (such as home birth, for example) is best done as a couple. Consider asking these questions:

>> **Where do you deliver?** Most doctors deliver at just one hospital — maybe two. If you choose a midwife, find out whether she delivers at homes only or also at hospitals, and make sure she can do it where you want to be. Many certified nurse-midwives deliver only at hospitals.

>> **What's your Cesarean rate?** The Cesarean rate in the United States and other developed countries is high. Although C-sections are often necessary and lifesaving, they have a higher risk of complications for your partner and the baby. A significantly higher Cesarean rate than your area's average is a warning sign that your doctor may be too quick with the knife.

>> **How many inductions do you do?** Nobody wants to be pregnant forever, or even nine months, but pregnancies were designed to end naturally. Some doctors do way too many inductions, especially on Friday mornings. Your convenience isn't always the goal when the doctor offers to induce labor. Also, induced labors have a higher Cesarean rate, and Cesarean deliveries cause more maternal and fetal complications.

>> **Who's on call?** Does the doctor come in when her patients go into the hospital or do residents manage labor? Early in labor, some doctors have the resident on call or the nurse check their patient and call them for instructions. This isn't necessarily a problem, but knowing it ahead of time keeps you from badgering the nurses about when your doctor is coming in. For midwives, find out whether she has an assistant or backup person to cover for her if she can't attend.

>> **How do you feel about [fill in the blank]?** If you have an unusual request, politely approach your practitioner with this line instead of demanding, "We want [whatever]." If you both want to spend labor in the hot tub naked, now would be a good time to get your practitioner's feedback on this idea.

REMEMBER

Make sure you and your partner agree on what you want *before* discussing plans with your practitioner, and discuss it well before labor starts. Arguing in front of the nurses and trying to talk your partner out of an epidural at 6 centimeters is considered really bad form by the hospital staff, and they may not let you use the coffee machine or show you their hidden stash of emergency snacks for fainting fathers if they don't like the way you talk to your partner!

Working with a midwife

A midwife delivery in the hospital or birthing center can be a wonderful option. Midwives really are committed to fewer interventions in labor and often give much more personal care. However, your partner may become so attached to the midwife that you feel a little left out. Don't let that happen; go to appointments and get to know the midwife yourself so she knows you're interested in being a real part of the partnership. Most midwives actually want you as an integral part of the birthing team.

TIP

If you and your partner are thinking about delivering with a midwife, check the American College of Nurse-Midwives (www. midwife.org) or the Midwives Alliance of North America (www. mana.org) for options in your area. Using a search engine or checking chat boards on sites such as www.mothering.com for information is often the best way to get other people's opinions and experiences on what using a midwife or having a home birth is like.

A personal interview is the best way to get a feel for not only the nuts-and-bolts information about a midwife's education and experience but also a sense of whether your personalities will mesh for the next nine months. When you interview a prospective midwife, ask the following questions:

>> **What's your training?** Some midwives have nearly as many degrees as your doctor, and others have no formal training at all. But don't necessarily reject a midwife because of a lack

of diplomas: Some people have a natural ability to deliver babies, love the work, and have all the knowledge necessary for a safe outcome, as long as they have medical backup nearby.

>> **How long have you been doing this?** The longer the better. You see everything if you work in obstetrics long enough.

>> **What's *your* backup plan?** If she says a backup plan isn't necessary, reconsider this person. Having a backup plan is always necessary; emergencies can happen to anyone.

Getting some additional help with a doula

Although the word *doula* may have you picturing some sort of metal-studded medieval torture device, a doula actually can be a soon-to-be dad's secret weapon — one that can take some of the pressure off your very tense shoulders. A *doula* is a person, generally a woman, with a comprehensive understanding of the birthing process. She is hired to provide emotional and physical support throughout labor. Think of her as your very own in-hospital, labor-specific Google search/motivational speaker who encourages you to participate in labor and delivery as much or as little as you're comfortable with. Services doulas offer include the following:

>> Offering your partner nutrition advice and tips on coping with pregnancy discomforts

>> Helping the two of you create a birth plan

>> Staying with you and your partner throughout labor and delivery (the doctor and nurses aren't present the whole time if you deliver in a hospital)

>> Facilitating communication of the birth plan and the decisions of the mother and father to the doctor/midwife and nurses

>> Giving light massage to your partner (and even you) during labor and delivery

>> Encouraging different positions to help advance labor

>> Helping your partner get baby latched on for the first breast-feeding post-delivery

If you think doulas are only necessary for deliveries in which the father isn't involved, think again. Labor is a complex process, and as it progresses you and your partner will be asked to make many decisions about procedures and medications for which you may not feel fully prepared. A doula can inform you about both the risks and benefits involved and help you explore other options that may better suit your birth plan.

Doulas also provide your partner constant support while giving you the opportunity to step out of the room to grab a quick snack or take a breath of fresh air. For long labors, a 15-minute nap can make the difference for a worn-out dad-to-be (coauthor Matthew experienced this revelatory occurrence firsthand). Doulas ensure that someone who understands the process and your birthing choices is with your partner at all times — even when your eyes are closed.

Working with a doula has a medical benefit, too. Research shows that couples who have a doula present during childbirth tend to have shorter labors with fewer complications and a reduction in the use of labor-inducing medications, forceps, vacuum extractions, and C-sections.

After your new family returns home, most doulas make a post-partum visit that provides support for mom and baby, and they also provide telephone support for a specified duration following birth. Some doulas work mainly with moms for the birth, while others specialize in helping out after you return home.

Talk to your doctor about having a doula early in your prenatal care if you're delivering at the hospital. Not all doctors — or all hospital staff, including nurses — welcome doulas with open arms. However, this is *your* delivery, and it's up to you to decide who gets to be there, within reason.

Not all doulas are created equal. Make sure to interview multiple candidates and ensure they're certified by DONA International. For more information about hiring a doula, visit the DONA website: www.dona.org.

Looking at Labor Choices

Standard labor practices vary depending on who's delivering and where you deliver, but no matter the situation, you and your partner have to make a number of decisions and can opt to make dozens of others if you have preferences. Educate yourselves on common procedures and their pros and cons by talking with your medical practitioner and doing some reading.

One of the biggest issues for women in labor is deciding whether to have an epidural or other pain medication. In this section, we discuss that decision and another big issue: water births.

Going all natural or getting the epidural

REMEMBER

Although you're welcome to have your say if you say it nicely, the decision about pain medication is really up to your partner. As long as she's not planning to do anything unsafe, she's the one who has to go through labor, not you, so the drug decision should be hers.

The *all-natural* method of childbirth, which avoids unnecessary pain medication and medical interventions such as episiotomies, seems to have peaked about the time the hippie movement went mainstream and started buying BMWs, but letting nature take its course in childbirth still has many proponents. Women have been having babies naturally since forever, and many women find going through labor without any medication empowering.

TIP

Classes that teach breathing and relaxation techniques as a natural way to deal with pain, such as the Bradley Method (see www.bradleybirth.com for classes near you), are available. A doula, midwife, or obstetrician who's supportive of natural childbirth can also be a good source of information on the pros and cons of delivering naturally and the classes available in your area. Some classes focus on specific breathing patterns (can you say, "Hoo hoo hee"?), whereas others stress learning to listen to your body, relaxation methods, and the benefits of staying upright during labor.

Around 71 percent of women in labor these days have an *epidural,* an injection that numbs the nerves from the abdomen down to the thighs. An epidural is usually given when labor is well established, around 4 centimeters, because contractions can slow down if it's given too early. Some doctors, though, order epidurals earlier and then start a labor-inducing drug called Pitocin if contractions slow down.

Epidurals are better than they used to be. They can be run as a continuous infusion on a pump so they don't wear off and need to be reinjected. Some hospitals even offer *walking epidurals,* where the dose given may still allow patients to walk, which is better for keeping labor going than lying in bed. However, this type of epidural may not work as advertised, and your doctor may want your partner to stay on the fetal monitor, so don't count on your partner being able to walk around untethered. If your hospital offers wireless monitoring, you might be able to get up and ambulate, with occasional pit stops for your practitioner to check your progress.

Some women turn down the epidural but receive intravenous pain medications to help with labor pains. One problem with IV medications is that they can depress the baby's ability to breathe after birth, so they can't be given too close to the time of delivery.

Taking it to the water

Water birth is delivery of the baby while the mother is in a large tub of water. The baby is delivered while under the water, which is considered by proponents of the practice to be less traumatic to the baby because he has spent nine months in water. Although water birth sounds like a warm, back-to-nature experience, no cultures actually practice it. This fact doesn't mean that water birth doesn't have some appealing possibilities, mostly for mom-to-be, who gets to spend most of her labor floating in a tub of water. Many women find that laboring in water reduces pain and aids in relaxation.

Babies have never been traditionally born into a vat of water, and although most babies don't breathe until they're out of the water, a few baby deaths have been related to water birth. Laboring in water and getting out for the actual delivery may be a safer option to consider.

The following women absolutely should *not* have a water birth:

>> Women giving birth prematurely. (See Chapter 7 for more on preterm delivery.)

>> Women with genital herpes.

>> Women whose babies have passed *meconium,* the first stool, before delivery. These babies need their mouth and nose suctioned as soon as the head is delivered to help prevent meconium aspiration into the lungs. Meconium is visible as a greenish color to the amniotic fluid or even as small fecal particles when your partner's water breaks.

Creating a Birth Plan

A *birth plan* is a document that outlines the procedures, medications, and contingency plans that you and your partner are comfortable with throughout labor and delivery. It details your ideal birth experience while acknowledging the unpredictability of the process.

A birth plan isn't a set of marching orders for your nurses, doctor, or midwife, so keep it simple and friendly. You share this document with your entire birthing team, and not all doctors and nurses are thrilled at the prospect of a couple telling them how to do their jobs.

Creating a birth plan requires that you and your partner discuss what you're comfortable with and make many important decisions prior to your arrival at the hospital. The last thing you want to do is leave life-altering, labor-changing decisions to be made during an emotionally wrought time. And for more ideas than what we share here, check out *Birth Plans For Dummies,* written by coauthor Sharon and Rachel Gurevich and published by Wiley.

Visualizing your ideal experience

Labor and delivery are like reading a choose-your-own-adventure novel; every decision you make can lead you to a slightly different outcome.

As corny as it may sound, you and your partner should spend some time with your eyes closed trying to picture what your perfect experience would look like. Try to be realistic — a pain-free, 60-minute labor is highly unlikely, and making that dream a reality is beyond your control. Instead, focus on the things you can control.

When creating a birth plan, consider the following basic questions:

>> What types of medication does your partner want to have administered?

>> Do you want to delay clamping of the umbilical cord until it stops pulsating rather than cut it immediately after birth? This is a hot birthing topic today. (See the sidebar "When to cut the cord" for more information.)

>> Do you want to cut the cord? Do you want to bank the cord blood?

>> Does your partner want final approval before the doctor performs a vacuum extraction? This involves a suction device that helps pull the baby out, which can cause painful tearing of the vagina and temporarily misshapen baby heads. It's a generally safe (and in some cases necessary) procedure, but many women want to have the choice as to whether it's performed.

>> Does your partner want constant or intermittent fetal monitoring? *Fetal monitoring* tracks baby's stress levels during childbirth, and constant monitoring limits your partner's ability to move freely during labor. In a hospital delivery, being monitored at least part of the time is probably a given.

>> Does your partner want to veto an episiotomy? An *episiotomy* is a surgical incision that enlarges the vaginal opening to allow the baby to come out more easily. It used to be a common procedure, but most studies show that letting the body tear naturally is a better option. An episiotomy is quite painful during recovery and not an attractive option for most women unless absolutely necessary for the baby's health.

>> Does your partner want to be able to get up and walk around while laboring? Keep in mind that pain medications and ambulation may be mutually exclusive.

>> Are you opting to forgo circumcision?

To make sure you both feel positive about your childbirth experience, you need to prepare answers to these important questions. Many procedures may be done as a matter of course that may not jibe with you and your partner's desires, so invest the time beforehand to avoid any regrets that you could have prevented.

TIP

Many prenatal classes include exercises that help you visualize your ideal experience, and some even offer help developing your birth plan. When selecting a class, ask the instructor whether these activities are included as part of the course. Having a third party involved, be it a doula or your prenatal instructor, may help you and your partner narrow down your list of what's truly important and turn those priorities into a cohesive, effective birth plan.

WHEN TO CUT THE CORD

Birth is full of hot topics, and when to clamp and cut the umbilical cord is currently one of them. Many practitioners cut the cord immediately because that's the way it was done when they went to medical school. Doing so also allows the nurse to take the baby to the warming table and make sure he's doing okay before bringing him back to your partner.

But if your partner wants to bond with the baby first or start nursing before the assessment is done, or even if you just want your baby to get the benefits of receiving the blood that's in the cord, you can ask your practitioner to delay cord-clamping and cutting until the cord stops pulsating, which usually happens within one to five minutes after birth. The World Health Organization recommends waiting one to three minutes before cutting the cord.

You may also have heard that there are benefits to waiting but you don't really know what they are, so here's a list:

- **The baby gets a little extra blood, which can also give him a little extra iron.** Some studies have shown that babies who experience delayed cord-cutting are less likely to be iron-deficient in infancy.

(continued)

(continued)

- **The baby gets an immune system boost and other health benefits.** Waiting to cut the cord could transfer stem cells and T cells that may help protect the baby against respiratory illness, brain hemorrhages, and other problems in infancy.

On the other hand, there are also concerns about delayed cord-cutting. The World Health Organization lists the following possible risks of delayed cord-cutting:

- **An increased risk of *polycythemia*, a condition caused by an excess of red blood cells.** Polycythemia may cause lethargy, seizures, tremors, stroke, apnea, and respiratory distress. Delayed cord-clamping can increase the risk of your newborn developing polycythemia or worsen it if he has congenital polycythemia.

- **An increased risk of jaundice from an increased red blood cell count.** In several studies, babies who had delayed cord-clamping were at higher risk of developing jaundice and needing phototherapy to resolve the condition.

Talk to your practitioner about the pros and cons of delayed cord-cutting well before the delivery. You may still have to remind your practitioner of your wishes at the time of birth because he is very likely to clamp the cord immediately out of habit. After the cord is clamped, unclamping won't get the blood flowing again because the blood in the cord will clot quickly.

Drafting your plan

After you and your partner decide what your ideal birth looks like, you need to put it into writing. Try to use language that's friendly, concise, represents your flexibility, and includes your absolute no-negotiation items.

Births don't usually go exactly according to plan, so allow wiggle room for the unexpected to make sure the nurses and doctors know that your priority is having a healthy baby. Here are some basic tips for crafting your birth plan:

>> Write a nice, short introduction that introduces who you are and thanks your team in advance for following your plan.

>> Include a brief overview that states your basic, overall desires for the kind of labor and delivery you and your partner want.

>> Break the main body into three sections: labor, delivery, and post-delivery.

>> Under each heading, make the major points into a bulleted list for easy reading.

Keep it to one page unless you know ahead of time that your labor and delivery will be complicated and therefore require more steps.

TIP

Because the majority of what you outline in the birth plan is up to your partner to decide and ultimately undergo, get involved in this project by letting her know you're interested in having some input. Make her favorite dinner and start a dialogue. Ask her questions about what she wants and tell her what you want, too. Take notes during your discussion and then start composing your birth plan together. Your birth plan will be a work-in-progress because your ideas may change during the pregnancy, but do at least get the dialogue started early in pregnancy.

Use the following birth plan as an outline for creating an effective, concise document for your team:

The Johnson Family Birth Plan

The Midwives at Methodist Hospital Family Center

Parents: Rachel & Evan Johnson

Doula: Holly Barhamand

We're looking forward to having our baby at Methodist Hospital with the midwife group and staff! We know you see a lot of birth plans, and we thank you for reading ours.

We anticipate a normal birth and would like to allow the process to unfold naturally. However, in the unlikely event of a complication, we'll cooperate fully after having an informed discussion with the birth team. We're also willing to sign release forms if legally required to avoid "routine" procedures we opt against.

Overall, we'd like no medication, exam, or procedure to be administered to mother or baby until it's explained to us and we've given our consent. Thank you in advance for all your hard work and excellent care!

Labor:

>> *I'd like to attempt labor without pain medication — I will ask (loudly, I'm sure!) if I feel I need something.*

>> *We prefer intermittent, external fetal monitoring to continuous or internal. We consent to admission strip monitoring.*

>> *I decline all vaginal or other internal exams except with my expressed consent at the time.*

>> *I prefer to avoid IV. If IV is necessary, please use a saline lock.*

Delivery:

>> *I'd like to have freedom of movement and position during delivery — squatting, hands and knees, and so on.*

>> *I very strongly prefer natural tearing to an episiotomy.*

>> *We very strongly prefer delaying cord-cutting until the cord has stopped pulsating (we'll consider consent for exception if baby is in distress or excess meconium is present).*

>> *We decline Pitocin, uterine massage, and pulling the cord.*

>> *If surgery is required, Evan and Holly (our doula) need to be present. I prefer regional anesthesia rather than general, except in case of an emergency. Please use double-layer sutures when repairing my uterus.*

Post–delivery

>> *Please place baby on mother's abdomen immediately. We'd like the baby to remain with parents at all times. We'd like to start breast-feeding as soon as possible and delay potential interruptions.*

We respectfully request the following:

>> *No routine suctioning of the baby's mouth and nose (unless needed)*

>> *No erythromycin eye ointment*

>> *No vitamin K injection (unless there is bruising or birth trauma)*

>> *No vaccinations to be given at this time*

>> *No blood to be drawn from baby; we consent to a PKU test and are happy to discuss desired timing of this test with the nursing staff*

Thank you for your sensitivity to our preferences and for bringing your knowledge and care to this great event in our lives.

REMEMBER

As important as this day is to you, you aren't a celebrity, and the staff won't meet unrealistic demands with a smile and a nod. Nor will your team take unnecessary risks that could harm mother or baby just to meet your birth plan's requirements. Keep your birth plan focused on the elements of the birthing process that can be controlled, take each hurdle one at a time, and if and when things begin to deviate from the plan, help your partner make the best decisions possible by getting as much information as you can about the risks and benefits from the knowledgeable members of your team.

Sharing your birth plan with the world

Unfortunately, labor usually doesn't begin on that imprecise due date you've been hanging your hat on for the last nine months. Babies can come early, and with so much to get ready for, you may find yourself putting off creating and sharing your birth plan. Make time to write your birth plan toward the beginning of the third trimester, which gives you plenty of time to share it with your birthing team and any inquiring relatives and friends.

Going over your plan with the birthing team

Have your birth plan in place far in advance of your due date so you can share it with your doctor or midwife during the seventh or eighth month of pregnancy. Doing so gives you time to discuss the plan and address any concerns your medical practitioner may have. If you're hiring a doula, schedule a prenatal visit to go over the document.

Upon arrival at your delivery room, give a copy of your birth plan to the nurse assigned to your room. Hang a copy on the front of your door, if permitted, so that anyone who enters your room can read it first. Also hang a copy on the wall in your room, preferably near where your partner will deliver. Giving your medical practitioner a visual reminder can't hurt. Don't go crazy posting your birth plan all around the room though. If your birth plan contains standard, routine, agreed-upon-in-advance procedures, festooning the room with your birth plan will undoubtedly be seen as slightly weird by the staff.

TIP

Getting off on the right foot is always a good first step. Deliver your birth plan to the nurses on duty with a plate of fresh-baked goodies. Making cookies or cupcakes can be a welcome distraction during early labor at home and can make the overworked, underpaid nurses more welcoming of your birthing decisions.

Informing family and friends of your plan

Choosing not to have an epidural, opting to use a midwife, or allowing a doula into your birthing room and not your partner's mom/sister/best friend can cause quite a stir. Anything you choose to do or not do that departs from other people's birthing experiences not only is "new and weird" but also can make them feel like you think the way they did it was wrong.

Conveying your plans early and often is key to getting everyone on the same page — or at least reading the same book — by the time the big day rolls around. Even if you can't get everyone to agree with your decisions, don't sweat it. Thank everyone for their concerns but assure them that you'd never make a decision that wasn't both educated and in the best interest of your partner and child. And, at the end of the day, after baby arrives, nobody will care how she got here.

REMEMBER

Unless you're openly soliciting advice from others in your lives, talk about the plan as if it were a done deal. Talking about considerations and decisions you're making with a larger group of people means that although you may get a wide spectrum of opinions, you'll also get an even wider spectrum of criticism when your decision doesn't adhere to everyone else's recommendations. However, you and your spouse have the right to decide the birthing option that works best for you. When your plan is in place, simply tell the people in your lives where, when, and how you plan on having the baby.

If you and your partner are worried about the reaction your in-laws will have to the news of your plans to have an at-home water birth, don't be afraid to share the news of your personal birth plan via e-mail or text. Or just be vague about your plans; other people aren't really entitled to know all the details of your life, although they may feel like they should. Also, the more unconventional your birth plan is, the more information your family and friends will want about your choices. In those instances, it's best to formulate a detailed, concrete birth plan before sharing the information.

REMEMBER

Many people are quite opinionated when it comes to whether to have a medicated labor or to circumcise. Don't feel the need to argue your position; the decision is ultimately yours, and what you want most is to do what's best for mother and baby in your eyes. Consider telling people that you plan on seeing how events unfold and that you'll address mom's and baby's needs as you see fit on delivery day. After all, nobody knows what your partner will need or want until she needs or wants it.

Get educated on your options and be honest with your friends and family. If all else fails and someone still insists you're wrong, have a confrontation. Arguments aren't enjoyable, but you'll be happier if you have it hashed out before the big day arrives.

Picking the Cast: Who's Present, Who Visits, and Who Gets a Call

Labor and delivery aren't the times for a family reunion. Having a baby is exhausting, emotional, and the one time in your lives when you need to focus on each other and your baby more than anything else in the world — which means you and your partner probably won't want many people in the room with you. To avoid any arguments or awkwardness at the hospital when you should be focusing on other matters, decide in advance who to allow in the room for delivery, who can visit at the hospital, and how to spread news of the birth to everyone who isn't present. Hospital rules, especially during outbreaks such as Covid-19, may limit visitors and make the decision for you.

Deciding who gets to attend the birth

Deciding who gets to be in the room is a big decision that's not yours to make. Your partner is the one nearly naked under a spotlight in a room full of people, so she gets to make the call on who's allowed in the room during labor and delivery. And gentlemen, let's face it — she just may not want your mother there, no matter how much your mother would like to be present. As labor progresses, most women don't care who sees what because they're so focused on birthing the baby, but it's still best for her labor to have only the people she wants to have present. Any stress or distraction in early labor can slow down the process.

In addition to you, the doctor or midwife, a doula (if applicable), and nurses, some women opt to have a sister or close friend in the room who can provide much-needed emotional support. Other women decide to have one or both parents present. Again, check with your hospital or birthing center to see who (and how many) they allow to be present for a birth.

WARNING

Telling family members or friends that they need to leave isn't easy, but if your partner doesn't want someone in the room, it's your job to politely ask the person to exit. (Or you can let your nurse play hatchet man; most have had years of experience dealing with out-of-control visitors.) For instance, if her father won't stop offering unsolicited stories about how painful his foot surgery was in comparison to her labor, and she's on the verge of clobbering him with forceps, pull him aside, thank him for being there to support you both, let him know that your partner sends her love, and then firmly explain that she wants silence in the room for the remainder of the delivery.

Of course, this message won't go over well, but it's not about other people at this point. Put your partner's needs first and worry about hurt feelings later. Besides, the moment baby arrives, nobody will remember anything other than how perfect and amazing your new bundle of joy is.

Planning ahead for visitors

Being inundated with visitors at the hospital may seem nice in theory, but in practice it can become overwhelming in a heartbeat.

You'll be tired, and your partner and baby will need rest, so make sure to take enough time for yourselves.

Also, having too many people handle your newborn only increases the risk of spreading illness. Invite only the most important people in your lives to the hospital and save the rest for a home visit in the following weeks. Thank anyone who offers to come and say that you look forward to spending time with the person in the coming weeks. Simply telling someone that your new family needs rest, not visitors, should do the trick.

TIP

If someone shows up unannounced whom you'd rather not have at the hospital, don't be afraid to tell her that you have to keep visits short — say five minutes or so — because your partner and baby need time to rest. Schedule a follow-up visit if you want. And if there's someone whom you don't want allowed into your room, for safety reasons or otherwise, be sure to alert the staff of the person's name and description.

There's never been a better time in your life to focus inward, so don't spend time worrying about what other people think about your decisions. If someone is offended, you can always make it up to that person later.

Spreading the news

Spreading the news far and wide can be both exhausting and time-consuming, and after a delivery, you and your partner likely won't be up for talking to everyone you know. Nor will you have the time! Nonetheless, everyone you know will request to be alerted within seconds after baby's arrival into the world. Although a group text will suffice for most of your friends and family, some people will want more information. Immediate family will want — and in most cases, deserve — a personal call so they can discuss all the details. Decisions about who gets called first and who calls the rest of the family to pass on the details can create situations that may be brought up during arguments years after the fact. Come up with a plan for who calls whom ahead of time and don't wing it. Hurt feelings over this can last for decades. They shouldn't, but they do.

ANNOUNCING BABY'S ARRIVAL VIA SOCIAL MEDIA

Sending an update to 500 of your nearest and not-so-nearest friends every time you have a witty musing about your favorite celebrity may be fun on the average day, but it may not be appropriate during labor and delivery.

Your partner may want you to keep the world abreast of the baby developments while she's in labor, but most women prefer that you focus on soothing them and not navigating your smartphone.

A word of warning: As easy as it is to communicate using social networking sites, sharing major news, such as the birth of your child, via Instagram or Snapchat will be offensive and hurtful to some of the more important people in your life. Finding out your best friend's baby arrived via a status update that already has 75 comments will leave those who truly love you feeling a bit cold. Take their feelings into consideration when making announcements throughout the pregnancy process. Make sure to hold off any major announcements until initiating your phone tree.

However, after news of the baby has spread through the appropriate channels to the appropriate people, social networking sites are a great way to show off your new bundle of joy to the adoring masses. Doing so may cut down on the number of visits and phone calls you receive when you're basking in the glow of new fatherhood.

3

Whoa, Baby! Labor, Delivery, and the First Days at Home

Get familiar with what happens in labor so you can avoid unnecessary runs to the hospital — yet get there in plenty of time when you really have to.

Understand options for delivery and why circumstances can change quickly in labor, leading to a change in your well-thought-out plans.

Review the characteristics of the typical newborn so you won't be shocked and say something you regret when you first see your baby.

Get to know your newborn in his first days of life by spending time with him and watching him begin to become an individual.

Learn how to give mom kudos for the job she's done and bolster up her confidence as she tackles a job she may be anxious to do but feel anxious about doing well.

Chapter **10**

Wowing the Maternity Floor: How to Be the Best Labor and Delivery Partner

No matter how many birth plans you write (refer to Chapter 9 for info on writing a birth plan) and how many times you suffer through a relative's birth story, labor always comes as a surprise. Labor may also be the first time you see your partner in real pain. Even worse, you know it's your fault — because she reminds you of that fact approximately every five minutes, although all will be forgiven as soon as the baby emerges. The end result is worth it, though, so fasten your seat belt and get ready for the roller-coaster ride that is labor and delivery.

No two labors are alike, so we can't say exactly what will happen in your partner's labor. The only thing most labors have in common is a beginning and an end. However, labor can begin in a number of ways and can end in an operating room, a birthing center, the back seat of the car (not to scare you), or in your own bedroom. Although details differ, knowing approximately how labor will go can reduce your anxiety by, well, maybe a little bit.

When It's Time, It's Time — Is It Time?

Although you may think you won't have trouble telling when your partner is in labor, you may. Contractions often get closer as labor progresses, but sometimes they don't. Some women are in a lot of pain in labor, and some aren't. All this confusion over the start of labor may have you leaping into the car every time your partner sighs during the last month of pregnancy; an actual moan may have you reaching for the phone to call 911.

REMEMBER

Go ahead and take 911 off speed dial and take a deep breath while you're at it. Although labor isn't always clear–cut, you can follow a few general rules when it comes to heading for the hospital:

>> **If your partner's water breaks, call your medical practitioner.** If you're having the baby in the hospital, your doctor will probably want your partner to come in, even if she isn't having contractions. However, many women prefer to go through early labor at home, even after the water breaks. Discuss this with your practitioner. After the water breaks, your partner has an increased risk of infection and a small chance that the umbilical cord can *prolapse* (fall below the baby's head, a medical emergency).

>> **If your partner is a beta strep carrier, go to the hospital as soon as her water breaks.** During pregnancy, women are tested for *beta strep,* common bacteria that can be carried in the vagina. The bacteria normally cause no harm in healthy women, but after the water bag breaks, beta strep can ascend up to the fetus and cause serious infection, so intravenous antibiotics need to be started right away.

>> **If your partner is in severe pain, even if the contractions aren't regular, call your medical practitioner.** Pregnancy complications such as the placenta separating from the uterine wall, called *placental abruption,* can cause severe pain and can be life-threatening.

>> **If bleeding like a heavy menstrual period occurs, call your medical practitioner.** A small amount of blood-tinged mucus is common when the mucus plug is passed, but heavier bleeding needs medical evaluation.

>> **When contractions are regular and getting closer, call your medical practitioner.** They don't have to be — and may never be — five minutes apart.

Avoiding numerous dry runs (yes, it's us again)

Calling your medical practitioner and following his advice before going to the hospital can save you many embarrassing excursions in and out of the labor and delivery ward. Think no one ever gets sent home without a baby? Think again. Think no one has ever gotten sent home ten or more times in a single pregnancy? Think again, again. And yes, the staff will remember you from last week, and the week before, et cetera, et cetera.

Many women have contractions in the last month of pregnancy. If your partner's contractions aren't becoming stronger or getting closer together, this probably isn't the real deal. Unless her water breaks, she's in severe pain, or she's bleeding, wait until contractions get stronger and closer together. Just being in the labor and delivery ward really doesn't speed up the birthing process.

Knowing when it's too late to head out

When your partner can't walk or talk through contractions that are progressively stronger and closer together, it's really time to go to the hospital. You'll know this instinctively when she says, "It's time to go *now*." But if by some chance she's a woman with short labors and says she feels pressure, has to have a bowel movement, or starts to push, dial 911 — unless you personally want to deliver the baby in the back seat or on the hospital lawn. (Coauthor Sharon has seen both situations.) Most emergency medical technicians have delivered babies before or at the very least have read the manual that tells them what to do.

REMEMBER

If the EMTs don't arrive in time, get your medical practitioner (or anyone's medical practitioner, actually) on the phone and follow his instructions. Rapid deliveries are usually uncomplicated, and your job may consist of calming your partner and not letting the baby fall on the floor. In addition:

>> **Don't pull on the cord or cut it.** Cutting the cord, dealing with the placenta, and worrying about vaginal tears should be done by someone who has been schooled in such things.

>> **Dry the baby off and keep him warm.** Skin-to-skin contact with mom with a blanket or towel over baby's back is ideal.

>> **If the baby isn't breathing, flick his heels.** Don't slap him or turn him upside down, even if you've seen it in the movies.

REMEMBER

Don't dwell too much on the possibility of an unexpected home delivery. The odds are very small that a first labor will progress so quickly that baby is born at home.

Supporting Your Partner During Labor

Women in labor need lots of support. Your partner needs to hear that she's doing well, that things are progressing as they should, and that she really can do this. Even if her mother, sister, doula, and five of her dearest friends are with her, she needs *you*. Support means different things to different women, though, and your job is to figure out what your partner needs while in labor and do it.

Figuring out what she needs from you

Your partner may not be in a talkative mood during labor, so asking her what she wants you to do may get you kicked out of the room. This is one time in her life when she wants you to think for yourself and take action. Take the lead by offering choices. Ask her whether she wants

>> A back rub

>> A massage

>> A hand to hold

>> You to sit behind her and support her back

>> An epidural

>> You to kick her mom out of the room

>> Ice chips

>> To get in the tub

>> Any of the other labor options you discussed before today

Not taking the insults seriously

Women aren't responsible for anything they say during labor, but you are, so don't get upset over any suggestions your partner makes about your anatomy or her comments on your ancestry. And she doesn't really mean what she said about your mother, either.

Pain makes people say things they don't mean and may not even remember, so don't file away her remarks for another day. Vocalizing the pain in this way is both healthy and normal. Because you're not in pain, you don't get the same privileges, so save the snappy retorts for another time.

Looking at What Happens During and After Labor

Although childbirth classes and books do their best to tell you what happens in labor, the reality is hard to describe in a book. But because it's our job to give you all the facts you can handle, the following sections describe what the normal stages of labor look like.

First stage

The first stage of labor encompasses the time between the first labor pain and complete dilation, when your partner begins to push. Because quite a few things happen during the first stage of labor, it's further broken down into three types of labor: early, active, and transition.

Early labor

Early labor is the time between the start of labor and dilation of the cervix to 5 centimeters. This is the longest part of labor, sometimes lasting a day or two. It's also the time when you're most likely to be sent home if you go to the hospital too early.

During the early stage, contractions are often far apart and irregular. In fact, they may start and stop more than once. These early contractions thin and dilate the cervix. In late pregnancy, the cervix is thick, and the opening between the uterus and vagina is closed.

Normally, the cervix thins before it begins to dilate, but there are no hard and fast rules. Many women are already somewhat thinned and dilated before labor begins.

Active labor

Things really start to move along during *active labor,* which is marked by regular contractions that become stronger and dilate the cervix from 6 to 10 centimeters. Active labor takes four to eight hours on average, although subsequent labors are often much shorter. A woman in active labor usually can't walk or talk through her contractions. She also may become a creature you haven't met before, one who knows words that may totally surprise you. If you're not already at the hospital or haven't called your practitioner if you're having a home birth, now's the time.

TIP

You need to be active in active labor, too. If your partner is doing natural childbirth, she needs help staying focused and breathing through the contractions. Don't just tell her to breathe; breathe with her. Some women want you to count off the seconds; others don't. Be guided by her responses, even if they're a little impolite at the height of a contraction.

If your partner is having an epidural, she'll also appreciate your help. See the later section "What to expect during epidural placement" for the do's and don'ts.

Transition labor

Transition, the hardest stage, is the last part of active labor. Transition lasts from 7 centimeters to full dilation, or 10 centimeters. If your partner has a good epidural, this stage will probably breeze by, but if she's going natural, transition can be difficult. Transition can last anywhere from a few minutes in someone having a second or subsequent baby to a few hours in a woman having her first child. Typical side effects of transition include

>> Intermittent urges to push

>> Shaking

>> Vomiting

Second stage

Second-stage labor lasts from the first push to the final delivery — anywhere from two minutes to three-plus hours. Women with epidurals often push less effectively, and medical practitioners may let the baby *labor down* — meaning that the baby descends through the birth canal under the force of the contractions, without pushing — if your partner is comfortable and the baby is doing okay.

Push, push, push!

Active pushing requires help from you, but don't actually push along with your partner or you may get hemorrhoids almost the size of the baby after delivery. The nurse may ask you to help support your partner's legs or to support her back slightly.

The people in attendance at the delivery usually do lots of enthusiastic cheering when mom starts pushing. You'll find it easy to be enthusiastic when the baby's head finally begins to appear, although a little apprehension about how that big thing is going to make its way out of your partner's body is also normal.

Not all women are into the cheerleading scene, though, and actually prefer just to hear a single voice (yours) offering encouragement or no loud noises at all. If your partner looks aggravated during the cheers (beyond the effort of pushing), ask her what she wants. Then do it, and ask everyone else to comply.

Most delivery rooms have mirrors near the foot of the bed so that your partner can see what's going on. Not everyone wants to see what's going on down there, but some women do. When your medical practitioner takes her seat at the end of the delivery bed or table, she may block the mirror, but most mirrors can be adjusted so your partner has a better view if she wants it. Make sure the mirror is where she wants it, even if where she wants it is out of view. Pushing is difficult with your eyes open, so she may not see much of the actual birth.

If you want to cut the cord or you and your partner have chosen to delay cord-clamping until the cord stops pulsing, make sure your wishes are known. Although many practitioners ask you automatically, it's safest to speak up. If you're turning a little green, don't feel like you have to cut the cord. In fact, if you're turning a little green, go sit on the floor or in a chair so the staff doesn't have to tend to you.

REMEMBER

Getting a little lightheaded during delivery is *not* a sign of weakness. Many guys don't eat enough while their partner is in labor and often have to stand for several hours helping her push. Deliveries are very messy; vomit, poop, and blood can make a pungent odor that can be hard to deal with, even for the most experienced labor and delivery staff. Try not to add to the mess by passing out and taking the delivery tray with you.

It's a miracle!

Birth is miraculous. There's no other way to put it. Even practitioners who've seen thousands of births are still awed by it at times. Watching a new human being come into the world is an amazing privilege, especially when she's *your* new human being.

Crying at deliveries isn't unusual. Of course, the baby usually cries, and family members often do too, but sometimes even the staff cries if they've gotten really attached to a particular couple. Don't expect your doctor or midwife to get all teary-eyed, although it does happen in some cases.

Don't be surprised if your first feeling upon seeing your baby is dismay, either. New babies aren't always the most beautiful of creatures. (We discuss newborn peculiarities in Chapter 11.)

If the baby is okay, your practitioner may give your partner the baby to hold and possibly nurse, if she wants to try immediately. Some centers prefer to dry off, weigh, and assess the baby before bringing her back to mom to nurse, but many postpone this for an hour or so, as long as baby and mom are stable. Either way, within the first 15 minutes, the baby will be dried off, weighed, and wrapped up so one or both of you can hold her or your partner can start nursing.

Wrapping things up after the birth

The placenta is usually delivered within 15 minutes of the birth. Contractions may accompany the loosening and passage of the placenta, but if your partner had an epidural, she may not notice. If the placenta doesn't pass within 15 minutes, some medical practitioners give additional medication to help loosen the placenta or gently tug on it. Both the medication and tugging can cause uncomfortable cramping. Other practitioners give the placenta more time to release on its own before starting medical interventions.

Very rarely, a condition called *placenta accreta* occurs when the placenta can't be removed from the uterine wall. In severe cases, a hysterectomy is performed because the placenta can't be removed, and severe bleeding often develops.

If your partner has a vaginal tear or received an *episiotomy* — a surgical incision (usually between the vulva and the anus) to give the baby a little extra room and avoid tearing — the wound needs to be closed after the placenta is delivered. Stitching everything back together normally takes about 15 minutes. Your partner receives an injection of numbing medication before stitches are put in unless she is still completely numb from the epidural. If she didn't have an epidural, passing the placenta and stitching may be mildly uncomfortable or annoying.

Many facilities now do delivery and recovery in the same room, so the staff will refresh the bed and change your partner's gown after the mechanics of the delivery are all taken care of. And she can eat! If she wants something special, you may be sent out to get what she wants, or better yet, you can send one of her friends or her mom out so you can stay to admire your new family.

Helping baby right after delivery

If the baby doesn't breathe well at first (many don't, so don't panic), the staff may take her right over to the warmer to give her a little oxygen. Don't worry; the staff will bring her back to your partner as soon as she's stable.

REMEMBER

As normal as it is to ask a lot of questions and want to know exactly what's happening, try to stay to the sidelines so you don't interfere with your baby's care. You want the staff to focus on taking care of the baby, not talking to you.

Most issues that affect babies right after delivery are related to breathing. Transitioning from not breathing inside the womb to breathing on one's own is hard, and some babies take a few minutes to get the hang of it.

Oxygen may be given by *blow by,* which means a tube is placed near the baby's nose but not too close to her eyes. If she needs extra help, oxygen is given with a bag and mask connected to an oxygen source; the mask fits over her mouth and nose, and the staff squeezes the bag to force oxygen into the lungs.

REMEMBER

If the baby doesn't pink up and start crying quickly, she may be taken to the special-care nursery or NICU (neonatal intensive care unit) for further evaluation. You're usually welcome to accompany her and find out what's happening, but don't forget your partner, still lying on the bed, feeling as confused and upset as you are and possibly getting stitches in her bottom at the same time. Make sure you keep her informed about what's happening and let her know you haven't forgotten about her. She may want you to follow the baby so you can report back and tell her what's going on.

Walking Through Common Labor Procedures

In the interests of making you familiar with all possible aspects of labor and delivery, some of the procedures you can expect to see during labor are detailed in the next sections.

Vaginal exams

Vaginal exams — when the cervix is checked for dilation — are often uncomfortable, especially when they're done during a contraction, but they're the only way to assess labor progression. Although your partner may not be overly fond of vaginal checks, you may love them because they give you new information to convey to friends and family in the waiting room or on the other end of your group text messages.

IVs

If you're delivering in a hospital in the United States, your partner will most likely have an *intravenous infusion*, or IV for short. The IV serves the following purposes:

>> **Supplying fluids:** Many hospitals restrict fluids when labor begins, and getting dehydrated is easy when you're working extra hard and not taking anything in. If an epidural is given, prehydration is necessary to avoid a drop in blood pressure, which can decrease oxygen flow to the baby.

>> **In case of Cesarean delivery:** With the percentage of Cesarean deliveries now more than 30 percent in the United States, there's a very good chance your partner will end up with a Cesarean. If the surgery is done as an emergency, with time being of the essence, having an IV already in place saves time.

>> **Covering the hospital's legal obligations:** If a woman has serious bleeding, an emergency Cesarean, or just about any complication, an IV is necessary to give fluids to replace possible blood loss and maintain normal blood pressure, which often drops if spinal anesthesia is given for the surgery. Many hospitals routinely give IVs before they're really needed because, unfortunately, we live in a litigious society, and in the case of a malpractice suit, the lawyers will want to know if she had an IV in place for just such possible emergencies.

After an IV is in place it shouldn't be terribly uncomfortable, so if it is, let your partner's nurse know. Sometimes just retaping the catheter so it's at a different angle helps with the discomfort. Women who want to walk without dragging around an IV pole or spend time in the hot tub can have the IV *hep-locked*, which means the end is capped off and the bag of fluid detached. If needed, the hep-lock is flushed with solution to make sure it's still working before the bag is reattached.

But despite all this, some women — and your partner may be one of them — really don't want an IV during labor, as long as everything's going well. It may make her feel like the birth is a medical procedure or she may just have a massive fear of needles. Obviously, IVs aren't necessary for childbirth; millions of babies around the world are born without benefit of an IV every day. For a normal, uncomplicated delivery, an IV is certainly an option, not an essential.

TIP

If your partner is adamant about not having an IV:

>> Talk to her medical provider ahead of time, both to get his views on the topics and so he can put a note in her chart, if he'll agree to forgo the IV.

>> Understand that pain medication is generally given via IV in the hospital because it acts more quickly and also disappears faster. Injected or oral medications stay in the system longer and can make your baby sleepy and less able to breathe well at birth. If your partner plans to write "Give me my epidural" on her forehead before going to the hospital, an IV is inevitable because epidural anesthesia causes side effects that IV fluid can counter, like a drop in blood pressure or a fever.

>> Realize that a medical emergency throws all previous agreements out the window; there may not be time to have an earnest discussion about the pros and cons of IVs. In a real emergency, the IV is in before anyone has time to discuss it.

Membrane ruptures

Although many women fear that their water will break somewhere embarrassing, like in church or in the middle of aisle three at the grocery store, only around 10 percent of women's membranes rupture before labor starts. Often the membranes are broken by medical personnel using what looks like a crochet hook to snag the membranes and tear them. This procedure isn't painful for your partner or the baby, although it might be slightly uncomfortable because it's done during a vaginal exam.

Your practitioner may rupture the membranes if she wants to check the fluid inside the sac for the presence of meconium, a sign of potential stress, sometime before or during labor. Between 6 to 25 percent of babies pass meconium before delivery; the older the meconium, the yellower and less particulate the fluid is. Newer meconium may be dark green, sticky, and form particles that can be sucked into the baby's lungs, causing respiratory problems at birth. The presence of either old or new meconium can cause respiratory problems at birth, so the fluid is always checked for meconium as soon as the membranes rupture.

Keep in mind, however, that meconium can be inhaled before birth; there's no way to prevent this from happening because babies take practice breaths while still in the womb. Most of the time, the baby clears the meconium from the lungs, and no problems ensue, but meconium inhalation can cause severe lung infection and problems with circulation that require mechanical ventilation until the lungs heal, usually within a few days.

The membranes may also be ruptured to

>> Try to speed up labor (even though labor doesn't always go faster after the membranes are ruptured)

>> Allow for the placement of internal monitoring devices (see the upcoming "Fetal monitoring" section for more about the ways your baby's heartbeat can be monitored before birth)

REMEMBER

Rupturing membranes can lead to harder, more painful contractions that don't actually speed up the process, so ask your medical practitioner why he wants to do this if you have concerns about it.

Fetal monitoring

Fetal monitoring devices record the fetal heart rate and the frequency and duration of the contractions. Sounds cool, right? Just don't let yourself become so enamored with the technology that you forget about the person at the other end! Many men love gadgets and start watching the monitor like it's the educational channel, but we guarantee that if you do that, your partner won't appreciate it.

Monitoring your partner and the baby externally

External monitoring systems consist of two recording devices fastened around your partner's stomach and plugged into a fetal monitor, which provides a continuous printout of the fetal heart rate and the contractions. The monitor records the duration of contractions and the time between them but doesn't tell you the strength of the contraction. Each contraction resembles a hill or a bell-shaped curve, starting low, rising slowly, and then returning to baseline. Because the device sits on your partner's abdomen, attached with a belt or under a belly band, her body shape and position can affect how the contractions look on the monitor. Contractions that look like very large mountains on the monitor don't always indicate really strong contractions, and tiny hills don't necessarily mean the contractions are mild.

The external fetal heart monitor tracks and records the fetal heart rate as well, but it has some limitations. Namely, it records an average of beats rather than the baby's exact heartbeat. External monitors can determine *variability*, the difference in heart rate over a certain time period, and beat-to-beat variability can help ascertain how well the baby is handling labor.

A heartbeat that stays the same with little variation may indicate that the baby is stressed. Short periods of decreased variability also occur when the baby is asleep. (And yes, babies do take short naps during labor!) The fetal heart rate may also have a short period of minimal beat-to-beat variability if your partner gets a dose of a narcotic pain medication.

The external monitor also can't always distinguish between mom's heart rate and baby's. If your partner has a rapid heartbeat because of fever, anxiety, or other reasons, or if the baby has *bradycardia* (an extremely low heart rate), it may not be obvious that the external monitor isn't recording the right heartbeat.

Monitoring internally

Internal monitors resolve the shortcomings of external monitors by giving more accurate information. Internal contraction monitors are inserted directly into the uterus, which makes them able to record the exact strength of each contraction. You may be disappointed to watch those huge mountains that appeared to be very strong contractions shrink down to little blips on the monitor, indicating that the uterus is contracting only mildly, or you may be excited to see the opposite.

Internal fetal monitors fasten a tiny wire into the baby's scalp that records the exact fetal heart rate. This ensures that the variability displayed is an accurate representation of the fetal heartbeat. An internal monitor can also differentiate maternal and fetal heart rates, if it's difficult to tell whose heart rate is recording on the external monitor.

Some centers use internal monitors routinely, whereas others use them only if they're having trouble picking up the heart rate or assessing the contractions. Internal monitor complications occur rarely and include infection at the site of insertion or *hematoma* (a large bruise).

Coping with Labor Pain

Although you and your partner discussed pain medication options before the big day (and we discuss making the decision on pain medication in Chapter 9), nothing is written in stone when labor actually starts. A staunch *au naturel* supporter may find herself asking for an epidural the minute she hits the labor floor, and a woman who was sure she's epidural material may find herself breathing through labor and deciding she'd rather do without one. Don't ever be surprised by the decisions of a laboring woman.

Enduring it: Going unmedicated

Going unmedicated was all the rage in the 1970s but fell out of favor when epidural anesthesia became available in all but the smallest hospitals. Unmedicated delivery still does have some advantages, and there are good reasons to consider it. Your partner may decide to go unmedicated for the following reasons:

>> Babies whose moms haven't received medication may be more alert and may nurse better. Medication does cross the placenta to the fetus before delivery.

>> Moving around during labor is easier if you're not medicated. Epidural anesthesia usually keeps you in bed, although "walking epidurals" are offered by some centers.

>> Pushing is sometimes more effective without an epidural, although some centers let an epidural wear down enough for mom to be able to push.

>> Water therapy can't be utilized if you have epidural anesthesia.

>> Going through labor unmedicated can be an empowering experience.

>> Some women have bad reactions to medications in general and don't want to take anything they don't really need.

One good thing about going unmedicated is that with a first labor, it's almost never too late to change your mind and request an epidural. If your partner decides she wants an epidural at 9 centimeters, in many centers, she can have one.

Dulling it: Sedation (no, not for you)

Sedation takes the edge off labor without numbing the lower part of the body. Typical sedatives given in labor include Demerol, Nubain, or Stadol, which can be given intramuscularly or intravenously. IV administration takes effect quickly and lasts one to two hours.

Sedation may be given if it's too early in the labor to give epidural anesthesia. Sedation can take the edge off the pain and help your partner get a little sleep, but it can also slow contractions in some cases.

Because sedation can reach the baby, narcotics and narcotic-type medications aren't often given if delivery is expected within the hour because the baby may not breathe well.

Blocking it out: Epidurals

Epidural anesthesia consists of medications given through a catheter placed in the spinal canal. The pro of epidurals is obvious: They decrease pain. They do have other benefits as well, in some cases. For example:

>> Epidurals can help a tense mom relax. Tension can slow labor; women who are especially tense may benefit from an epidural to help them relax.

>> Epidurals provide continuous pain relief. In many cases, a continuous infusion of medication prevents the medication from wearing off.

Medications used in epidurals

Several different types of medication are used in epidural anesthesia. Anesthetics such as lidocaine or bupivacaine may be combined with narcotics such as fentanyl or morphine. Narcotics decrease the amount of local anesthetics needed to achieve adequate comfort. Narcotics given in an epidural don't cause drowsiness the way sedatives do.

What to expect during epidural placement

An epidural can be given at any stage of labor but usually isn't given in very early labor because it can slow progress. Some doctors will start oxytocin, a drug used to induce labor, when epidural anesthesia is given in early labor.

A large amount of IV fluid, approximately one bag, is infused rapidly to offset the drop in blood pressure that may occur with epidural anesthesia. This infusion can be uncomfortable because the fluid is at room temperature and feels cold.

Dads are very much in demand during epidural placement to give mom a person to lean on so she can get into the proper "curled shrimp" position for catheter placement (see Figure 10-1). The epidural catheter is placed into the epidural space on the mid-back by inserting a metal needle into the epidural space and then threading the catheter through the needle. Only the soft plastic catheter remains in the back. She must remain sitting up and still, even through contractions, for a period of five to ten minutes while the catheter is placed.

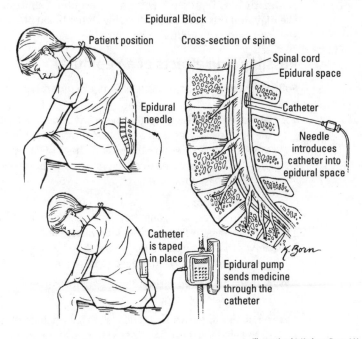

Illustration by Kathryn Born, MA

FIGURE 10-1: Placement of the epidural catheter requires remaining curled up and still for a short period.

After the catheter is taped in place, the anesthesiologist assists her back to a lying down position and assesses her blood pressure and comfort level for several minutes. In many centers, the epidural catheter is attached to an infusion pump that delivers a continuous infusion during labor to help maintain adequate pain relief.

WARNING

If you feel at all shaky or nervous while your partner receives the epidural, or if you start to get lightheaded from standing in one position too long, ask someone else to take over supporting mom so you can sit down before you fall down.

Sometimes placing the catheter is difficult because of your partner's anatomy, and more than one needle stick may be necessary. This isn't anyone's fault, and getting the catheter placed correctly is important. You can help by staying calm and keeping your partner calm, too.

When the catheter is in place, a test dose is given, and your partner's blood pressure is carefully assessed because epidural anesthesia can cause blood pressure to drop. She has to wear an automatic blood-pressure cuff on her arm for a short period, and she may find this very uncomfortable. If her blood pressure is low, she may be tilted slightly to her left side.

Possible side effects of an epidural

Following are some of the side effects of epidural anesthesia:

>> **Difficulty urinating:** Most women can't urinate well after the epidural is given, and a full bladder can get in the way of the baby's head and slow the pushing stage of labor. A Foley catheter may be placed to drain urine or the bladder may be emptied intermittently.

>> **Hot spots:** Sometimes women have an area that doesn't "take" to the epidural, and they need to change positions so that the anesthesia goes to a different area and numbs the nerves that haven't been numbed well. In the worst-case scenario, the epidural may need to be re-placed.

>> **Nausea and/or vomiting:** These symptoms may also occur in labors without epidurals.

>> **A rise in temperature:** It's difficult to tell whether infection or the epidural is causing a rise in temperature, so

intravenous antibiotics must be given to avoid complications in case an infection is present. Any time mom runs a fever, the fetus may also develop one, from the increase in womb temperature.

>> **Shivering:** The fluid infusion or the epidural can cause shivering. Your partner will appreciate extra blankets, especially if they're straight out of the warmer.

Deviating from Your Birth Plan/Vision

Everyone has some vision of how labor is going to go, even if it isn't committed to paper. But most labors don't follow the book or the birth plan. Knowing this ahead of time helps you avoid serious disappointment. Consider the birth plan as a guideline of what you would like to happen, with the proviso that mom's and baby's well-being come first.

Some women feel guilty about taking pain medication in labor if they were gung-ho to go unmedicated. If your partner wants to take pain medication but is hesitating because she feels like she's letting the birth plan — or you — down, encourage her to follow her instincts. Remind her that no one knows what labor is like until she's in it and that most women do end up taking pain medication in labor. After all, labor hurts!

On the other hand, your partner may have gone from au naturel woman to "give me the drugs!" seemingly in the blink of an eye, and you may be the one having a hard time with it and trying to encourage her to stick to the plan. Don't do it. Encouragement is fine if she's just going through a rough spot in transition, for example, but if she's made her decision, your job is to support her in it. You may have devised the birth plan together, but she's the one going through labor, not you.

REMEMBER

If your practitioner participates in a call group and baby comes at night or on the weekend, you may have a different practitioner for the actual delivery. After having established a relationship with a doctor over the past nine months, having a stranger do the delivery can be frustrating, especially if your partner specifically chose a doctor for her approach to labor. However, rest assured that whoever delivers your baby will do everything she can to ensure a safe and smooth delivery. Discuss this possibility with your practitioner in advance to find out what to expect.

If your partner ends up having a C-section or if the baby has any type of problem, large or small, she may feel that something she did in labor caused the problem. Assure her that this is not the case (because it isn't). Things go wrong in labor that are no one's fault; they can't be predicted or, in most cases, prevented. Your job is to tell her that she did exactly what she should have and that she has no reason for regrets. And if you have any niggling doubts about the wisdom of her labor choices, keep them to yourself.

Having a Cesarean

Cesareans now comprise more than 30 percent of all deliveries in the United States, so the odds of having one are high. Although Cesareans are major surgeries, they're generally safe for your partner and the baby. However, babies born by C-section may retain more fluid in the respiratory tract than babies born vaginally, and the fluid can be aspirated into the lungs, causing breathing difficulties.

WARNING

Maternal complications such as infection, anesthesia complications, blood clots, and excessive bleeding can also occur, as with any surgery.

Scheduled C-section

You can schedule a Cesarean ahead of time if you know your partner's going to need one. Knowing she's going to have a Cesarean ahead of time helps you get things ready for her homecoming, knowing that she's going to be extremely sore as well as tired. Your partner may not want to navigate stairs for the first week afterward, and she won't be able to drive for several weeks. You'll know she's ready to get behind the wheel again when she can stomp her feet on the floor without any pain, which generally takes about two weeks.

Reasons for planned Cesareans

Reasons for a scheduled Cesarean include previous Cesarean delivery and abnormal fetal position, such as *breech* (feet first) or *transverse* (sideways) lie. Most of the time, but not always, these are determined ahead of time, but babies have been known to switch positions just days before delivery.

WARNING

Occasionally, women ask for a medically unnecessary Cesarean delivery. Some doctors perform these procedures, but having surgery you don't need is never a good idea. Cesarean delivery is riskier for the baby because fluid doesn't get squeezed out of the lungs during the birth, setting up potential respiratory difficulties.

Multiples are almost always delivered by Cesarean, even though twins who are both *vertex* (head down) can certainly be delivered vaginally. However, after the first twin is delivered, there's an abundance of room in the womb, and the second twin may flip or turn sideways with the joy of having all that space to himself, necessitating a Cesarean for baby B. No mother wants to experience both a vaginal delivery *and* a Cesarean with all the attendant discomforts on the same day, so most twins are scheduled for C-sections, although some doctors will consider a vaginal delivery, depending on how the babies are positioned.

Setting the date

Choosing your baby's birth date can be exciting, but consider the following caveats:

» Don't choose a weekend day. Most practitioners don't schedule surgery for the weekend.

» Don't expect to bypass the last three weeks of pregnancy with an early delivery date. Practitioners shouldn't schedule Cesareans or induce labor prior to 39 weeks unless it's medically necessary. For first-time moms, the recommendation is 41 weeks.

» Understand that the baby may come before your scheduled date. The baby hasn't read your birth plan and doesn't know that you want him to be born on an auspicious date, and he may decide to show up a week earlier.

» Realize that having an 8 a.m. surgery time scheduled doesn't always mean your surgery will be at 8 a.m. Emergency cases can bump you off the schedule, which is understandable, so don't get too upset if you're delayed because someone else's Cesarean needs to be done first.

Unplanned Cesarean delivery

A large percentage of Cesareans are unplanned, with the most common reason noted as "failure to progress," which means labor wasn't progressing as expected. This can mean a baby is too large for the pelvis, an unusual maternal anatomy, or a practitioner who's getting antsy about how things are going.

If labor goes on too long, complications such as infection become more likely, and doing a C-section is often less stressful than waiting for the situation to possibly deteriorate. And as all too many practitioners are well aware, the decision to do a C-section is less likely to be attacked in court than a delay in action that leads to problems with the mother or baby.

Fetal distress is an undeniable reason for an unplanned C-section, although true fetal distress is different from potential fetal distress that could possibly worsen if labor goes on.

>> True fetal distress is marked by a run down the hall at top speed, minimal surgery prep, and often general anesthesia, because it's the quickest way to put mom to sleep.

>> Potential fetal distress or mild distress usually results in a more leisurely trip to the operating room and a much calmer atmosphere because the baby isn't in any real danger yet. And because you don't want her to reach that point, a C-section can be the best option. Trust your practitioner; if he says you need to do a C-section, do it.

REMEMBER

Choosing a medical practitioner whose philosophy on Cesareans fits with yours is essential. Doctors do have different tolerance levels for deviations from the norm, and doctors who have a low tolerance for deviance generally have higher Cesarean rates because they're less likely to watch and wait for a short time before performing surgery.

What to expect before the operation

Certain procedures must be done before Cesarean delivery. Normally, a Foley catheter is placed to keep the bladder empty so it won't be injured during the surgery. If your partner already has an epidural, she won't even feel the catheter placement; if she doesn't, she may be mildly uncomfortable during the procedure. In some hospitals, the Foley is placed after the epidural or spinal is placed.

A preparatory mini-shave is done (if she hasn't already done it herself) to eliminate hair where the incision goes. Most Cesarean scars are known as a bikini cut, a horizontal lower abdominal incision (see Figure 10-2). Occasionally, a vertical skin incision is done if the baby lies in a position that makes him difficult to reach or if the surgery has to be done very rapidly.

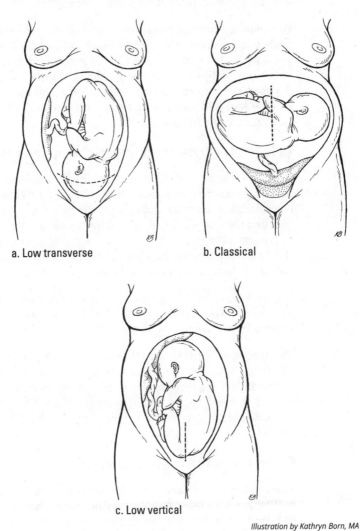

a. Low transverse

b. Classical

c. Low vertical

Illustration by Kathryn Born, MA

FIGURE 10-2: Most Cesarean incisions are done just above the pubic hairline.

Your partner may be given medications to reduce the chance of nausea and to neutralize stomach acids in case of vomiting and possible aspiration into the lungs. She'll also be given an intravenous line if she doesn't already have one. If spinal anesthesia is used for the procedure, fluid will be quickly infused, which can feel very cold. Also, an adequate amount of fluid is necessary to keep blood pressure from dropping after the Cesarean.

Your partner may be taken into the operating room by herself while you get dressed in a sterile outfit. When you're allowed in, you'll probably be given a seat right near her head so you can talk to her and support her without getting in anyone's way. Keeping the operative area sterile is extremely important during surgery, and the staff will take care to make sure you don't inadvertently contaminate anything.

What to expect during the surgery

When the surgery actually gets underway, removing the baby takes between five and ten minutes. You won't be able to see much because a sterile drape is placed between your partner's head and the rest of her body. When the baby is delivered, she may be brought close to your wife so she can see her, but she won't be able to nurse immediately or do any type of skin-to-skin contact because of the sterile operating field.

If general anesthesia isn't used, your partner may feel tugging during the surgery. This is normal, but she may need lots of reassurance that it's okay.

Because babies born via C-sections have an increased risk of complications, a pediatrician or special-care nursery personnel may be present for the delivery. You'll be allowed to walk over to the warmer to see the baby, and in many hospitals, after the baby is weighed and cleaned, she'll be given to you to hold next to your partner.

Getting past disappointment

When you have the baby, you have him; it doesn't really matter how he got here. Your partner may not see it that way, though, and she may mourn the loss of the "perfect" labor and delivery and feel like she failed the labor test. With so many women having Cesareans today, this feeling of failure is less common than it used to be, but if you and your partner had your hearts set on a certain labor scenario, a deviation from the script can be upsetting.

AS LONG AS YOU'RE IN THERE . . . THE TUMMY TUCK OPTION

As long as your partner is having a Cesarean birth, she may ponder whether she could have a few inches of excess skin or fat removed at the same time. (Obviously, this isn't something you should, under any circumstances, suggest that she ask the doctor about.)

Although a full tummy tuck is probably out of the question — unless you're a famous Hollywood star — your partner's doctor may be willing to do a mini-tummy tuck, removing some of the excess skin and any previous Cesarean scars.

The trouble with a tummy tuck when you're nine months pregnant is that everything is stretched, so a doctor can't optimally see what he has to work with. He may take off too much or too little. The other problem is that obstetricians aren't plastic surgeons; tummy tucks aren't their area of expertise.

Additionally, full tummy tucks are usually done under general anesthesia; after you've waited nine months for your baby, your partner probably won't want to be asleep when she arrives. And if she has general anesthesia for the procedure, you probably won't be allowed in the operating room.

Waiting until all the pregnancy swelling and stretching has subsided and having a tummy tuck then is a better option.

You can be a big help by accentuating the positives in the situation: reminding her how well she handled the change in plans and how she put the baby's needs before her wishes.

REMEMBER

Understanding why certain procedures were necessary can be very important in helping new mothers "grieve" the loss of a perfect delivery. Request a time to speak with the person who delivered your baby so you and your partner can ask lingering questions about why the delivery went the way it did.

Chapter **11**

Caring for Your Newborn

Walking out the hospital door with a newborn who's still basically a stranger to you can be an intimidating experience. Getting to know your baby is a process that takes time. Fortunately, you'll be putting in lots of time with this demanding stranger, and before you know it, you'll feel as if you've known this marvelous little person all your life. In this chapter, we walk you through the seemingly mundane tasks that help you build a lifetime relationship with your new baby.

Getting Your First Look at a Typical Newborn

Newborns don't look anything like the smooth-skinned, dimpled, smiling babies on TV. A new baby emerges from nine months in a dark, watery environment, and her skin shows it. She squints like she's just emerged from a cave. Although your newborn may not look exactly like the baby in your idealized dreams, she'll look perfect to you — at least after you get used to her in a day or two.

Examining your newborn

What should you expect when your newborn is put into your arms for the first time? Not the Gerber baby, that's for sure — although your baby will be, your partner will assure you, the most beautiful creature she's ever seen. You may seriously wonder about her taste in human beings because newborn babies have the following characteristics:

>> **Small:** The average baby is around 7 pounds and 20 inches long. The reality of how small and fragile a newborn is won't hit you until you hold him.

>> **Red and covered with — what's that white stuff?** Newborns are amazingly red. They come out a dark red and then turn a lighter red, which gradually fades to a normal skin color over a few days. Many newborns are coated, especially in the creases, with *vernix,* a creamy substance that protected baby's skin in mom's amniotic fluid.

>> **Wrinkled and peeling:** Because he just spent nine months immersed in water, baby's entire skin has the equivalent look of dishpan hands, and as soon as he begins to dry out, his skin wrinkles because it's no longer waterlogged. His skin will crack and peel, especially around bendable joints such as the ankles and wrists.

>> **Cone-headed:** If your partner pushed for any amount of time or if the baby was delivered by vacuum extraction, his head may be pointed at the back or he may have a little cone cup, like a jaunty little hat, to the side of his head. His head will become round in a week or so. (Cesarean babies may escape the cone-head look, unless your partner pushed for some time before the C-section.)

>> **Spotted, dotted, and blotched:** Newborns often have a variety of blotches, splotches, whiteheads, and other marks that fade over time. *Milia* look like little whiteheads on the baby's nose, chin, and forehead. Don't squeeze these; they'll disappear on their own. The majority of black, Indian, and Asian babies have what look like black and blue marks on their legs or buttocks, called *Mongolian spots,* which fade with time. Red blotches on the back of the neck, eyelids, and between the eyes, called *stork bites,* are immature blood vessels that also disappear with time.

>> **Not very well put together:** Newborns often seem like they may fall apart if a strong wind comes along. Their heads wobble alarmingly, and their arms and legs shoot off in all directions when they're startled. No wonder nurses wrap them up tight in blankets.

>> **A bit, uh, out of proportion:** You may be saying, "That's my boy!" but baby boys may have overlarge genitals due to fluid retention, trauma during delivery, and hormonal influences. This condition is temporary. Girls often have swollen genitalia as well, but it's less noticeable. Also, girls may pass a few drops of blood from the vagina. Hormones cause this somewhat disconcerting event also.

>> **Swollen breasts:** Because of maternal hormones, both baby boys and girls often have swollen breasts that may actually produce a few drops of milk. This condition disappears within a few days

>> **May have no family resemblance:** Before you start getting suspicious that the baby isn't yours, rest assured that many newborns look slightly Asian, even if their parents aren't. Puffiness and swelling around the eyes make them appear Asian, and the yellow tinge of jaundice that many babies have after the first day or two may have you convinced that someone has a lot of explaining to do. The puffiness will improve daily, and by the end of the week, you won't be able to stop telling everyone how much the baby looks like you.

Rating the reflexes

Newborns are active from the minute they're born. Your baby will yawn, grimace, and even seem to smile a little. (Yes, the smiles are really caused by gas at this stage, just like your mother says.) Babies also have certain reflex actions that are normal at birth. Your medical practitioner will assess the baby to make sure these reflexes are present. Lack of normal reflexes can indicate a problem that you need to investigate.

Here are the normal reflexes newborns exhibit:

>> **Babinski reflex:** When the bottom of baby's foot is stroked, her big toe rises, and the other toes fan out. The Babinski reflex lasts for around two years.

>> **Grasp reflex:** If the baby's palm is stroked, she closes her fingers, a reflex that lasts several months.

>> **The Moro, or startle, reflex:** Your baby tremors slightly, throws back her head, and flails her arms and legs away from her side in response to a sudden movement or a loud noise. The Moro reflex lasts five or six months before disappearing.

>> **Rooting reflex:** Stroking the corner of the baby's mouth makes her turn toward the touch; this helps her find the breast or bottle for feeding.

>> **Step reflex:** When her foot touches a solid surface, she appears to step, lifting one foot and then the other. This doesn't mean she's an athletic prodigy or even that she'll walk early, however.

>> **Sucking reflex:** When an object touches the roof of the baby's mouth, she begins to suck. This reflex doesn't develop until around 32 weeks of pregnancy and isn't fully developed until 36 weeks, which is why preemies often can't take a bottle well or breast-feed easily.

>> **Tonic neck reflex (TNR):** If the baby's head turns to the side, her arm on that side stretches out, and the opposite arm bends at the elbow, making her look like she's fencing. The TNR lasts six to seven months.

Feeding a Newborn

Every baby needs to be fed, but the sheer number of choices to make about feeding may have you begging your partner to consider nothing but breast-feeding for at least the next year. However, although breast-feeding is best for the baby, it may not be best for your partner.

REMEMBER

Even though your opinion is probably valued, the final decision about breast-feeding is absolutely, unquestionably your partner's. Many women just aren't comfortable with breast-feeding, and a woman who isn't comfortable usually doesn't do it well, leading to a stressed-out mom, hungry baby, and (often) bewildered dad. Rest assured that bottle-feeding is a perfectly fine method of feeding your newborn if your partner can't or doesn't want to breast-feed.

A number of considerations go into the decision to breast- or bottle-feed. If your partner has even the slightest interest, breast-feeding for the first few days so the baby receives *colostrum*, the first fluids produced, is a good way to start. Colostrum contains many nutrients and antibodies that are good for the baby. If your partner hates it, she can stop at any time, but she may love it! If she stops breast-feeding, though, getting the milk flowing again is hard, but not at all impossible. See Chapter 12 for more on making the decision to breast-feed and read on for the basics on baby-feeding methods.

Breast-feeding basics

If your partner decides to breast-feed, you may be breathing a sigh of relief that the nighttime duties won't fall to you, but not so fast! Breast-fed babies usually eat more frequently than bottle-fed babies because they digest breast milk more easily. If you're co-sleeping or even if the baby is across the room, you'll probably be awake at 12 a.m., 3 a.m., and 6 a.m., too.

Even if you normally sleep like the dead and wouldn't wake up if the Titanic floated through your bedroom, getting up and offering support for at least one of the night feedings can be a wonderful contribution to your partner and make you feel closer to your baby. Get your partner a drink, help her get into a comfortable position, and talk to her if she wants conversation. Late-night talks provide time and space for you and your partner to have discussions you may not be able to during the day.

If you're working full-time, getting up in the night is hard but worth it. Getting to know your new little person and your partner better is worth the sacrifice, and this time too shall pass, faster than you can imagine.

Getting started

Although breast-feeding seems like it should be easy and natural, it isn't always. Many women today have no role models for breast-feeding; their moms may not have breast-fed, their friends may not be doing it, and you're not much help, either. Most hospitals have lactation consultants to help new moms get started breast-feeding. Some also offer at-home visits if needed. If you have a doula, she'll be invaluable in helping with issues that arise. And of course, books like *Breastfeeding For Dummies* (Wiley) cover everything you need to know and are available for consultation day and night.

With all that said, it does help to know about the most common breast-feeding problems:

>> **Latch-on problems:** Women with large or flat nipples often have a difficult time getting the baby to latch on. This is frustrating for mom and baby alike and often ends with both

in tears. If the baby isn't properly latched, he won't get enough milk. A baby who doesn't latch on well can also cause bleeding, cracked, and painful nipples.

Patience can often conquer latch-on problems. Sometimes, though, additional assistance from a nipple shield is necessary. A *nipple shield* fits over mom's nipple to give the baby something to grasp onto if her nipples are very flat.

>> **Parental anxiety:** Many new parents are obsessed with their baby's weight. Breast-feeding can frustrate parents who want to know exactly how much milk the baby is getting at each feeding. However, you can still measure his intake if you have a baby scale and really have to know; just weigh the baby before and after a feeding and compare. Don't change his clothes — not even his diaper — or the weight won't be accurate. A baby scale can save the sanity of weight-obsessed parents. But if your baby is producing wet diapers six to eight times a day, along with a poopy diaper at least every other day, he's most likely getting enough.

>> **Supply issues:** Most women have ample milk supply starting around the third day after delivery, but some need supplements to increase milk supply. Drinking plenty of fluids, getting enough rest, and taking herbs such as fenugreek can help increase supply. (Talk to a lactation consultant first about doses, benefits, and drawbacks.) Before a good milk supply is established, supplementing the baby's diet with formula or pumping rather than nursing is discouraged, because sucking increases the supply. Pumping isn't as effective as a baby's suck at stimulating milk supply. Breast milk is the original supply-and-demand system.

Supplemental bottles

After your partner's milk supply is well established, you can give baby supplemental bottles of formula or pumped breast milk. Bottle-feeding is a nice way for you to feed and bond with the baby occasionally, and it gives your partner a chance to get out of the house or actually take an uninterrupted shower. Decreasing the number of nursing times a day reduces the milk supply, though, so don't overdo the supplemental bottles. Most likely mom will still have to pump and save the milk for a later feeding.

Don't be surprised if the baby doesn't quite understand what to do with the bottle at first. Bottle-feeding and breast-feeding require completely different tongue positioning and techniques on the baby's part. Some babies refuse supplemental bottles, which can be a problem if your partner gets sick or for some reason can't breast-feed. Although you can feed a recalcitrant breast-feeder with an eyedropper, the process certainly isn't fun for either of you. Some medical practitioners recommend an occasional supplemental bottle after nursing is well established so the baby gets used to taking an occasional bottle. Check with your pediatrician.

Many dads are a little envious of the closeness of the breast-feeding relationship and enjoy skin-to-skin contact while they feed the baby. Others find this just too weird. Whichever camp you're in, supplemental bottles can give you time to study your baby's face in detail and revel in the miracle you've created.

Pumping

Pumping to fill a supplemental bottle or if your partner goes back to work is easier than it used to be. Your partner can use an electric pump that's more efficient than the old bicycle horn–type pumps. A really good pump can be really pricey but is worth it if your partner is going to use it a lot. Insurance companies must reimburse the cost of renting or buying a pump under the Affordable Care Act. Pumping is nowhere near as efficient as nursing is, so the amount produced may be much less than you think it should be. This difference is normal and not a sign that the baby isn't getting enough milk.

TIP

Store pumped milk in feeding-sized amounts, especially if you're freezing it, because you don't want to thaw out more than you'll use at one time. Use plastic or glass containers with well-fitted tops, but avoid anything containing bisphenol A (BPA), a chemical that can be toxic to infants. Collection bags made specifically for freezing breast milk are ideal.

WARNING

Don't use plastic baggies or bags from disposable bottles to store frozen breast milk because they may leak or contain substances that affect the milk's nutrients.

You can store breast milk at room temperature for up to six hours, in the refrigerator for up to eight days, and in the freezer for up to 12 months.

Bottle-feeding basics

Bottle-feeding has never been more complicated. Not only do you have to choose a formula and a nipple type, but you also have to worry about the materials from which the bottle is made. Recent reports about the high levels of BPA (a chemical used in plastics) released when bottles are heated in the microwave or dishwasher led the FDA to ban the use of BPA in all baby bottles and sippy cups. Microwave warming can also cause hot spots that pose a burn threat in the heated formula, so it's not recommended in any case. At least you no longer need to sterilize bottles on top of the stove — ask your mom or grandma about how much fun that used to be!

Winning the bottle battle

Once upon a time, all baby bottles were made of glass. Then parents got tired of being beaned with glass bottles, and everyone worried about glass bottles breaking when babies threw them out of the crib, so plastic bottles were invented about two minutes after the invention of plastic. Not only were they lighter and unbreakable, but they also came in pretty colors.

Then bottle manufacturers decided to mix things up a bit. Now bottles and nipples are no longer interchangeable, and bottle "systems" sometimes include plastic liners and inserts that reduce air intake and, hopefully, colic. Every bottle has to be used with its own system, and parents have to decide which one works best for their baby.

WARNING

Studies have shown cause for concern about plastic bottles releasing the harmful chemical BPA when heated. Some parents have switched back to glass, but manufacturers now create BPA-free plastic bottle systems. If you have older bottles and they're not BPA-free, get rid of them. Spending more money on another whole bottle system is painful, but it's better than worrying about poisoning your child every time you warm a bottle.

Choosing a formula

After you pick your bottles, you can start worrying about which formula to use. The array is truly formidable. For starters, you have to consider powder versus concentrate versus ready-made. Then you may want to consider your pediatrician's preference. Following are the advantages and disadvantages of each type:

>> **Ready-to-serve formula** can be very convenient for travel if you use one container at a feeding. However, it's out of the question for everyday use for most people because a month's supply is equal to the national budget of a small European country.

>> **Concentrate** comes in small cans, and you dilute it with water before feeding. It's easy to use but more expensive than powder, though it's cheaper than ready-to-serve.

>> **Powder** is the cheapest of the three options. If you're out of the house, it's easy to put the powder in a bottle and just fill with warm water when the baby's ready to eat. However, powder comes in ginormous cans that take up half your kitchen countertop. Powder also clumps and takes more effort to shake smooth, a consideration at 4 a.m. when any effort seems like too much. Shaking the bottle to mix increases the bubbles and air inside the bottle, which can cause gassiness, so if your baby is already prone to gas, powder formula may not be for you.

After you decide on the form of your formula, it's time to choose one. This won't be easy; about a hundred different formulas are on the market, all claiming to be the best (although most grudgingly acknowledge that breast–feeding is also very good). Following are the general categories of formulas:

>> **Regular:** Regular formula is made from cow's milk and contains 20 calories per ounce. Regular formula is usually fortified with iron. Some are also fortified with long-chain polyunsaturated fats that they claim enhance eye and brain development, but these claims aren't well substantiated.

>> **Enhanced:** Enhanced formula, often used for premature or failure-to-thrive babies, contains 24 calories per ounce. Don't use this kind unless your doctor recommends it.

>> **Soy:** Soy-based formulas may be used by parents wanting to avoid animal proteins or because they think their baby has a cow's milk allergy. But some babies with cow's milk allergy also have a soy allergy. Besides, soy contains estrogen, and some studies show that too much soy can be harmful to infants and children. Make sure to do your research before using soy formula.

>> **Hypoallergenic:** Babies who are allergic to lactose or soy may need protein hydrolysate formulas, which are easier to digest. Nutramigen and Alimentum are examples of protein hydrolysate formulas made by different companies. These formulas are ridiculously expensive and also smell bad, so use them only if your doctor recommends them.

>> **Organic:** Regardless of the kind of formula you buy, there's likely an organic option available. It will cost significantly more but will meet FDA guidelines for organic foods. The ingredients are mostly the same; what you're paying for are ingredients that haven't been knowingly exposed to pesticides or chemicals and contain no genetically modified organisms.

Preparing a bottle

The hardest part of preparing some bottles is putting the "system" together. Some bottles have inserts to put in; others have little bags to put in place that hold the formula. Unless you want to add new frustrations to your life at 4 a.m., pick a simple system.

To make a bottle, read the instructions on the formula label. For powder, you mix a certain number of scoops with a certain amount of water, sometimes a foggy concept in the middle of the night. You usually dilute concentrates 1:1, and you don't need to dilute ready-to-serve formulas at all.

WARNING

Never try to "stretch" formula by adding more water than usual or by adding water to ready-to-serve formulas. You may deprive your baby of essential nutrition by doing so. Also, cow's milk and plant-based milks are not suitable for babies and can cause severe illness and even death if used in place of formula or breastmilk.

Many parents prefer to use distilled water, sometimes labeled as *nursery water*, rather than tap water, but if you have city water, it's probably not necessary. Boil the water from the tap if you're concerned about it, and use cold water rather than hot, which may contain more lead from the pipes. Let the water run for 30 seconds to reduce lead and other mineral contamination.

If you want to use well water, have a sample of it tested to make sure it doesn't contain high levels of nitrates or other minerals. Boiling well water concentrates nitrates instead of removing them, so it isn't recommended.

Knowing how much formula is enough

When your baby is brand-new, she probably won't take more than 2 or 3 ounces at a time. The most important thing about bottle-feeding is not to try to force the last drop down your child's throat. Keep in mind that *you* made the decision on how much to put in the bottle — your baby didn't ask for that much. Let her make the decision about how hungry she is. With childhood obesity at an all-time high and a major health concern, the last thing you want to do is overfeed your child from an early age.

On the other hand, if she drains the bottle and acts like she's still hungry, give her a little more. Babies aren't machines, and they don't take the same amount of formula at each feeding. When she stops sucking and tries to push the bottle out of her mouth, she's had enough.

Changing Diapers

Changing diapers is the task new parents are probably least excited about. If you and your partner find yourselves playing rock-paper-scissors to determine which of you gets stuck changing the runny yellow poop that has overflowed out of the diaper and on to the sleeper, your shirt, and the new leather sofa, you're normal.

Diaper duty isn't fun, but it's necessary an appalling number of times a day when your baby is new, so rest assured you'll both get plenty of experience.

Cleaning baby boys

Boys and girls really are different when it comes to diaper changing. When dealing with a baby boy, the worst part is projectile urination. You can easily avoid it if you remember to keep the penis covered at all times. Don't worry if you forget, though. A few good shots to the eye will reinforce your memory quickly.

Boys who've been circumcised (see Figure 11-1a), which means that the foreskin covering the tip of the penis has been removed, need extra TLC at first. You may need to wrap Vaseline-coated gauze around the tip for the first few days, depending on your practitioner's instructions. Change the gauze every time you change his diaper.

When you remove the gauze around the circumcision, you may be horrified to see that the skin is a yellowish color. This is normal healing for a mucous membrane. If the area is oozing or has pus or a foul odor, call your medical practitioner.

Uncircumcised boys are a little harder to clean, and the foreskin (see Figure 11-1b) needs to be kept loose. The foreskin doesn't retract or pull back easily before the age of 1 or even longer. Up to this point, you should clean only the outside of the foreskin. When it can be retracted, gently push it back as far as it will go, which isn't going to be very far, and clean with water (no soap or other products!). Return the foreskin to its normal position afterward. If the foreskin becomes red or swollen, have your medical practitioner take a look to make sure baby boy doesn't have an infection.

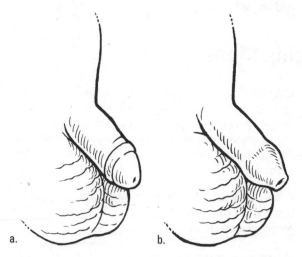

Illustration by Kathryn Born, MA

FIGURE 11-1: A circumcised penis (a) and an uncircumcised penis (b).

Cleaning baby girls

Baby girls aren't likely to spray the room when you remove their diaper, but they have their own set of problems. Keep these points in mind when changing a baby girl:

>> Girls have lots of nooks and crevices, and getting all of them clean is difficult. A runny, poopy diaper goes everywhere. Use moistened wipes or cotton balls to make sure you remove all the stool.

CIRCED OR UNCIRCED? MAKING THE DECISION

Circumcision is a procedure in which the foreskin of the penis is removed. For Jewish parents, circumcision is a religious ritual usually done in a ceremony called a *bris*. For other parents, whether to have baby boy circumcised is a personal choice. Twenty years ago, nearly all baby boys were circumcised, but today, more parents are questioning whether a surgical cosmetic procedure is necessary in a baby's first days of life. Around 50 to 60 percent of baby boys in the United States are now circumcised each year, but the percentage varies quite a bit from one part of the country to another.

The main benefit to circumcision is ease in cleaning and avoiding the need to have the foreskin removed at a later date for medical reasons. Boys who are circumcised also have fewer urinary tract infections. Uncircumcised males are more likely to contract sexually transmitted diseases later in life. Some dads just want their son circumcised so they'll "look the same."

>> Girls are more likely to have urinary tract infections because of the proximity of the anus and vagina to the urethra, so it's really important to make sure the whole area is clean.

>> Always wipe from front to back. Doing so helps to avoid introducing fecal matter into the vaginal area, which can cause infections.

>> Don't be too gentle. Make sure to thoroughly wipe the opening of the vagina or it can close up. If that happens you have to apply a steroid cream to help reopen it, or, even worse, have it surgically reopened. Don't worry too much about this, though — it's not a common problem.

Bathing Your Squirming Bundle of Joy

Few things strike fear into the hearts of inexperienced parents like the first bath. Take a squirmy baby, soap him all over to make him incredibly difficult to hold on to, and then put him in a tub of water. Sounds like a recipe for disaster, or at the very least, parental heart failure, but it doesn't have to be. Many hospitals now do a "trial run" bath to make sure you won't drown the poor child right off the bat, but even the least experienced new dad can learn to give baby a bath. Fortunately, you don't need to give your baby a bath every day; doing so can dry out his skin. Every other day is probably enough for both of you.

Here's how to bathe your newborn:

1. **Get your supplies ready first.**

   Nothing makes a bath more difficult than getting the water drawn, the baby undressed, and the towel laid out and realizing you forgot to get the soap, or the lotion, or the diaper. No, the baby doesn't wear the diaper into the bath, but you need it ready the minute you take him out, especially if your baby's a boy, unless you want an eyeful of urine.

2. **Put the baby in a comfortable spot.**

   Undressing him on the toilet lid may seem like a good idea if you're bathing him in the sink or on the counter if you're bathing him in a little baby bath, but those surfaces are cold and hard, even with a towel over them, and they may be riddled with germs. Get him ready on the changing table or bed; take off everything except the diaper (urine, remember?) and bring him into the bathroom wrapped in a towel.

3. **Hold the baby and fill the tub, or have your partner handle one of those jobs.**

   Baby's bath water should be 90 to100 degrees. You can monitor the temperature to make sure it isn't too hot or too cold with cute little floating bath toys that have built-in thermometers. If you're using a sink, pad it by lining it with a towel. A towel also helps reduce the slipperiness of a baby bathtub.

4. **Before putting the baby into the bath, wet a washcloth and squirt baby soap onto it.**

   This way you don't have to do it while you try to hold the baby in the water at the same time.

5. **Undo the diaper tabs, whip off the diaper, and put the baby in the water.**

   Don't give him time to do anything dastardly.

6. **Don't expect the baby to enjoy this new experience at first.**

   Yes, he spent nine months in water, but he's forgotten already, and your inexperienced hands aren't supporting him as well as the womb did. Some baby tubs have a little sling or are curved to support the baby. Otherwise, support his head and neck with your hand or the crook of your arm if you're well coordinated.

7. **Wash the baby with the soapy washcloth, starting at his head and working your way down.**

   Yes, just like you'd wash the wall or the car. The genitalia should be the last part you wash. When you get to the bottom (literally), use a clean washcloth if it seems more hygienic to you.

8. **Rinse him off with a clean washcloth.**

9. **Lift him out of the water and wrap the towel around him.**

   A towel with a little hood helps keep him warm and makes him look like an adorable elf. Don't admire him too long, though, because you need to get his diaper back on — quickly.

10. **Carry him to the changing surface, where the fresh diaper is already laid out. To keep him warm, keep the towel over the top half of his body while you put the diaper on.**

11. **Dry him off gently and dress him.**

    Babies have delicate skin, so don't rub too hard with the towel.

12. **Do a little baby massage if you have enough energy left for it.**

    Just put some lotion on your hands and gently massage your baby's arms, legs, chest, and back. He'll learn to loosen up, and it may just relax him enough so that he'll take a nap.

13. **Now collapse on the couch — you've earned it!**

Holding Your Baby

Newborns demand to be held a lot, and their brains thrive through touch. You're going to find yourself carrying the baby around quite a bit during the first few weeks. Babies who are colicky (cry a lot) are often more comfortable if you keep moving, and moving also helps dispense your tension and anxiety when you're on hour two of a colic episode. You can hold babies in several ways, and yours may have a definite preference. Try these tried-and-true baby holds:

>> **Cradle position:** Cradle the baby's head in the crook of your arm. Most people hold the baby on the left side, but go with what works for you.

>> **Football hold:** In this hold, baby's head rests on your hand looking up, her body lies on your arm, and her feet are pointed at your elbow.

>> **Over the shoulder:** Some gassy babies feel better with pressure on their abdomen, so slinging them up onto your shoulder may help get the gas out. However, spit-up-prone babies and vomiters also like this position, so have a burp cloth on your shoulder at all times. A big one.

Whichever position you choose to hold your baby in, use it often! Nothing is better for dad and baby bonding than time spent in close proximity — except maybe hands-free holding. Having baby strapped to you allows you to get more in tune with baby's movements, noises, and facial expressions. As a bonus, wearing baby allows you to complete daily tasks and chores around the house that won't get done as quickly and easily otherwise.

Most men enjoy using a baby carrier that straps onto their body like a backpack and is easily worn on the front, side, or back. Wraparound slings can be used almost immediately, but they're generally more popular with women because of their more feminine aesthetic. That said, they're comfortable and soothing, and any man who's comfortable with his masculinity should give it a shot. Buy black or another neutral color to share with your partner.

More popular with men is the pouch sling, a tube of fabric that turns you into a human kangaroo, which can be used beginning at four months of age — usually when baby can hold up her own head. Soft-structured carriers, such as the über-popular BabyBjörn, are comfortable and easy to use but are best used starting at four months of age.

Figure 11-2 shows you how to carry your baby in a carrier, if you're interested in doing so. Whichever carrier you use, always make sure baby has an unobstructed airway. Also, just because you're hands-free doesn't mean you're baby-free. Don't bend over at the waist or baby can fall out of the carrier. Yes, it happens.

Front pack   Sling   Backpack

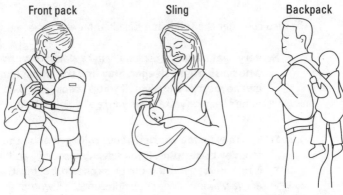

© John Wiley & Sons, Inc.

FIGURE 11-2: A baby carrier lets your baby see more of the world and keeps your hands free in the process.

WARNING

One last thing, and it's a big one: Make sure your baby's head doesn't fall forward so her chin touches her chest in a sling. This position can make it difficult for your baby to breathe.

Co-sleeping Pros and Cons

Co-sleeping, or sleeping with the baby in your bed, goes in and out of vogue. Right now co-sleeping is popular with many parents, although it comes with a twist in some cases: The baby may sleep in a little sidecar, or co-sleeper, that attaches to your bed. You get the whole bed to yourself, but the baby is right nearby.

If you're not comfortable sharing the bed with baby, traditional bassinets, small playpens, and baby beds also work well. If you're still debating about keeping the baby in your bed or even in your room, consider the following advantages:

>> **Co-sleeping is convenient if your partner is breast-feeding.** Breast-feeding is much easier if you don't have to get out of bed to get the baby.

>> **You hear the baby as soon as he starts stirring.** Although this itself has pros and cons, the benefit is that he doesn't have a chance to work himself into a crying frenzy before a feeding.

>> **It can give you a sense of closeness as a family.** To hear your baby's soft breathing is reassuring and also enjoyable.

Also consider the following disadvantages:

>> **Very light sleepers, especially light sleepers with a baby who's also a light sleeper, may find the whole family awake most of the night.** If you're keeping the baby awake or he's keeping you awake, you're all going to be excessively cranky.

>> **You may be too worried about rolling over on the baby to enjoy co-sleeping.** If you sleep very soundly and the baby is right next to you, this can be a concern, but most parents are very aware of the baby's presence. If it worries you, a bassinet or other sleeping arrangement in the room may be better for you. The American Academy of Pediatrics recommends keeping your baby in your room but *not* in your bed because the bedding in an adult bed poses a suffocation risk to an infant; it advises using a co-sleeper that attaches to the bed instead.

>> **If one of you works odd shifts, you may worry about getting in or out of the room without waking the baby.** However, babies usually aren't disturbed by normal noises and probably won't even hear you come and go.

>> **When you put the baby in your bed, you eventually have to put him out.** Your child may prefer to stay in your bed until he goes to college, but you may want your bed back in a few years. Some children don't go quietly into the dark night and put up quite a fight about sleeping in their own rooms.

REMEMBER

Even if you don't want the baby in your room with you, baby monitors make it possible to hear the slightest stirring from another room.

Back to Sleep: Helping Baby Sleep Safely and Comfortably

Once upon a time, almost all babies slept on their stomachs. The babies preferred it, they had less gas, and if they spit up or vomited, they were less likely to choke. Then, in 1992, the American Academy of Pediatrics (AAP) released new recommendations about placing babies on their backs rather than stomachs to sleep, claiming new studies that showed that babies were less likely to die of sudden infant death syndrome (SIDS) if they slept on their backs.

The "Back to Sleep" campaign went into full swing in 1994, heavily promoted by pediatricians. Within a few years, almost all babies were put to sleep on their backs, at least while they were in the hospital. Since the back-sleeping movement was launched, the incidence of SIDS-related deaths has dropped by more than 50 percent, from 3 deaths per 2,000 live births to 1 per 2,000 in 2013. In the United States, 80 to 90 percent of babies sleep on their backs, according to 2013 reports.

WARNING

A baby who is used to sleeping on her back but is placed prone (on her stomach) to sleep, possibly by a caregiver not familiar with the benefits of back sleeping, has an 18-fold increased risk of SIDS, according to the AAP.

Side positioning was originally considered a viable alternative to back sleeping, but more recent recommendations from the AAP are that side sleeping also increases the risk of SIDS, as well as the risk of the baby moving from a side to a prone position. To further reduce the risk of injury or death, keep soft fluffy blankets, pillows, and mattress pads out of the crib as well. A firm sleeping surface is best.

Coping if baby hates being on his back

Many babies truly hate sleeping on their backs. They don't sleep well, their parents don't sleep well, and everyone is miserable. What should you do if you and your baby are both desperate to get some sleep?

>> **Rock the baby to sleep first.** If he's asleep before you lay him down, he may stay asleep when you place him on his back.

>> **Tough it out.** This is really hard to do, but a good night's sleep isn't worth the risk of SIDS.

>> **Use a pacifier.** Even if you hate them, pacifiers really do soothe some babies. The AAP recommends using one at bedtime because pacifier use also decreases SIDS risk.

Swaddling your little one

Some parents find their newborns are calmer and sleep better when they're tightly wrapped in blankets so their arms and legs can't go flying off in every direction whenever they're startled. Nurses swaddle newborns in the hospital for this reason (and because it makes them look adorable). Even the most fumble-fingered dad can do this at home, even though it won't look at all like the nurse's version at first. To swaddle, follow these instructions and also refer to Figure 11-3:

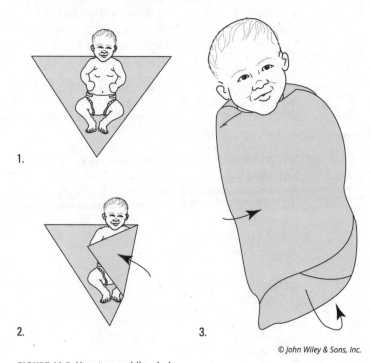

1.

2.   3.

© John Wiley & Sons, Inc.

FIGURE 11-3: How to swaddle a baby.

1. **Put the blanket on a flat surface like a diamond, with a point up.**

2. **Fold the pointy end at the top down about 6 inches.**

3. **Put the baby on the blanket, with her head just above the folded-down edge.**

4. **Pull one of the pointy ends on the side across the baby, covering her arms, and tuck it behind her back.**

5. **Bring up the bottom point to the baby's chin.**

6. **Repeat Step 4 using the remaining point of the blanket.**

   Make it tight enough to make the baby feel secure, but not tight enough to cut off her circulation!

Realize that the baby isn't going to lie perfectly still during this procedure. It'll take you at least a few tries to get it right.

Preventing the flat-head look

In addition to sleeping on their backs, babies nowadays also spend hours with their heads back in swings, bouncy seats, and car seats. No wonder so many of them have flat heads. A flattened back or side part of the head, called *plagiocephaly*, can be more than just a cosmetic problem. Though 20 percent of infants today have flat heads, according to the AAP, all but 8 percent will round out naturally without treatment by 24 months.

You can help prevent plagiocephaly in your child by following these suggestions:

>> **Give baby lots of tummy time.** Babies need to spend some time on their stomachs when they're awake to strengthen their neck muscles. This time also gives the back of the head a chance to round out.

>> **Carry the baby.** Don't always plop the baby in a swing or bouncer when he's awake; carry him around with you so he gets to see more of the world and doesn't put pressure on his head.

>> **Change the room around.** If possible, move the crib from one side of the room to the other from time to time so the baby sleeps with his head turned a different way. Or leave the crib in place and turn the baby, moving him from one end of the crib to the other. Plagiocephaly is treated by

molding a custom helmet that exerts pressure on the baby's head and gradually changes the shape as the baby grows. The helmet is worn 23 hours out of the day and is adjusted as the baby's head begins to round out.

Having your baby wear a helmet 23 hours a day for several months is understandably upsetting for parents. It's possible to make helmet-wearing more fun — for you, not the baby — by painting the helmet or applying decals to cute it up. Having the plaster mold of their head done will probably annoy your child far more than the helmet will.

Soothing Baby Indigestion

All babies fuss from time to time, and many have a short fussy period every single day, usually around the time when you're the busiest and have the least patience for it. Although all screaming seems pretty much the same to you, fussiness can be caused by one end or the other of the gastrointestinal tract.

Colic

Colic can send a parent around the bend in no time at all. It's defined by the Mayo Clinic as "three hours of crying a day at least three days a week for three weeks or more in a well-fed, healthy baby." Colic affects around 40 percent of infants and generally starts between three and six weeks of age and ends by three months of age. They may seem like the longest three months of your life.

No one really knows what causes colic, but colicky babies often pull their legs up to their stomach and act as if they have a belly ache, so perhaps they do. Breast-fed and bottle-fed babies both get colic, and changing the formula rarely helps. Things that help calm a colicky baby include:

>> **Car rides:** The motion of the car calms down many colicky babies. With the price of gas, this can be an expensive solution, but believe us, you'll try anything after the first two hours.

>> **Decreased stimulation:** Some babies can't handle any handling or stimulation when they're colicky and do better in a quiet, dark room.

>> **Exercise balls:** Some babies love lying on an exercise ball, with you holding them in position. These big balls can do double-duty in pregnancy and labor, when moms-to-be can squat on them or lean over them.

>> **Position changes:** Some babies like pressure on their abdomen, so letting her dangle over your arm while you walk around may work. Putting her over your knee, face down, and patting her back may work, too. See Figure 11-4 for help.

>> **Vibration:** Vibrating chairs or swings calm some colicky babies. If you don't have either of these, you can do what many a desperate parent has tried: putting the infant seat on the dryer and turning it on. Whether it's the motion or the noise, something about it calms some babies. (Make sure to remain next to the baby to make sure she doesn't fall off of the dryer, and always attach the safety belt, even if she's sitting on the floor in the chair.)

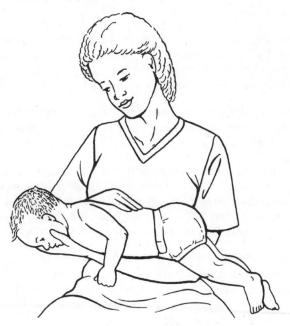

FIGURE 11-4: Try this position if your baby is colicky.

Illustration by Kathryn Born, MA

Gas

Babies often need help to get gas out of their stomachs after they eat. Some babies burp it up spontaneously, but others need to be patted between the shoulder blades for a few minutes to get the gas out.

TIP

If the baby falls asleep at the end of a feeding without burping, don't put him down without getting a burp up. He'll give you just enough time to fall asleep or get involved with something before he wakes up with that piercing cry that means a bubble is stuck. Take a few extra minutes and get him to burp; you'll be glad you did.

Reflux

Although many babies spit up after feedings, gastrointestinal reflux disease (GERD) is a whole different entity. Gastrointestinal reflux (GER — not the same thing as GERD), or normal spitting, occurs in more than half of all babies, but it's usually worse between the ages of 1 and 4 months and disappears by 6 to 12 months.

TIP

Keeping the baby in an upright position for half an hour or so after feedings helps reduce GER, and then keeping her at a 30-degree angle for sleep may help. Some parents elevate one end of the crib to keep the baby's head higher than her feet.

Despite what you may be told, studies show that thickening the formula with cereal doesn't help, and it may worsen respiratory problems in children with GERD.

GER is annoying and potentially ruinous to your clothing and the baby's, but GERD is a more serious problem. Babies with GERD fail to gain weight, may have respiratory difficulties from milk aspiration, and may have feeding aversion, which is understandable because food so often brings them discomfort.

Breast-fed babies are less likely to develop GER or GERD because breast milk digests more easily and empties out of the stomach twice as fast as formula. Medications to reduce stomach acid or to keep stomach acid from entering the esophagus may be prescribed to treat GERD.

KEEPING YOUR COOL DURING BABY MELTDOWNS

Babies sense stress, and an already stressed-out, screaming baby is made unhappier by a stressed-out, screaming parent. To help maintain control in difficult situations, try these ideas:

- **Leave the house.** You and your partner can take turns getting out of Dodge for a short time.

- **Close the door.** For periods of time when you can't leave the house but truly can't take it anymore, put the baby in her room and close the door for a few minutes.

- **Get help.** When a crying baby brings you to the brink, you may be shocked at how quickly your anger escalates. Anger management courses can help you tame an out-of-control temper. Learning to do it now rather than later is beneficial, because this child will be doing things to drive you crazy for the next 50 years. (No, parenthood isn't easier when your children are adults — just ask your own parents!)

Scheduling Immunizations

Immunizations have become a divisive topic today — one that many parents have vehement opinions about. Although studies have shown no connection between vaccinations and the rise in the number of children diagnosed with some form of autism, a brain disorder that now affects 1 in 105 babies in the United States, many parents worry about the number of vaccines given in the first year of baby's life.

The number of injections a baby receives in his first year can seem overwhelming, but studies have shown immunization schedules to be safe for your baby. Table 11-1 shows the average newborn schedule of immunizations (some of the series are continued after the first birthday).

TABLE 11-1 Average First-Year Immunization Schedule

Vaccine	Before Leaving Hospital	2 Months	4 Months	6 Months	1 Year
Hepatitis B	x	x		x	
Rotavirus		x	x	x	
Diphtheria/ tetanus/pertussis		x	x	x	
Haemophilus influenzae type B		x	x	x	x
Pneumococcal		x	x	x	x
Inactivated poliovirus		x	x	x	
Influenza				x	
Measles/mumps/ rubella					x
Varicella					x
Hepatitis A					x

Skipping some shots?

Immunizations are so controversial in some circles today that you may consider giving the baby some but not all of the recommended vaccines, possibly skipping influenza, hepatitis, and chickenpox vaccines and splitting the measles-mumps-rubella injection into three separate shots. Talk seriously with your pediatrician about the advisability of this, and check with your local board of education, because some schools may require certain immunizations before your child is allowed to start school. See the upcoming section "Taking a stand on the vaccination debate" for more on the controversy over what diseases to vaccinate for — and when.

Spreading them out

Many parents compromise on the immunization question by spacing the immunizations over a longer time period than that recommended by the AAP. Taking more time may necessitate more visits to the pediatrician than are normally scheduled but can make it easier to determine which injection is causing a reaction if a problem occurs.

Pediatrician Robert Sears published an alternative vaccination schedule in his book *The Vaccine Book* (Little, Brown and Company). Be aware, however, that the AAP has vigorously protested his alternative schedule and continues to support the current guidelines. Discuss alternative schedules and the pros and cons thoroughly with your medical practitioner before making up your mind about vaccination.

Taking a stand on the vaccination debate

If you decide not to vaccinate your child — and only around one percent of American parents forgo all vaccinations — it's important to know the potential risks of taking this stand. The incidences of certain nearly eradicated diseases, such as *pertussis* (better known as whooping cough), have skyrocketed in the last few years. In 2012, there were 48,277 reported cases of pertussis in the United States, the most since 1955. Cases dropped back down to just under 20,000 in 2019, still far over the low number — less than 2,000 cases — in the 1970s. Around 50 percent of babies under 12 who develop this disorder need hospitalization. The incidence of other potentially serious diseases, such as measles, have also risen in the past decade.

Even common and considered-mild diseases such as chickenpox can cause serious illness. Before the chickenpox vaccine, more than 100,000 people — mostly children — were hospitalized each year from chickenpox complications, and around 100 died.

When you choose not to vaccinate your child, you're depending on herd immunity — also known as community immunity — to keep your child from getting a common disease. *Herd immunity* means that a high percentage of the community is immunized, which decreases the risk of transmission to those who aren't immunized. This protects your child only as long as a high percentage of children around you are immunized.

If you live in an area where more children aren't immunized, your child has a much higher risk of developing a communicable disease. Outbreaks of pertussis and other infectious diseases have occurred in these types of areas.

To vaccinate or not is your choice as a parent. Weigh all the facts carefully — not just the hype, of which there is plenty on both sides of the debate — before making your decision.

MARKING THE MILESTONES

Baby books are a wonderful invention; it's a shame more parents don't use them throughout their child's infancy. Nearly every baby shower includes one as a gift, and most parents start out with great enthusiasm, recording every pregnancy symptom, movement, and ultrasound. But when the actual baby arrives, time is precious, and the baby book is often neglected, although an occasional guilt trip may result in copious recording for a week or so.

Make every attempt to record your baby's milestones somewhere. You don't have to use a baby book; you can use baby calendars, your own journal, or a blog to keep track of your baby's first tooth, word, or step. You may think now that you could never forget such important milestones, but the sad truth is that you can, very easily. And if you have more than one child, trying to remember who had croup and who had chickenpox gets to be impossible. And when you have grandchildren, many years from now, you can prove to their parents how much more advanced the grandchildren are compared to them at the same age!

IN THIS CHAPTER

» Doing the dirty work around the house

» Being supportive during breast-feeding and dealing with any issues

» Helping your partner recover from a C-section

» Providing emotional assistance when your partner's hormones are haywire

» Dealing with changes and establishing a new "normal"

Chapter **12**

Supporting the New Mom . . . and Surviving Yourself!

A new baby is a celebrity, with every coo, smile, and gurgle met with a flash of the camera. A doting parent or grandparent is always ready to meet baby's every whim, and your protective nature makes you feel like you could uproot a mighty sequoia if it somehow threatened the well-being of your baby. Unfortunately, baby's time in the limelight comes at the expense of the woman who just spent the better part of a year carrying that child and hours (or days!) in labor. She suddenly goes from living as an A-list celebrity to feeling like an out-of-work actress working for tips at the local diner.

This is your chance to step up and shine, new dad, by making sure your partner feels every bit as adored, pampered, and attended to as that new bundle of joy. This means taking care of tangible needs, like making sure the litter box is clean and dinner's on the table, as well as less-tangible needs, like emotionally supporting your partner, limiting guests, and getting by on less sleep.

We know that the upheaval of a new baby can be a difficult adjustment for new dads, too, but rising to these challenges has long-term benefits for the health and happiness of your whole family. This chapter helps guide you through your partner's post-partum needs and teaches you how to be a hero for the new mom in your life.

Handling Housework during the Recovery Phase

New moms and dads both experience the stress of adapting to a new little person who's still a stranger, but moms have the added burden of uncontrolled hormones and physical recovery from the delivery. Your partner's energy needs to be directed at keeping herself together right now, not worrying about the house — or you.

REMEMBER

While your partner recovers, gets her hormones back together, and works into her new routine as a mom, she needs you to pick up the scut work around the house without being told what to do. You may not know exactly what that entails, but that's why we're here: to help you with all the things that need to be done. The following sections may look like a list of chores, but remember that a happy mom means a happy baby — and a happy next six months for your new family.

Getting the house in order

TV commercials make it appear that men are only good for making messes and that women derive joy from cleaning up after them, but in the real world, making sure the home is in tiptop shape is everyone's job. Except that now that your partner is limited to lifting nothing heavier than a baby for the next six weeks, cleaning has just become your full responsibility.

TIP

You don't have time to clean every part of the house every day, so ask your partner point-blank what tasks are most important to her, and then carry out her requests word for word — even if they seem irrational. For example, if she wants the bathroom cleaned every day, then grab your toilet brush and get scrubbing. She'll be spending a lot more time in there following labor because of postpartum bleeding, which can last anywhere from two to eight weeks, so a clean environment may help her relax and keep her from feeling embarrassed when visitors — who always seem to use the bathroom — unexpectedly appear.

Speaking of visitors, well-wishers come bearing a lot of stuff, which means clutter can get out of control very quickly. Because mom is trapped indoors with a baby who's feeding around the clock, feeling suffocated by balloons, flowers, and stuffed animals may only increase her anxiety. Make sure to find a new home for everything that comes into the house.

Doing the dishes, vacuuming, and taking out the trash are additional obvious tasks that need regular attention, but what about the less-obvious tasks? The following sections guide you through some of the more unexpected tasks you're about to become intimately acquainted with.

Battling baby's bottomless laundry basket

Laundry may seem straightforward, but like all things related to babies, it's complicated. If you're already accustomed to the ins and outs of laundry, you'll have ample opportunity over the next few weeks to put these basic skills into action. But laundering baby's things is a bit different. We break down the important points for you here:

>> **Wash brand-new infant clothes prior to first use to remove any chemicals or germs in the fabric.** As new clothes arrive, be sure to remove all price tags, stickers, and plastic tag holders.

>> **To avoid exposing your baby to dyes and chemicals that can irritate his delicate skin, wash baby clothes in dye- and chemical-free detergent.** Generally, any detergents labeled as dye- and chemical-free are okay to use. Using organic is always best but can be quite pricey. Several detergents, such as Dreft, are designed specifically to wash baby clothes.

>> **Use the delicate cycles on your washer and dryer.** Using the delicate cycle helps keep the materials in baby clothing from shrinking, which they tend to do. And baby clothes are outgrown fast enough without adding shrinkage to the mix.

>> **Be sure to treat stains — and you'll have stains, on your clothes and baby's alike — prior to washing.** Rinse away or wipe off any detritus from the article of clothing or blanket, and spray on the treatment of your choice. Most off-the-shelf stain treaters aren't especially gentle, so you may want to try a natural solution such as a blend of vinegar and water or lemon and water.

Couples opting to take the eco–friendly route of cloth diapers find the mounting laundry pile an even taller task. Follow these steps to take care of this particularly dirty laundry:

1. **Rinse the diapers.**

   Consider installing a sprayer attachment on your toilet to help with loose stools and urine. It allows you to rinse the diapers and flush without having to dunk the diaper into the toilet. As baby ages and poop becomes more solid, shake off poops into the toilet and flush them.

2. **Pretreat cloth diapers by placing them in a pail, sprinkling stains with baking soda, and covering the pail to keep smells at bay for no more than three days.**

   Place an air freshener inside the pail to help control odors, too. Another option is to place dirty diapers in a laundry-safe wet bag, zip it shut to contain the smell, and then wash the bag.

3. **Gather a load of no more than two dozen diapers. If you're using hook-and-loop diapers, fasten all tabs on each diaper to keep them from sticking to one another.**

4. **Use a quarter to half the amount of laundry detergent you would for a normal load.**

   Using a normal amount can lead to detergent buildup in the fabric. Diapers are designed to absorb, after all, and they're not discriminating about it.

5. **Wash on a cold/cold cycle.**

6. **Wash a second time, using a hot/cold cycle to kill any remaining bacteria.**

If you opt for the new cloth diapers that fit into reusable inserts, make sure you fully understand which part gets washed; what, if anything, gets thrown out (sometimes there's a disposable inner liner for the messy parts); and how to wash the rest. These diapers are pricey, and you don't want to add another hit to your budget by throwing out the vital parts.

Dealing with pet duty

Animals require a delicate transition when baby arrives. To help reduce the shock of a new human roommate, prior to bringing baby home from the hospital, wash your pet's bed or favorite toys in baby laundry detergent to get her used to what baby will smell like. You can also prepare your pets by inviting over friends with babies so your animals adjust to the sounds of babies. Enroll your dogs in an obedience course to make sure they're well trained and will lie down on the floor next to you on command.

REMEMBER

No matter how well trained or prepared your pets are, take care when introducing them to your baby. When baby comes through the door, be prepared to deal with any jumping, clawing, growling, or roughhousing your pet may engage in with both mom and baby. Keep animals separated from mom until she's healed enough to endure any unexpected pet reactions. When you trust that your pet won't react wildly, have the animal sit next to you while you hold the baby. Reward your pet with treats as you interact with the baby to begin making a positive connection between the two. Never hold your baby in your pet's face, as this can cause a possibly dangerous reaction from the animal.

In addition to mediating interactions between your partner and rambunctious pets and baby and *all* pets, it's also your responsibility to complete all pet-related tasks. That means changing the kitty litter, taking the dog for walks, grooming, and playing. Making sure your pet's life stays as normal as possible eases everyone's transition. For example, if your dog enjoys playing catch, make sure to play catch with her as often as you did before so she doesn't make a negative association between the new baby and your lack of attention.

REMEMBER

After contact with your pets, make sure to wash your hands with soap and water before handling the baby.

Becoming the errand boy

Grab the keys and get rolling, because driving duties are up to you for a while. Doctors recommend that women who have a vaginal birth don't drive for two weeks following delivery. That time could increase for a Cesarean delivery; follow your partner's practitioner's instructions. Some suggest that she be able to pick up her foot and stomp on the ground without any abdominal pain before driving.

TIP

Use the hours you spend driving to the grocery store and the post office (to mail thank-you notes, of course!) to recharge your batteries. Alone time is hard to come by these days.

Don't forget to extend an invitation to mom and baby, too. Many women begin to feel trapped in the house, so start including your partner in outings whenever she feels up to it. If she doesn't feel up to it or can't come along for the ride, bring her back some flowers or another favorite treat to make her feel loved and cared for.

THE WEIGHT GAME

Your partner may not be ready to get back into her pre-pregnancy jeans the moment she gets home from the hospital. Some women do lose a considerable amount of weight shortly after delivery, but some actually put on weight because of fluid retention. And as with all weight loss, unfortunately, losing pounds put on during and after pregnancy requires time and hard work.

Exercise helps the body recover from pregnancy (and has also been linked to decreased occurrence of depression), but even with exercise, it takes an average of two or three months before a woman gets back to her normal body weight. And even then, things will have changed. Stomachs get softer, body parts seemingly shift, stretch marks appear, and your partner is likely to feel like a stranger in her own body.

You can help her improve her body image and fitness by reminding her how beautiful you think she is and by planning activities that get you both moving together. A nice walk around the park or the neighborhood is always an enjoyable activity for the whole family, and following a normal childbirth, women can begin light walking a few days after returning home. If the gym is her scene, ask her if she'd like you to hire a personal trainer with knowledge of post-pregnancy fitness. If the yoga studio is her style, she may enjoy a mom-and-baby yoga class.

Whatever her desires, make sure her OB-GYN clears her prior to beginning any workout routine. She'll likely be advised to stick with activities that she engaged in before having the baby. She needs to start small, and you need to make sure she's comfortable. Remind her to exercise at a slow pace with moderate effort, especially during the first weeks. If she experiences an increase in bleeding, shortness of breath, or extreme fatigue, have her wait a few days before trying again.

Most important, let any new exercise regimen be her idea. Suggesting that a new mom join a gym will put you squarely in the doghouse.

Taking care of meals

For the first few weeks following delivery, you need to manage the meals because your partner is likely too physically drained — and too busy feeding baby — to think about cooking. Whether you're the guy who likes to take charge in the kitchen or the type who routinely forgets to add the cheese packet to macaroni and cheese, making sure you and your partner are well nourished is one of your most important roles.

Understanding what she needs

REMEMBER

Breast-feeding women need to consume an additional 400 to 600 calories more than they would when eating a normal diet. That's because breast-feeding burns about as many calories as a 30-minute run. New moms need to eat energy-packed, nutritious foods to help their bodies recover from labor and delivery. And with all the extra work you're doing on reduced sleep, you need these same foods too! Keep the following nutrition do's and don'ts in mind when grocery shopping and preparing meals:

>> **Do stock up on milk, yogurt, and other dairy products, if your partner can tolerate dairy.** Vitamin D and calcium are especially important for new moms. Some women are forced to eliminate dairy from their diets because it can cause excess gas and fussiness in the nursing baby. To get her the nutrients she otherwise would get from dairy, stock up on plant-based milk substitutes, such as soy or almond milk, which are fortified with vitamins.

» **Don't bring home a lot of foods that are high in sugar, carbohydrates, and fat.** Nothing is forbidden here, but don't go overboard. Not only is it bad for her waistline — and yours — but all the refined sugars, flours, and artificial fats are hard to digest and aren't ideal postpartum nutrition for baby or mom. As hard as it is to deny a new mother anything, try to talk her out of those cravings for an all-day diet of snack foods.

» **Do make sure she gets enough water.** If she's breast-feeding, she needs to drink at least 72 ounces of water each day to aid in milk production. If your tap water doesn't taste good, pick up a filtration pitcher or faucet attachment.

» **Don't let her (or you!) drink too much alcohol.** A glass of wine or a beer is okay, especially as a way for the new mom to clear her head and relax. But nursing moms should keep in mind that because alcohol enters the bloodstream, it enters the breast milk too, so moderation is essential. Non-nursing moms, and dads for that matter, still must be responsible caregivers, and alcohol lowers inhibitions and decreases sound judgment. Always drink responsibly.

In addition to taking her nutritional requirements into account, make sure to ask her what sounds good before doing any grocery shopping. Just like during pregnancy, many women find certain foods unappetizing and/or nauseating following childbirth.

Putting food on the table

Because you'll be getting less sleep and doing more work around the house, you may not be eager to strap on the apron three times a day. To make the task easier on yourself, cook meals that you can eat multiple times or freeze for future consumption, such as easy-to-assemble casseroles or pots of soup. If time allows, this can be a great nesting activity with your partner prior to delivery, too.

Another great idea that only requires a little work on your end is to make a bunch of peanut butter sandwiches, put them back in the bread bag, and store the bag in the fridge, so that she can just grab one quickly. This is especially helpful for a mom who is home alone during the day, when making good eating choices may be next to impossible with a baby whose needs come first.

Make sure mom has plenty of nutritious foods around that she can just grab and eat without either of you having to prep. Keep yogurt, nuts, fruit, and precut, precleaned raw veggies on hand as quick energy boosts that require no cooking.

When friends and family ask you what they can do to help, ask them to bring you a meal in a freezer-safe storage container in lieu of flowers. Having prepared homemade meals on hand helps you avoid the temptation to order takeout or fast food, which is high in sodium and fat and not the most nutritious for mom and baby.

Calling in backup

Not every new dad has the luxury of taking ample time off work to attend to the needs of his partner, which means your partner may be facing a lot of alone time with baby at a very early stage.

Leaving a new mom alone while you're off at work isn't a good idea. Many women, especially those who deliver via C-section, need physical and emotional support during the daytime for several weeks following delivery.

Talk to your partner about the needs and desires she has while you're at work, and help her find the appropriate support from friends, family, and neighbors. Make chore lists for daytime helpers so your partner doesn't feel burdened by having to ask for help.

If financially viable, hire a cleaning service. It will be the best gift you can give to your partner . . . and yourself.

Following the birth of their grandchild, your parents and your partner's parents may want to visit and help, especially when you go back to work. Before agreeing to visits, however, make sure your partner wants them around. All the advice and constant companionship from a parental figure may cause her more stress. She also may want a chance to go it alone without anyone's help. If she does want them around, try to stagger the visits to provide a longer duration of coverage — and a little more sanity for you and your partner.

Supporting a Breast-Feeding Mom

Breast-feeding is a full-time job, especially in the first few months, and although it may be more fun and rewarding than changing poop-filled diapers, it's still a lot of responsibility. To the untrained eye, it may look like your partner is simply sitting in a rocking chair holding your baby, but she's actually working very hard to develop a complicated feeding relationship. The next sections show you how you can help mom and baby be as successful as possible.

TIP

If you feel really lost on this subject, check out coauthor Sharon's *Breastfeeding For Dummies,* coauthored with Carol Vannais and published by Wiley, for more in-depth encouragement.

Making the decision to breast-feed

If your partner is physically capable of breast-feeding (some medical conditions prevent women from doing so), the decision is ultimately hers. It's her body, her time, and her commitment. Prior to the arrival of baby, discuss this topic so you can both research the benefits of breast-feeding and decide whether to do it and, if so, for how long. Keep in mind, though, that it's her prerogative to change her mind about any decisions after the baby actually arrives.

The U.S. Department of Health and Human Services says that breast-feeding is an important health choice and recommends that any amount of time spent breast-feeding benefits both mom and baby. Breast-feeding is a natural process, and the milk contains disease-fighting cells that help protect infants from germs, illness, and even SIDS (sudden infant death syndrome — turn to Chapter 11 for more info). Infant formula, while meeting the requirements of basic nutrition, doesn't include the human cells, hormones, or antibodies that fight disease.

For the new mother, breast-feeding — when it works — is a wonderful bonding experience that has been shown to decrease the risk of postpartum depression and lessen its impact. It also causes more *afterpains,* which are spasms that help shrink the uterus back down to normal size. Producing milk also burns anywhere from 200 to 600 calories a day. Studies also show that breast-feeding decreases a woman's risk of breast cancer and increases her bone density after baby is weaned, reducing her chances of developing osteoporosis.

The health benefits for baby and mom are good reasons to breast-feed, but be sure your partner considers the following details when making the decision:

>> **Ability:** Breast-feeding isn't possible if your partner had breast reconstruction surgery that cut the ducts.

>> **Comfort:** Some women aren't comfortable with the idea of breast-feeding. If your partner is one of them, don't blame her. This discomfort may be due to a culture that makes breasts into sex objects rather than feeding machinery.

>> **Convenience:** Breast-feeding is much more convenient at home than bottle-feeding, but it can be awkward when you're out and about. Although many shopping centers, museums, and amusement parks have nursing stations, not all do, and your partner may not be comfortable nursing in public. That's why nursing covers were invented.

>> **Schedule:** If your partner is going back to work in a few weeks, establishing nursing may seem like too much trouble. But nursing for even a short time is better than not nursing at all. Encourage her to try, even for a short time. Just don't be pushy about it.

REMEMBER

The American Academy of Pediatrics recommends breast-feeding for the first year of a child's life, and the World Health Organization recommends breast-feeding for the first two years. However, the benefits of breast-feeding continue for as long as mother and baby do it, whether it be three days or three years. The more you support your partner in breast-feeding, the more unparalleled health benefits your baby will receive.

Whether you start off baby with formula or switch after a period of breast-feeding, do your research about the best, safest formula for your child. Many breast-fed babies resist the transition, so be patient. Then again, you're probably used to that by now.

Offering lactation support

LeBron James makes dunking a basketball look as simple as flushing a toilet, but that doesn't mean you can do it. If your partner chooses to breast-feed, keep in mind that it's not as easy as it looks, especially at first. Issues will arise, and although you can't be the one to solve those issues, your support is a major factor in her success. Be positive and upbeat, listen to your partner when she talks, and thank her profusely for making such a wise decision for both the baby's health and hers.

The most important role for dad is to stay informed about the process of breast-feeding. Many complications can arise, and the more you know about how to help your partner through those issues, the more likely mom and baby will be able to work through them. One of the most common reasons women have for ceasing breast-feeding is that it's uncomfortable or painful. Breast-feeding *should not hurt* after mom and baby establish the correct feeding positions and *latches* (how baby attaches her mouth to the nipple).

Some of the most common breast-feeding issues are

>> **Sore nipples:** This problem is usually temporary during the first few days as mom adjusts to breast-feeding. For some women, the pain increases, and the nipples become chapped or cracked. This is most commonly a result of a bad latch and can be treated by correcting the latch.

>> **Pain from breast engorgement:** *Engorgement* occurs when the breasts fill up with milk. It can be eased by massage, milk expression, and warm compresses.

>> **Clogged ducts:** This occurs when the breast hasn't been completely emptied and it becomes clogged, causing a small lump to form inside the breast. Heat packs, massage, and increased feeding from the clogged breast can treat it.

>> **Mastitis:** *Mastitis* is a breast infection that a small percentage of breast-feeding women get. It can cause fevers, tiredness, and a hard lump in the breast. Treat with warm compresses, acetaminophen (Tylenol), and a trip to the doctor for a round of antibiotics.

REMEMBER

Remember that it's the mother's decision to quit breast-feeding if she so chooses; it should never be your suggestion. If lactation issues arise, don't tell her to throw in the towel and go buy some formula, no matter how frustrated or tearful she becomes. Listen to her concerns, help her find resources to correct problems, and ultimately, be supportive no matter what she decides.

BREAST-FEEDING 911

If your partner experiences discomfort or suffers from a low supply, know where to go to get her the help she needs. Many hospitals employ lactation consultants and may also provide free breast-feeding support groups your wife can attend. Some lactation consultants also make home visits to help mom and baby work out their issues. Here are a few resources to contact when your partner needs guidance:

- La Leche League International: phone 800-525-3243; website www.llli.org.
- International Board of Lactation Consultant Examiners: phone 703-560-7330; website www.iblce.org.
- International Lactation Consultant Association: phone 919-861-5577; website www.ilca.org.

Whenever your partner decides for any reason to stop breast-feeding, thank her for the time she has invested in doing so and congratulate her for her achievements. You both should be proud of the hard, rewarding work you've done.

Including yourself in the process

REMEMBER

Just because mom does the actual breast-feeding doesn't mean you can't be involved, too. An important role for dad is to serve as mom's arms and legs while she breast-feeds, especially in the early stages, while your partner's mobility is severely limited by a baby who eats at frequent intervals all day long. Let your partner know that you're happy to get her anything she needs and thank her for breast-feeding the baby. The more you can anticipate her needs, the better. Always have a drink and snack at hand, as well as the TV remote and something to read.

Many women feel frustrated by not being able to do things for themselves. Reassure her that baby's constant eating schedule is only temporary and that it won't be long before he eats less often and her mobility returns. Until then, make sure to bring your partner everything she asks for without hesitation.

TIP

Sometimes, fathers of breast-fed babies feel as though they're missing out on an important, unparalleled bonding opportunity. Remember that breast-feeding is about the well-being of your child, and although you can't ever experience what your partner does, you can join in on the skin-on-skin bonding by letting baby rest on your bare chest post-feeding. You can also occasionally give baby supplemental bottles of pumped milk. (See Chapter 11 for more on supplemental bottles.)

Dealing with Post-Cesarean Issues

Not only is the hospital stay longer for a C-section (three to four days total) than for a vaginal delivery (one to two days total), but the recovery time upon returning home is extended as well. A Cesarean delivery is classified as a major surgery, which means that even if everything goes smoothly, you have to care for a woman who has been through nine months of pregnancy followed by a serious operation. You also need to be on the lookout to make sure no complications arise while your partner is recovering.

Helping with a normal recovery

Give your partner additional physical support for the first few weeks following a C-section. She shouldn't engage in vigorous exercise or household chores or even climb a lot of steps. If you have to go back to work during the first two weeks postdelivery, find a family member or friend who can come to your home and provide all-day support for your partner.

Emotionally, it's important for the new mom to sit and bond with her baby following a Cesarean procedure. Some women experience feelings of disappointment and can even struggle to bond with a newborn when unable to give birth vaginally. Most, however, have no trouble bonding after spending some time together.

If the operation was unexpected, many new dads and moms need some time to decompress following the stress of the situation. Following the birth, discuss the events leading up to the Cesarean with your partner. Some new parents find it helpful to discuss the events with the obstetrician to help deal with any negative feelings they have about their birth experience.

Pain management is important following a Cesarean. When not properly managed, pain can reduce the chances of successful breast-feeding and increase the chances of postpartum depression. Encourage your partner to ask her doctors about appropriate pain relief medication and how it will affect her breast milk.

Knowing when to call the doctor

Most women who deliver via Cesarean recover quickly and without incident. However, watch out for these warning signs and contact a physician immediately if your partner

>> Incurs a fever in excess of 100 degrees

>> Notices pus discharge from the incision

>> Suffers a swollen, red, painful area in the leg or the breast, possibly accompanied by flu-like symptoms

>> Complains of a painful headache that doesn't subside

>> Experiences abrupt pain in the abdomen, including abnormal tenderness or burning

>> Has a foul-smelling vaginal discharge

>> Experiences an unusual amount of heavy bleeding that soaks a sanitary pad within an hour

>> Feels abnormally anxious, panicky, and/or depressed

Riding the Ups and Downs of Hormones

If feeling physically normal while exhausted and still carrying a few pounds of extra baby weight wasn't hard enough for a new mom, along come the hormones to make it all even worse. As her body recovers from childbirth, a woman needs several months for her hormone levels to completely even out. The following sections touch on the many changes your partner may experience and how to deal with them.

Thinking before speaking in the sensitive postpartum period

If you've ever put your foot in your mouth, then you know you can accidentally hurt your partner's feelings via your own thought-lessness. After delivery you need to be even more careful of what you say, because your partner's emotional sensitivity may feel like uncharted, shark-infested waters.

TIP

Avoid using leading statements — such as "why don't you just" and "why didn't you" — when your partner is upset. You don't have all the answers, and she's not looking for answers, anyway. What she's likely seeking is a listening ear and an understanding hug. The last thing you ever want to tell a tearful new mother when she confesses feelings of isolation is, "Why didn't you just go out today?" She likely has worked very hard all day taking care of herself and the baby, and flippantly suggesting that she should have done more than she did can make her feel like a failure.

To show support, ask her questions that show you're listening, such as, "What would make you feel better?" and "What can I do to help you?" If your partner responds with "I don't know" or "Nothing will help until the baby is older/sleeps more/cries less," then tell her you want to help in any way possible. If she has trouble expressing what she needs, you may find yourself becoming frustrated with your inability to fix the problem. Until she can express her needs, plan some time away for her that doesn't force her to make any decisions but instead pampers and caters to her needs and shows her how much you care.

REMEMBER

When your partner is upset about something you said, keep in mind that hormones are at play, but don't suggest to her that hormones are the reason she's being sensitive. (That will go over about as well as telling her she's moody because "it's that time of the month.") The last thing you want to do is imply that her feelings aren't legitimate. Simply apologize for any and all offending statements and let her know that you understand where she's coming from. And remember — your hormones are at play, too, and your emotions will be all over the map. Offer the same grace and validation you want from your partner.

TIP

Many new moms also become sensitive to anything involving hurt or neglected children, which can make TV programs, movies, and books potential minefields. To the best of your abilities, do research about the contents of your entertainment. If the movie you want to watch involves a child death, botched childbirth, kidnapping, or the destruction of the earth, move it down in your queue for later viewing.

Shedding light on physical symptoms

Body-drenching night sweats are very common for new moms, and you can't do much to help except to set up a fan near the bed. Sudden hair loss is another physical effect of surging hormones. In the first few months following delivery, most women begin to notice a lot more hair coming out in the shower and on the hairbrush. Reassure your partner that this is normal and that her hair will go back to normal by nine months after delivery. If it doesn't, have her seek treatment from a dermatologist.

Getting through the "baby blues"

Nearly every new mom experiences the *baby blues*, emotional mood swings and mild depression triggered by hormone changes after delivery. And although you didn't have to deliver the baby, many of these same issues can and will affect you. Symptoms of the baby blues include

>> Anxiety or feelings that she's not doing things "right"

>> Crying for no reason — at least for what seems like no reason to you

>> Difficulty concentrating

>> Irritability

>> Mood swings

>> Periods of sadness

>> Trouble sleeping

WARNING

The baby blues normally last no more than two weeks after giving birth, so if symptoms last longer or seem more severe, get your partner to her medical practitioner for help. Many women don't recognize the severity of their own symptoms or don't have the emotional energy to deal with them, so you need to have her back. If you suspect your partner may be dealing with a more serious postpartum mood disorder, check out Chapter 13 for advice.

Sleeping (or Doing Without)

Surprise! It's a baby who doesn't sleep through the night. Depending on your newborn, you may be woken every hour on the hour for feedings and comforting. Or you may be one of the lucky parents catching hours and hours of uninterrupted sleep. Every baby is different, but one thing is constant: Sleep is a precious commodity for new parents.

Babies' sleeping habits change frequently, but the average newborn sleeps about eight hours during the day, waking up every hour or so to eat. They generally sleep another eight hours during the night, again waking frequently to eat. Newborn sleep cycles are shorter than those of adults, and they spend more time in light sleep than adults do, which accounts for the frequent disturbances.

REMEMBER

The common rule of thumb is to sleep when your baby sleeps. You may be tempted to tackle one of the million chores that need to be done around the house or to enjoy an hour watching tennis in peace, but close your eyes instead. If you nap during the day when you have a chance, you'll be in much better shape to deal with a baby who's ready to party when you're ready for pillow time at night. You can take turns with your partner throughout the night, alternating who gets up each time or switching nights. Use a schedule that works for you both.

Many babies wake up for good before the sun has a chance to hit the horizon. If you're routinely jarred from sleep at an obscenely early hour, alternate days of getting up early with your partner so at least one of you can get some additional sleep. That way, when the early riser's energy wanes later in the day, the other partner can step up to help out.

A baby's internal sleep clock begins to mature between the ages of six and nine weeks and starts to become constant between three and five months. By ten months, the average baby's sleep cycle is constant, and she'll go to bed and wake up at the same time every day. If you're still awake by that time and haven't become addicted to caffeine, congratulations. Your sleep cycle will start getting longer, too.

FERBER VERSUS NO-CRY

Different schools of thought have varying theories about how to help a baby sleep through the night. Many parents opt to use the Ferber method, created by Dr. Richard Ferber. Commonly referred to as *Ferberizing* your baby, this is the classic cry-it-out system that offers limited comforting for a baby in an effort to teach her how to fall asleep by self-soothing.

An increasing number of parents are beginning to use alternative no-cry methods that address an individual baby's sleep issues and offer parents tools to help babies put themselves to sleep without so many tears. Generally, a no-cry method encourages a slow, steady process to segue from co-sleeping to crib sleeping that involves building a positive association with the crib for your baby instead of letting her cry until she falls asleep. Research all your options and decide which method suits your parenting style.

Many babies begin sleeping through the night between four and six months. Then again, many babies begin sleeping through the night at one year of age. Both are normal. Consult your pediatrician if your baby's sleep pattern is unmanageable for you and your partner.

Coping with Company

Family and friends will be vying for any opportunity to get their hands on your baby. Being surrounded by love is important at this time, but mom, dad, and baby also need to get plenty of rest and have sufficient time to bond as a family. And getting plenty of rest and private family time helps keep you from lashing out at your mother when she offers yet another "helpful pointer" about the proper way to fold bath towels.

Try not to schedule multiple visitors at a time, and limit the number of visits to two or three per day. Now is also the time in your life when it's okay to cancel or say no to visits. If Aunt Sarah is scheduled to drop by in the evening and your partner just needs to catch some shut-eye, put your partner's needs first. Reassure Aunt Sarah that she'll get to see the baby in due time. If she's offended, she'll get over it the moment she holds your baby for the first time.

You and your partner should decide together when it's a good time to have people over and when you need some peace and quiet. However, she may feel guilty about saying no, even when you know very well that having an empty house is in all your best interests. Don't be afraid to turn people away without asking your partner so she doesn't always have to feel like the "bad guy."

As visitors cycle through your home, make sure they all wash their hands or use an alcohol-free hand sanitizer to avoid spreading germs. If someone is sick, it's your duty to keep him out of your home. Thank him for his support but let him know that exposing newborns to illness is dangerous.

Baby will be passed around a lot when company is visiting and often only handed back to the new mom for feedings. Make sure your partner gets plenty of nonfeeding time with the baby to avoid having her feel like a milking cow.

Dealing with grabby grandmas

Sharing isn't easy — especially for new grandmas. And as they'll gladly tell you (again and again), someday you'll understand when you have a grandchild of your own. Until then, you need to manage everyone's needs for the next 20-plus years without offending anyone.

The best way to handle a too-hands-on grandma is to be honest and respectful. If you want to hold your baby and your mother or mother-in-law is reluctant to give up the wheel, reach for the baby and say something like, "I just can't hold this little one enough. I've been waiting for this moment my whole life." There's nothing like a display of paternal love to remind a grabby grandma how important bonding is between parent and child.

Don't be passive-aggressive in your approach. Avoid asking questions like, "Mom, do you think I could hold the baby now?" You don't want to imply you think grandma is being overbearing, thoughtless, or disrespectful of your time. On the other hand, you don't want your mom to think that you have to ask permission to hold your own baby, either!

If the problem persists, speak to the offending grandparent in private. Thank grandma for her love and support, and use only *I* statements (such as, "I've really been feeling the need to spend more time bonding with my baby right now, and even though it may not be what everyone would want, I really need this time") to convey how much you want to spend time with your baby.

Managing unsolicited advice

One of the first things to raise the ire of a new parent is a pushy, well-meaning advice giver. It makes parents feel like they're the heroes in a zombie movie who turn around and see a horde of the undead ready to rip them to shreds. Everyone seems to have opinions when it comes to how to care for your baby, and if you start paying attention to everyone, you'll find yourself completely overwhelmed. So just run. Run far, far away and don't look back.

REMEMBER

Whether the advice is on how to hold him, how to burp him, or even how to soothe him when he's on a crying jag, try to internalize the fact that most people are reaching out with advice because of the love they feel for your newborn. When advice comes across as criticism of your parenting skills, shrug it off. You and your partner know your baby's needs and preferences better than anyone else. Defer to your instincts. Every baby is different, and what works for one may cause another one fits of hysteria.

REMEMBER

That being said, you may find some advice helpful, so be open to listening to what others who have parented before you have learned. Don't be afraid to reach out to others if you have questions, but never take someone's advice as gospel. Take the time to do your own homework and decide what works best for your family.

Don't feel the need to explain yourself, however. If your Uncle Robert thinks you're somehow failing your child by picking him up every time he cries, don't be afraid to push back. Say something like, "I guess the beauty of being a parent is getting to decide how you want to raise your own child."

Handling hurt feelings when you want to be alone

At some point you'll need time to yourself, and so will your partner. Baby love is all-encompassing, but you can't let it overtake your individuality. Even though visitors travel from afar and people want to shower your new family with affection, you have to put on your own oxygen mask first, so to speak. Whether you're a runner or an avid video gamer, don't feel guilty about taking time to do what you need to relax.

REMEMBER

Never under any circumstances utter the phrase, "I just need a break." Your partner won't like to hear that because nobody deserves a break more than a new mom. Let her know that you really need to blow off some steam to continue being the best caregiver you can be. If she's angry, tell her you understand how she feels and offer her the same amount of time upon your return. Even the breast-feeding mom can enjoy a brief walk or a quick run to the store just to have some time to be on her own again.

Make sure to schedule time for your mental well-being because it probably won't seem like a priority until you're raving like a madman because you just need a second of solitude. Keep a calendar and block out times in different colors for family time, dad time, mom time, and visiting hours.

If family or friends take offense when you say no to a visit or an invitation to attend a family function, don't change your mind to save their feelings. You deserve time to bond as a family and to unwind and just be yourself. Thank them for the offer, be honest about why you can't commit to that time, and plan a get-together for a later date that suits everyone's schedule.

Rediscovering the Physical and Romantic

Sexual relationships are likely what installed you in your new-found role as parents. Now that you are parents, that part of your life will be paused for at least six weeks, and it will be altered and tricky for the foreseeable future. It's important to understand going into it that for many couples, getting your sexual groove back takes time, attention, patience, and — perhaps most importantly — a sense of humor. But before you can start thinking about sex again, it's vital to start thinking about connection and communication.

Prioritizing love and romance

Sex is only a small part of connection in relationships. In fact, a strong mental and emotional connection is the foundation for a good sex life — especially life after baby. During this time, make sure to prioritize your partner's love language and speak it often. Whether it's affirming words, gifts, physical touch, or quality time, the new mom in your life will feel connected to you the more you provide for her needs during this time. Also, remember some of the ways you wooed her during your early dating life and drop a few love notes or flowers from time to time. Most importantly, learn to be a good listener. Nothing builds emotional connection like feeling seen and heard. Read a book or take a course on how to be a strong, empathetic communicator. Validation goes a long way toward connection.

Waiting at least six weeks for sex

Hang tight, fellas. It's gonna be a while. The earliest a woman can have sex is six weeks following delivery, and that's only after getting clearance from her medical practitioner. Your hormones may be raging, but you need to remember that your partner's genitalia have been through the wringer, so to speak, and intercourse can severely jeopardize her healing process.

Understanding changes in body and libido

In addition to needing time for physical healing, most women don't feel all that sexy for a while. Hormones are the major culprits, but a lack of sleep, breast-feeding, and the difficulty of straddling the roles of mother and sexual being are also hurdles. As hard as it is to internalize, remind yourself that her lack of physical interest in you has nothing to do with her feelings toward you. Her absence of desire isn't personal; it's physical.

Some women find their sexual desires return by the time their medical practitioner okays sex, but for many it can take between 6 and 12 months. Some new fathers also experience a diminished interest in sex when adjusting to the role of dad.

Learning to be patient and give grace

Even after your partner has healed and her desire returns, she may experience discomfort when returning to a normal sex life. Be prepared to take it slow. You may need several attempts before you actually have sex to completion. Time will also be at a premium, and baby just may wake up before you finish. Don't focus on orgasm being the outcome of sex right now. Yeah, it sounds counterintuitive to everything you've known before, but in reality sex is about connection, openness, and fun. It's adult play time, and if you focus on the end result only, you're setting yourself up for frustration and disappointment. This is an adjustment period, so allow yourself and your partner the time needed to adjust.

TIP

Time will also be at a premium as you work around baby's schedule, so as unromantic as it sounds, schedule sex with your partner and slowly ramp up to a frequency that works for both of you. With so much on your plates, scheduling can give you both the security of knowing the "when" and the excitement of thinking about the "how."

Birth control also needs to be a talking point for you and your partner. Many people believe that breast-feeding women can't get pregnant, but although breast-feeding does often delay a return to regular ovulation, some women do ovulate while nursing. Many breast-feeding women prefer not to go on birth control pills because of changes in milk supply, so condom usage is common for new parents returning to active sex lives. You can speak with a doctor to help you both determine a birth control option that fits your needs.

When to seek help

For some couples, the road back to a healthy sex life isn't manageable on their own. Due to pain, lack of desire, postpartum depression, or even bad communication during stressful times, couples often find it difficult to reconnect sexually after they become parents. Don't expect the problem to resolve on its own. Talk to your partner about your concerns without blaming her or the baby. Don't talk about what you're not getting in the bedroom — talk about what you want and how you feel. Work with a couples therapist, sex therapist, or find an online program to help guide you back to each other. Chances are, it will have the added benefit of improving your communication and, likely, the overall quality of your relationship.

4

Under Pressure: How to Worry the Right Way about the Big Stuff

Handle difficult issues that can arise after delivery. Be proactive in watching for potential problems and addressing them promptly.

Prepare yourself for the inevitable bumps, bruises, falls, and fevers of infancy and beyond. Brush up on your first-aid skills so you know the difference between when you need to seek professional help and when you should just reach for the bandages.

Run the numbers on what baby will cost you over the next few years, get your budget in order, and check your insurance plans to make sure you're all covered for the future.

Make plans for baby's future now by creating a savings plan that will help her get to Harvard — or anywhere else she wants to go in life.

Chapter **13**
Dealing with Difficult Issues after Delivery

N ot everyone goes home to perpetual roses and lollipops after baby is born. In fact, hardly anyone does. But serious issues in baby or mom are rare, so when they occur, they can really knock you for a loop. In this chapter, we describe some of the serious complications that can arise after delivery and how to handle them. You can skip this chapter if you don't need it — and we hope you never will.

Coping with Baby's Serious Health Problems

Approximately 1 in 33 babies born in the United States has a birth defect, according to the Centers for Disease Control and Prevention. Developmental delays, serious illnesses, and sudden infant death syndrome are problems no one wants to contemplate when having a baby, but they can and do happen. The following sections give you an overview of the most common serious health problems.

Congenital defects

Congenital defects, defects that exist at birth (also simply called *birth defects*), are common. Some are minor issues that no one but the parents would ever notice; others are more serious. The most common birth defects include

>> **Heart defects:** One in 100 to 200 babies has a heart defect, which can range from mild to severe. Heart defects comprise one-quarter to one-third of all birth defects.

>> **Down syndrome:** One in 800 babies is born with Down syndrome, which causes distinct physical features and mental retardation. The percentage is higher in older mothers and lower in mothers younger than 35.

>> **Cleft lip and/or palate:** One in 700 to 1,000 babies has deformities of the lip and hard palate.

>> **Neural tube defects:** One in 1,000 infants has neural tube defects, which affect the brain and spinal column. They include *spina bifida,* an abnormal opening in the spine, and *anencephaly,* an absence of part of the brain.

Sixty percent of the time, the reason for the birth defect is unknown. Inherited disorders, on the other hand, can be anticipated and often checked for before delivery if you know you have a family history of certain problems.

Some of the most common inherited genetic disorders include

>> **Cystic fibrosis:** A disorder that causes thick secretions in the respiratory and gastrointestinal tract, cystic fibrosis is the most common inherited genetic disorder in Caucasians in the United States, affecting 1 in 3,000 babies. Both parents must carry the defective gene for a child to have the disease; it's estimated that 12 million people in the United States are carriers.

>> **Sickle cell anemia:** An autosomal recessive disease that causes deformities of the red blood cells, sickle cell anemia affects mostly people of African and Middle Eastern descent. Approximately 2 million African Americans carry the sickle cell gene. Both parents must pass on the gene for a child to have sickle cell disease.

Minor birth defects are much more common than serious defects. Eye, ear, and limb defects; extra digits; abnormal development of the intestines; and birthmarks may not be life-threatening in most cases, but they can still be devastating for parents. It's normal to be upset and concerned about birth defects, especially visible ones.

Developmental delays

Many parents keep baby books that chronicle their baby's progress and eagerly await each milestone: the first smile, the first step, the first word. When milestones aren't met when books say they should be or when your friends' babies are meeting them but your baby isn't, doubt, concern, frustration, and a cold fear may begin to creep into your days.

REMEMBER

Moms are usually the first ones to recognize a problem, so if your partner voices concerns, don't belittle them, even if the baby seems fine to you. Verbalizing fears about your baby's development takes a lot of courage.

When babies are very young, physical milestones are very important. Babies, after all, don't dazzle you with their small talk or charm you with their recitation of *The Iliad*. If they lift up their head, it's a big deal. Rolling over for the first time merits phone calls to relatives all over the country, and the first gurgle — the one that startles the baby almost as much as it does you — earns your undivided attention for the next hour as you try to catch a command performance on video.

If your baby isn't keeping up with the other babies on the block (whether in your mind or in fact), discuss your concerns with your doctor. He may tell you that all babies are different and that you're making yourself crazy. Or he may nod and take notes, which is really frightening, because even when you know something's wrong, having someone else verify it makes it all too real.

Before you call in the cavalry because you suspect that your baby isn't meeting developmental milestones, take a deep breath and consider the following facts:

>> **Babies really do develop at different rates.** Milestones happen at an average age, and an average is just that: 50 percent of babies achieve the goal at a younger age, and 50 percent don't meet it until they're past that age.

>> **Babies all have different abilities.** Some are more physically oriented; others are more verbally inclined. Because physical milestones are all you have to go on at a young age, children who will shine verbally later but who will never make the track team — or pass through the kitchen without tripping over the linoleum — may seem to be behind early on, even if they're really not.

However, talk to your doctor if your baby doesn't meet the following milestones:

>> Turns her head in the direction of a voice or sound shortly after birth

>> Smiles spontaneously by one month

>> Imitates speech sounds by three to six months

>> Babbles by four to eight months

If your baby does have developmental delays, she'll need your help — and possibly the help of medical professionals such as physical therapists — to achieve normal milestones. Getting help early is the best thing you can do for her.

Illnesses

Infant illness can be *acute* (severe but brief) or *chronic* (long-lasting or recurring). Both are terrifying, especially if your baby has to be hospitalized. A sick baby, especially a chronically sick baby, changes your family dynamic in major ways and can become the focus of the entire family — an unhealthy situation in more ways than one. The following suggestions can help you deal with an illness in your infant, whether acute or chronic:

>> **Absolutely, positively avoid any hint of the "blame game."** Even if something one of you did caused the baby to get sick, it's over and done with, so pinning blame on your partner only makes you both feel worse. Babies can't be raised in a bubble, so getting sick is, unfortunately, a fact of life.

>> **Don't let yourselves get overtired.** Especially if your partner delivered not too long ago, she really needs to get enough rest. Take turns staying at the hospital or being up with the baby at home or one of you could get sick, too.

> **If your partner is breast-feeding, help her keep pumping.**
> Stress is hard on milk supply, and pumping isn't nearly as
> effective as a nursing baby for stimulating the supply, but
> encourage your partner to do her best. As long as she keeps
> it going in the interim, the supply will build up when the baby
> is nursing again.

SIDS

Sudden infant death syndrome, or SIDS, has decreased since pediatricians began recommending that babies sleep on their backs with the "Back to Sleep" campaign, but it's still the third most common cause of death for infants up to 1 year old. More than 7,000 babies in the United States succumb to SIDS each year.

Identifying the causes and debunking myths

The causes of SIDS still aren't clear. However, doctors know that the following are *not* causes of SIDS:

>> Choking

>> Immunizations

>> Infections

>> Suffocation

>> Vomiting

SIDS is considered to be *multifactorial,* meaning it doesn't have just one cause. Several factors must all be present for SIDS to occur, including abnormalities in the brain, respiratory system, and possibly the heart.

Understanding what increases the risks

The following factors increase the likelihood of SIDS:

>> The baby was born prematurely.

>> The baby is male.

>> The baby is of black, Native American, or Native Alaskan ethnicity.

>> The baby is between two and three months of age.

>> The baby is overheated or overdressed. Too many clothes or an overly heated room may increase the risk of SIDS. SIDS occurs more often in cooler fall and winter weather, when babies get bundled up.

>> The baby has a sibling who died of SIDS.

>> The baby was/is exposed to tobacco. SIDS rates are higher in babies whose moms smoked during pregnancy or who smoke around the baby.

>> The mother used cocaine, heroin, or methadone during pregnancy.

>> The baby recently had a respiratory infection.

>> The baby sleeps on his stomach, especially if he's switched from back to stomach sleeping or is overheated and sleeping on his stomach. (Side sleeping may seem like a compromise if your baby hates being on his back, but many side sleepers roll over onto their stomachs.)

Research also indicates that babies who are breast-fed and those who suck on pacifiers may have a lower risk of SIDS. Additionally, placing a fan in the window or even just opening a window has also been shown to decrease the risk of SIDS in at least one study, possibly because better ventilation may decrease carbon dioxide buildup.

Watching Out for Mom's Postpartum Mood Disorders

Female hormones are a jumbled mess right after delivery, which is why women are so emotionally fragile after giving birth. Add sleep deprivation and insecurities about parenting ability, and it's amazing that your partner can function at all. And yet women come home and often jump right in to full-time child care while they're still in healing mode with fluctuating hormones. Men would crumple under the strain — which is why women have babies.

Mood swings and depression are normal for the first few weeks or even months after having a baby, but sometimes more serious problems can arise. One of your jobs is being aware of the signs of a serious problem and making sure your partner gets help if needed. The following sections examine two of the more concerning postpartum mood disorders: depression and psychosis.

Taking a look at postpartum depression

Postpartum depression, a more serious form of the typical "baby blues" described in Chapter 12, occurs in between 9 and 16 percent of women. Some of the symptoms of baby blues and postpartum depression overlap, but postpartum depression is more pronounced, lasts longer, and includes serious signs that need immediate medical evaluation.

Recognizing the symptoms

Women with postpartum depression may have the following symptoms:

WARNING

>> **Anger and irritability:** Her anger may go far beyond a few swear words when she drops a quart of milk, and it can be frightening.

>> **Difficulty bonding with the baby:** This is a major red flag. If your partner pushes the baby off on you or other family members or says she's not a good mom or that the baby would be better off without her, get medical help.

>> **Disinterest in normal activities, including sex:** Seeing old friends, going out, and even everyday activities like cleaning the house, doing laundry, and watching TV may all go out the window. You may at first think she's just tired, but a deeper reason may be at the root of her continued lack of interest in life that lasts for several months after delivery.

>> **Guilt and shame over her negative thoughts:** Again, because she may not verbalize her thoughts, recognizing what's going on may be difficult. Statements like "I'm no good" or "Someone else would be a better mom to this baby" are warning signs.

>> **Loss of appetite:** Losing interest in eating is often an early sign of depression.

>> **Sleep difficulties:** She may not be able to sleep, even when you know she's exhausted, or she may want to do nothing but sleep.

>> **Thoughts about harming herself or the baby:** She may not verbalize these thoughts, so they may be hard to recognize. She may want other people to handle the baby because of her fears that she'll hurt him, accidentally or on purpose.

If you believe your partner is depressed, tell her that you're concerned about her health, allow her to discuss her symptoms and how she's feeling, and let her know that what she's dealing with is a serious medical condition. Postpartum depression doesn't mean she's a bad mother or a weak person; good people can suffer from it. Don't let her brush the issue aside by saying that it's just a matter of feeling sad and that she'll "snap out of it," because she won't. Postpartum depression can last up to a year, which can interfere with maternal child bonding and seriously disrupt your family.

Children of moms with untreated depression also suffer the consequences, with a higher incidence of behavior problems, sleeping disorders, feeding problems, hyperactivity, and language delays.

REMEMBER

A depressed new mom needs to be treated by a medical professional immediately, so work with your partner to schedule a session with her medical practitioner or call to discuss matters with her practitioner if your partner is not forthcoming

Knowing who's more at risk

Any woman can have postpartum depression, but the chances of this developing increase if

>> **She has a history of depression.**

>> **She's recently undergone major life changes.** These changes can include a move, a death, job loss, illness, pregnancy complications, or trouble between the two of you.

>> **She doesn't have a good support system.** Family and friends make a big difference in the life of a new mom. Postpartum depression makes reaching out to others difficult, so a woman who doesn't have pushy friends and family who check in on her even if she doesn't call them is very isolated.

>> **The pregnancy was unplanned or unwanted.**

Treating the disease

Treatment for postpartum depression may include

>> **Antidepressants:** Make sure the doctor knows whether your partner is breast-feeding so he can prescribe an antidepressant safe for use by breast-feeding moms.

>> **Counseling:** Talking things out with a professional is very helpful for some women.

>> **Hormone therapy:** Estrogen replacement to offset the rapid drop in estrogen after giving birth may be helpful for some women.

Taking care of yourself

If your partner is suffering from postpartum depression, a large part of her normal chores and responsibilities may fall on you. If you're trying to hold down a job, make sure your partner's okay, make sure the baby's okay, and run the household on top of it all, you may start to feel a little stressed yourself.

TIP

Though rushing in to take over a short-lived crisis is easy, a situation that drags on for months can take its toll on your mental and physical well-being. Take care of yourself by making sure you do the following:

>> **Call in the troops to help.** You may not have readily available family and friends, but if you do, enlist their aid. Send them to the store or have them come over and clean. This is a fine line because you don't want to give your partner the impression that she can't do all this stuff, even when she can't. If you call in your mom to clean or cook, your partner may view it as a judgment against her abilities and a sign that you feel your mom is more capable than she is. Sometimes hiring help for household chores is a better idea.

>> **Consider taking a leave of absence from work.** Some companies offer paid time off for dads or let you use vacation or sick time. You can also use Family Medical Leave Act (FMLA) time for up to 12 weeks of time off, but this will probably be unpaid time, unless you work for an extremely generous company. Dipping into savings or borrowing from your 401(k) isn't ideal, but if it gets your family through a difficult time, it's worth it.

>> **Eat right.** You'll feel better and be better able to handle situations if you're not eating junk food.

>> **Get enough sleep.** Sleep deprivation makes everything look worse. The very worst time to pore over your worries is the middle of the night; everything looks insurmountable at 3 a.m.

Acting fast to treat postpartum psychosis

Postpartum psychosis is an extremely dangerous psychiatric disorder that occurs in around 1 to 2 percent of women, usually in the first few weeks after giving birth. Women with bipolar disease or a history of postpartum psychosis are more likely to develop the condition. Onset is sudden and includes the following symptoms:

>> Bizarre thinking

>> Delusions

>> Hallucinations

>> Insomnia

>> Irritability

>> Paranoia

>> Rapidly changing moods

>> Restlessness

WARNING

Left untreated, postpartum psychosis can be lethal; the risk of suicide or infanticide is high. If your partner displays any of these symptoms, don't try to talk her out of it or persuade her to see her doctor. She almost certainly won't recognize her behavior as abnormal and in fact will probably consider you to be an adversary. Call 911 immediately.

Managing Grief

Grief is intense sorrow due to loss. The loss of the perfect child, the perfect partner, or perfect family can cause grief. The most important thing to remember about grief, no matter what the cause, is that it takes time to work through. Don't be hard on yourself or your partner when you're grieving, and don't expect you'll be in the same stages at the same time. Everyone works through grief differently.

Going through the stages of grief

Grief can be caused by many different scenarios, but the widely acknowledged five stages of grief, described by Elisabeth Kübler-Ross, include similar phases whatever the cause.

Whether you've found out that your baby has a long-term problem, your partner is suffering from serious postpartum illness, or your baby has to be hospitalized, expect to experience the five stages of grief:

1. **Denial:** The first stage of grief is often a feeling of "This can't be happening to us."

2. **Anger:** The second stage of grief is anger, often directed at God or other people.

3. **Bargaining:** Trying to make secret deals — "I'll donate our savings to this hospital if my baby's heart surgery saves her" — often with God (even if you don't believe in God!) is common in the bargaining stage.

4. **Depression:** When reality sets in and you realize that this is happening to you, fair or not, depression often follows.

5. **Acceptance:** Eventually you get through the other stages and settle down to deal with what you have to deal with, but you may still go in and out of earlier grief stages at different times.

Stages may not follow this exact pattern, and not everyone goes through every stage. Yo-yoing back and forth between several stages is also common.

TIP

Grieving is important during the entire pregnancy process. Even if your baby is born without incident, you'll be going through a lot of changes. Allow yourself and your partner to discuss the many things you're giving up to bring this child into the world. Even something as silly as giving up your daily latte to buy diapers can become a source of resentment over time. As a general rule, talk openly and honestly about the changes that affect you and support each other.

Also, cut yourself a break — parenting isn't easy, and it's perfectly natural to miss having nights out with friends or even being able to eat an entire meal before it gets cold. Grieving over the little things doesn't mean you don't love your baby; it means you're dealing with change in a healthy manner.

Why, why, why? Getting past the question

When grieving, getting bogged down in why a particular thing has happened to your partner or child is easy to do. However, it's not particularly good for you, especially if there's no way of deciphering exactly why something happened, and most of your thoughts are purely speculative.

REMEMBER

Unless knowing the reason why your problem happened can prevent a recurrence or change a situation, asking "why" doesn't help. Wanting a reason is a way of imposing control on a situation, but it doesn't help you move forward in helping your child.

Grieving together and separately

Everyone needs time to grieve a loss in his own way. Grieve together with your partner, certainly, but take time to grieve separately as well. Don't feel bad about needing to be alone with your thoughts occasionally. At the same time, the following tips can help you and your partner get through your grief, both together and on your own:

>> **Arm yourself with knowledge.** Knowledge really is power. Especially if your baby has a genetic or long-term condition, learning all you can about it helps you be your baby's best advocate and can help you and your partner feel like you're doing something productive in a frustratingly out-of-control situation.

>> **Don't get upset with your partner.** One day you or your partner may be raging at the world, and the next day the other one may take a turn. Listen to each other without taking things personally, trying to make it all better, or reproving your partner for her feelings.

» Expect to be discouraged at times. All people have moments when things look much worse than they really are, usually because they're tired, hungry, or just plain stressed. Identify the situation for what it is: temporary discouragement, not a new permanent negative outlook on life.

» Find a support group. If you're coming to terms with a birth defect, your child or partner is ill, or you're dealing with a loss, talking to other parents dealing with the same thing can be a lifesaver. When relevant, a support group can also be a really good source of information on specialists, educational programs, and other outside help.

» Get help for yourself. If you find yourself mentally overwhelmed, seek counseling, either with your partner or alone. Often just being able to talk through a situation with a person not involved helps you sort things out.

» Keep a journal, if the thought appeals to you. Journals are good for privately venting feelings and fears that you and your partner don't want to share with each other. They're also good for looking back later and realizing how far you've come.

» Stay physically close. It helps you feel less alone, keeps you centered on still being a couple, and helps keep your relationship going in a situation that could easily break it apart. Even if you don't feel like it, make the effort to hold hands, cuddle on the couch watching TV, and have sex regularly.

» Tell people when you're not up to something. Another baby's christening, a big family party, or a holiday celebration may all be beyond your or your partner's ability to handle at first. Don't be afraid to say no to things that you feel would strip you raw right now. People who love you will understand, even if they're disappointed.

Determining when grief has gone on too long

Grieving can take a long time, but sometimes grief takes on a life of its own, and a situation called *complicated grief* can become permanently entrenched in your or your partner's life. Although everyone has times when the sadness of circumstances becomes overwhelming, normally these feelings don't affect every aspect of life after the first few weeks or months. Complicated grief may be taking over after a period of time if you or your partner

>> Are preoccupied and bitter about what's happened

>> Are unusually angry, irritable, or agitated most of the time

>> Can't perform normal tasks, go to work, or participate in normal social functions

>> Feel that life has lost its meaning

>> Make rash decisions or do things you normally wouldn't do, such as drinking too much

>> Still feel numb and detached

REMEMBER

When grief becomes complicated, it becomes self-perpetuating. This is a time for intervention, either with medication or therapy. Talk to a grief counselor, psychologist, psychiatrist, or other mental health professional about your feelings and symptoms. Antidepressants have been found to help in some cases.

Talking to People about Your Child

Accepting a child's health problems is challenging enough for parents, and an emotionally sensitive situation is made even more difficult by the fact that eventually you need to inform other people of the problem. In time you may become accustomed to the comments of well-meaning but blundering family members and rude strangers, but at first you'll likely be uncomfortable and upset. The following sections give you guidelines for getting through these situations.

Telling others

Telling other people that your child has a problem can be gut-wrenching and can almost feel like you're hearing it for the first time yourself. When you tell other people your child has a problem, try the following tips:

>> **Keep it positive.** Maybe your child won't be able to be all you ever hoped for him. Actually, no child ever can! Remember that your child will be able to have a happy life,

no matter what his disability, and you can enjoy him no matter what his issues. That positive outlook will express itself in your message.

>> **Keep it simple.** Especially if your child has an ongoing medical problem, giving out information a little at a time may make it easier for others to digest.

>> **Keep it straightforward.** You may be tempted to sugarcoat a situation when explaining it to others, but there's no reason to give them hope that a child will grow to be something he won't. Be honest about the situation from the beginning.

Handling insensitive remarks

Unfortunately, people do notice when a child has a birth defect or development delay, and sometimes you hear them whispering to each other or pointing at your child. As devastating as this is, use it as a teaching experience if you can. If your child has a visible birth defect, comments *are* going to come your way — and your child will hear and understand those comments as she gets older.

REMEMBER

Openly discussing your child's disability as something not to be hidden or ashamed of sets a positive example for your child. This doesn't mean that you have to freely discuss your child with every obnoxious person who asks pointed questions. But addressing questions with an open, accepting, positive attitude tells your child — and everyone else — that she's a great kid and that you're happy with her just the way she is.

Sometimes you won't have the patience to deal with questions, and you don't have to educate every person who crosses your path. But when your mood allows it, try the following suggestions when confronted with insensitive remarks:

>> **Address an adult's comments in a nonjudgmental way, if you're up to it.** Most insensitive remarks are made out of ignorance, not malice, and even if they were made out of malice, addressing them politely can take the wind out of a person's puffed sails and, with any luck at all, shame the person into better behavior in the future.

>> **Answer a small child's questions.** Children, having no discretion at all, often ask their parents about people with visible problems (and often do so at the top of their lungs). Introduce yourself and use this opportunity to teach others about your child's disability.

>> **When your own relatives say inappropriate things, address it firmly and in a non-negotiable way.** Offer to teach them anything they'd like to know, but make it clear that this is your child, and you won't tolerate certain comments.

IN THIS CHAPTER

» Surviving illnesses and accidents

» Staying cool and handling emergencies

» Giving medicine, taking temperatures, and monitoring diapers

» Helping your child cope with teething

» Recognizing vaccination reactions

» Exploring reactions to vaccines, medications, and food

Chapter **14**

Survival Tips for Bumps, Boo-Boos, and More

N othing in fatherhood gets your adrenaline flowing like a "thump" from the other room, followed by a scream, or worse, by silence. Nothing, that is, except endless vomiting, a seizing child, or a fender bender with baby in the car.

Fatherhood often seems like a series of frightening moments, but most of the time, babies survive parental ineptitude and concern. No one gets through babyhood and early childhood without a few accidents, sicknesses, and spills and thrills along the way. If your child never has a bruise or bump, you're probably protecting him too much, and a child who never gets sick never develops a good immune system. So take heart when dealing with heart-stopping situations: They're an inevitable part of parenthood. In this chapter, we review the most common sources of parental anxiety, tell you what to do when they occur, and reassure you that, 99 times out of 100, baby — and you — will be just fine.

Handling Inevitable Illnesses

Most babies are now vaccinated — more about the vaccination reactions later in this chapter — against the most common illnesses, but plenty of illnesses can still infect your baby. And no matter how hard you try to protect your baby from illness-causing germs, you can't protect her from them all — and that's okay. Although hand washing, careful food handling, and cleanliness do help reduce germs, some germs are necessary. In fact, recent studies indicate that people who keep the bacteria around them at too much of a minimum are more likely to get sick than people who share their abode with a few stray germs. Go figure.

BREAST-FEEDING WHEN MOM IS SICK

Moms aren't allowed to get sick — it's in the code of parenthood. But if your partner does get sick while breast-feeding, you both may wonder about the wisdom of continuing to nurse.

If she's already sick, the baby has already been exposed to the germs before the sickness became evident, so there's no reason to avoid the baby. Very few illnesses require mom to stop breast-feeding. In fact, moms who develop colds and other common illnesses develop antibodies that they pass on through the breast milk, so nursing when sick may actually help the baby. Toxins such as E. coli, salmonella, botulism, and other gastrointestinal bugs stay in the GI tract and don't affect the milk, so breast-feeding is safe.

Your partner should check with the baby's doctor if she's taking heavy-duty cold medication that has a sedative effect, and she should avoid cough syrups with alcohol contents higher than 20 percent. Nasal sprays for sinus congestion can dry up her milk, so use them sparingly.

When your partner's sick, she's likely to require higher than usual amounts of fluid to stay hydrated — and a double dose of TLC to keep her going through nighttime nursing sessions. Getting up yourself and giving a bottle of pumped breast milk for a night or two so she can sleep will buy you bonus points as a helpful dad.

You can be sure your baby will catch something in her first year, no matter how carefully you clean the shopping cart handles. In the following sections, we fill you in on the symptoms, causes, and treatments of common illnesses so you'll feel prepared when the inevitable happens.

Dealing with common childhood diseases

Babies have immunity to many illnesses for their first six months because of antibodies passed on during pregnancy, but after six months, it's open season for germs. Following is a rundown of the illnesses you're most likely to encounter in baby's first year.

Common colds

The common cold is so common that it comes in more than 100 varieties, which is why having a cold this month doesn't mean you won't get another one next month. And because your baby has never had any of them, he's likely to have at least one case of the sniffles in the first year. In fact, the Mayo Clinic says that the average baby has eight to ten colds in the first two years of life, and each one lasts seven to ten days, no matter how many decongestants you buy.

For most babies, colds aren't serious, although they are messy. Typical symptoms of a cold include

>> Coughing

>> Decreased appetite (young babies may find it hard to nurse or drink from a bottle because of nasal stuffiness)

>> Irritability

>> Low-grade fever up to 100 degrees

>> Runny nose, which may start with clear, thin secretions that turn thicker and yellow or green

>> Sneezing

Children under the age of 2 shouldn't be given decongestant medications at all, according to the latest FDA findings that they don't work in young children and can have harmful side effects, besides. Infant acetaminophen or ibuprofen is fine to help the baby feel better. Running a cool-mist humidifier — hot mist can present a burn hazard — can also help clear clogged little noses. You can also use a little nasal saline and a bulb syringe you got from the hospital to suck the gunk out of little noses, or invest in newer "suckers" that look funny but actually do a better job at removing boogers.

Although colds aren't usually serious, babies younger than three months old who develop cold symptoms need to visit a medical practitioner. Babies that young are more likely to develop pneumonia or other complications from a cold.

Respiratory syncytial virus (RSV)

Respiratory syncytial virus (RSV) is a lower respiratory illness that infects most children at least once before age 2. Symptoms include lethargy, poor feeding, cough, difficulty breathing, and fever. RSV is the most common cause of pneumonia in children under 12 months, according to the Centers for Disease Control and Prevention. Although most cases are mild, severe illness requiring hospitalization can occur in children under 12 months, those with chronic health issues, and premature or otherwise compromised infants.

For less severe cases, which occur far more frequently, acetaminophen or ibuprofen helps with discomfort. Like most viruses, this one needs to run its course. If there's a reason to determine whether an infection is RSV, your medical practitioner can take a nasal swab and test for the virus.

Wheezing

Wheezing often follows a cold and doesn't always mean a baby is going to have asthma. Children younger than 2 who wheeze with respiratory infections are no more likely to develop asthma than children who don't wheeze, according to a study published in 2002 in the *American Journal of Respiratory and Critical Care Medicine*. Children who start wheezing at an older age are more likely to develop asthma.

Wheezing can be scary for parents and may require prescription bronchodilators that are breathed in as a mist, using a nebulizer, to open the narrowed airways and make it easier for the baby to breathe. Wheezing always requires a call to the pediatrician, especially if the baby doesn't have a cold or cold symptoms. An object stuck in the throat or more serious medical conditions can also cause wheezing. Some children wheeze with every upper respiratory infection and may need nebulizer treatments whenever they have bad colds.

WARNING

A child who's limp and exhausted, who has a bluish tinge around the lips, or who's struggling to breathe needs immediate medical attention. Call 911.

Ear infections

Between 5 and 15 percent of babies with colds develop an ear infection, which just prolongs the misery. Around half of all babies have an ear infection in the first year of life, with or without a cold. Contrary to popular opinion, tugging on the ears doesn't always indicate an ear infection, although it can. Other ear infection symptoms include the following:

>> Head shaking

>> Irritability

>> Mild fever

>> Refusal to nurse or take a bottle

>> Trouble sleeping

The thinking on treating ear infections has changed during the last few years. Ear infections may not require antibiotic treatment because more than eight out of ten heal without treatment. Some doctors treat and others wait, depending on the symptoms and the infection's severity. Regardless, infant pain relievers such as acetaminophen help with discomfort.

Vomiting

Small children and babies vomit more easily than adults when they're ill. Vomiting once at the beginning of an illness is common and requires no special treatment, but repeated vomiting requires medical evaluation because of the risk of dehydration.

WARNING

Signs of serious dehydration require medical treatment. A sunken *fontanel* (the soft spot on the top of an infant's head), extreme lethargy, sunken eyes, or sunken skin that remains raised after you pinch it deserve an immediate call to the baby's doctor.

Pediatricians often recommend giving vomiting children younger than six months an oral balanced-electrolyte solution such as Pedialyte in place of formula, starting with a few teaspoons or half an ounce every 15 minutes or so. Don't give plain water to any child younger than 1 unless your pediatrician specifically recommends it. A medication syringe often works better than a spoon for giving fluids if your baby refuses to drink. Gradually increase the amount you give each time if the baby isn't vomiting it back up.

WARNING

Don't give a volume more than you normally would. For example, if you normally give 4 ounces of formula every four hours, don't exceed that amount.

If no vomiting occurs after 12 hours, slowly start to reintroduce formula, but stop if vomiting occurs again. Breast-fed babies should continue to nurse because breast milk is more digestible than anything on the planet. However, if vomiting continues, call your doctor.

Some medical personnel recommend following the BRAT (bananas, rice, applesauce, and toast) diet during and after a vomiting illness for children older than 1, after they haven't vomited for eight hours or so, because these foods are easily digested. Others say to give children whatever they want and can keep down. Either way, go slowly and don't introduce any new foods until all vomiting and stomach upset have passed.

WARNING

Babies who suddenly start vomiting after every feeding even though they appear healthy and still have an appetite may have *pyloric stenosis*, a narrowing between the stomach and small intestine. Pyloric stenosis requires surgery but has no aftereffects; when it's fixed, it's fixed.

Infectious diseases

Many infectious diseases of old (30 years ago!) have been eradicated, or nearly so, because of vaccines (see the later section "Reacting to Medicines and Vaccines"). However, vaccines haven't been developed for everything, and sometimes a baby is exposed to an infectious disease before she gets the vaccine for it. Chicken pox, measles, mumps, and rubella (German measles) vaccines, for example, aren't given until age 1, and roseola, a common infectious disease in infants, has no vaccine. Being viruses, most common childhood diseases have no specific treatment beyond treating the symptoms and keeping the child comfortable.

WARNING

You should never give aspirin to treat fever or discomfort because of the possibility of Reye's syndrome, a rare disease that develops in children recovering from a viral infection. Taking aspirin increases the risk of developing Reye's syndrome, which can affect the brain and liver. Acetaminophen or ibuprofen are fine if your child is uncomfortable; follow your pediatrician's instructions on dosing.

Many infectious diseases are accompanied by rashes, so any time your child has a rash and fever, call your medical practitioner for advice. He may want to see your child, but then again, in some cases, he may not want you bringing your infectious child into the waiting room! If the disease is highly contagious and fairly evident from the type of rash, such as chicken pox, he may give instructions over the phone without seeing the child. Following are some common infectious diseases with rashes:

» **Chicken pox:** Chicken pox is unmistakable: small red spots that form blisters that break and crust. A mild temperature and respiratory symptoms often accompany chicken pox. In rare cases, chicken pox can cause *encephalitis*, brain inflammation that can have long-term consequences. There's no way to shorten the duration of the disease, but cool baths and anti-itch lotions help with discomfort.

» **Hand, foot, and mouth disease:** Although this sounds like some ghastly disease only ranch hands would catch, hand, foot, and mouth disease is a common virus that causes blisters on the — yes, you guessed it — hands and feet and in the mouth. Mild fever can also occur, and the mouth sores can make it hard for a child to eat.

» **Measles:** Also called *rubeola*, measles was once a common disease, but until recently it was all but conquered in America. In 2008, only 131 cases were confirmed in the United States, but in 2019, that number jumped to 1,289, with most cases not vaccinated or with unknown vaccination status. This increase is directly related to the number of unvaccinated children and adults in the U.S. Measles rarely occurs before six months of age because of maternal immunity being passed to the fetus. Children with measles usually appear quite ill and have a rash and high fever.

» **Mumps:** Mumps causes pain and swelling in the parotid glands, resulting in the classic "chipmunk" appearance.

Mumps, like measles and rubella, has become rare in developed countries thanks to the mumps vaccine. Mumps can cause painful testicular infection in males and affects sterility less than previously believed.

>> **Roseola:** Roseola has few complications but often results in frantic calls to medical personnel because the first symptom, which lasts for several days, is a high fever. Around day four the fever breaks and a rash appears. A telltale sign of roseola is that even with a fever as high as 104 degrees, the child doesn't appear ill. Roseola has no treatment and generally doesn't cause a great deal of discomfort.

>> **Rubella:** Rubella, sometimes called *German measles,* is a mild infection that causes a rash. Although not serious for infected children, rubella poses serious risks for pregnant women, causing a number of birth defects and pregnancy loss. Vaccination has made rubella rare in the United States.

Staying alert for scarier diseases

Some major-league bacteria and viruses can infect infants, but the signs are usually pretty obvious: Your baby looks and acts sick, refuses to eat, cries, and sleeps too little or too much. Rest assured that if your baby is seriously ill, you'll recognize the signs. In the following sections we tell you what to watch for.

Meningitis

Meningitis, an inflammation of the tissues that cover the brain, can require hospitalization. Meningitis can be bacterial or viral and is caused by a number of organisms. Vaccination for *Haemophilus influenzae* type B, also known as *Hib,* which is given starting at 2 months of age, reduces the chance of meningitis. Symptoms include fever, irritability, poor feeding, rash, seizures, a high-pitched cry, and stiff neck. In infants, the soft spot at the top of the head may be bulging rather than flat. Signs of meningitis need immediate treatment to prevent complications.

Diarrhea

Although diarrhea may seem like more of a nuisance than a serious disease, severe diarrhea can cause life-threatening dehydration in an infant within a day or two. Diarrhea accompanied by fever, vomiting, or refusal to drink fluids needs immediate treatment. Diarrhea is most often caused by bacterial or viral ill-nesses, including food poisoning.

The following symptoms indicate serious dehydration that needs a doctor's treatment:

>> Extreme lethargy

>> Sunken eyes

>> Sunken fontanel (the soft spot on top of baby's head)

>> Sunken skin that remains raised after you pinch it

Loose, frequent stools aren't always diarrhea; see the section "Deciphering Diaper Contents" later in this chapter for ways to distinguish diarrhea from normal stool.

Protecting Baby from Common Accidents — and Handling Them When They Happen Anyway

Because newborns aren't all that mobile, you may think they don't have a lot of accidents, but they most definitely do. In this section, we go over the most likely scenarios and tell you how to handle them.

Taking care of baby after a fall

Even a newborn can scoot well enough to fall off the changing table or bed, which is why you're not supposed to leave a baby unattended, without your hand on him, for even a second. Babies usually bounce pretty well and rarely break bones in a fall, but the parental guilt may be enough to put you in a rest home for a week.

Even worse is the "I was holding the baby on the couch and the next thing I knew there was a thump" fall. Most common in the first sleep-deprived weeks of parenthood, the "I dropped the baby" fall devastates guilty parents. Avoid the guilt by not lying down on the couch holding the baby — and don't sit up holding him if you're feeling really sleepy, either.

Parents rarely drop babies when they're walking, but a trip on the sidewalk or over a misplaced toy can send you and baby sprawling. Whenever the baby goes to the ground, watch for these signs that a medical evaluation is in order:

» **Gaping cuts:** If he falls on a metal object and comes up bleeding, see whether the wound's edges are close together or gaping. Gaping wounds usually need stitches, glue (no, this is not a do-it-yourself project!), or butterfly bandages. Take your baby to a doctor or hospital.

» **Huge bruises:** Foreheads are famous for developing immense bruises after a bump. Bruises alone aren't concerning, unless they're accompanied by other signs, such as sleepiness, or if they keep growing. Bruises that bleed excessively can be a sign of other diseases, such as hemophilia, a disease that affects the blood's ability to clot, and need to be evaluated.

» **Inability to move a body part:** Baby's bones are still made of mostly cartilage, which bends easily, so he's unlikely to break a bone in a fall. If a mobile baby refuses to crawl or use an extremity, have it checked out.

» **No crying:** Obviously, if your baby is completely unresponsive after a fall, call 911 immediately. Give him a minute, though; he may be too stunned to cry for a few seconds.

» **Prolonged crying:** Every baby cries after a fall, if for no other reason than that landing on the ground is startling. Besides, you're crying, so baby thinks he should be, too. However, crying that lasts more than a few minutes may indicate an injury that should be checked out.

» **Repeated vomiting:** A baby who falls with a full stomach may spit up, but repeated vomiting can indicate a head injury.

» **Sleepiness:** This is one of the trickiest judgment calls of parenthood: What do you do when the baby falls right before bedtime? Keeping a tired baby awake is nearly impossible, and you shouldn't wake him up every few minutes just to make sure he's still responsive. Watch him for an hour and keep him awake if possible, but don't stress if you can't. If it's nap time or the middle of the night, let him sleep, but assess his breathing and color for any changes every few hours and watch to make sure he's moving normally in his sleep. Breathing that becomes very heavy or deep may indicate a problem.

Staying safe in the car

Car accidents are a fact of life, and you can't always prevent other drivers from driving badly or from running into your rear end at a stoplight. This is why a properly fitted, age-appropriate, approved car seat is absolutely essential.

WARNING

Don't *ever* hold a newborn in a moving vehicle — not in the front seat, the back seat, or anywhere else. Numerous studies have proven that you can't hold on to an infant in an accident; the baby will fly out of your arms and straight out the front or side window into the street or will be tossed around the car like a rag doll. Yes, this warning is meant to create a vivid picture that will scare you into never riding with your child in your arms. Babies die this way every year because they were taken out of the car seat to be fed or soothed for a moment. A moment is all it takes.

REMEMBER

Following is essential car-safety information for your baby:

>> **Put newborns and small infants in a car seat designed for their weight.** Never put a newborn in a seat designed for an older child, or vice versa.

>> **Never put infants and small children in the front seat, even if they're in an approved car seat.** The front seat is much more dangerous for your child if you're in an accident. Put them in the back, no matter what.

>> **Use rear-facing car seats for children up to age 2.** Riding facing backward is safer in the event of a crash, and pediatricians now recommend keeping children rear facing to the weight limits of the seat they're in. Children don't mind riding backward, even at 2 or older, and you can place a mirror so you can see them.

>> **Don't use a car seat beyond its expiration date.** Yes, car seats have expiration dates, usually found on a sticker on the side of the seat. The plastic can degrade over time, making the seat unstable in a crash.

>> **Don't reuse a car seat that has been in an accident.** The car seat may have been weakened or damaged in the accident — even if it was a minor one — and may not perform as expected if you have another accident. It's worth the extra money to get a new one.

>> **Don't borrow a car seat unless you know the expiration date and know it's never been in an accident.** Don't take chances on a car seat that may be damaged in any way, even if it looks fine.

>> **Read the instructions so you install the seat correctly.** A huge percentage of car seats are found to be incorrectly installed when checked at car seat clinics.

>> **Keep the car seat straps tight-fitting by taking your baby's heavy coat off in the car.** The straps need to fit tightly to her, not her jacket, to keep her in place in the event of an accident.

>> **Don't add after-market car seat covers, covers that zip over the car seat, head positioners, or any other added items that didn't come with the car seat, no matter how cute they are or how well they match your car's décor.** The materials may not fit well enough to the seat to stay on in case of an accident, which could cause your baby to slide around and not be fully protected. The items also may not be flame-retardant.

>> **Don't carry dangerous loose items in the car, like shovels.** They become missiles in an accident.

>> **Always wear your own seat belt!** It sets a good example and helps you maintain control of the car in an accident, not to mention keeps you from flying around the car, possibly landing on the baby.

If you get in an accident, check the baby carefully for bruises and cuts, especially if the car seat is dented or banged up at all. Remove the car seat from the car with the baby in it if you can so you can check for signs of injury without causing more injury to the infant's neck or back.

Be assured that if your child is in a safe car seat, the chances of her getting injured in an accident are low. If you don't think you can afford a car seat, talk to your medical provider or health department; some organizations offer help with money for car seats.

Managing Medical Crises at Home

Staying calm while talking about what to do in an accident is much easier than staying calm if your child actually gets hurt. In this section, we give you hints on how to stay calm and effective if your child needs help.

Don't panic! Don't panic!

Panic is inevitable when your child is injured, but try not to show it because even babies can sense your alarm and respond to it with a few alarms of their own. Try to remember the following guidelines when your child crashes into the coffee table or experiences some other medical crisis:

>> At first glance, it always looks like more blood than it actually is. Because blood is red, you notice it immediately. The injury probably isn't as bad as it first looks.

>> Head and face wounds can bleed copiously because of the large number of blood vessels there. Clean up the area and you may find just a tiny cut or scrape.

>> Spurting blood can indicate a cut artery. Hold firm pressure over the wound with something clean. This injury requires medical attention because arteries, unlike veins, don't stop spurting on their own quickly enough to prevent significant blood loss. Call 911.

>> Any injury to the eye should be seen by an ophthalmologist. If your child has something stuck in his eye, don't pull it out; you may make things worse. Call 911.

>> If you suspect a neck injury, don't move your child. Call 911 for help.

Calling the doctor

In an emergency, thinking clearly is very difficult. Sometimes you may even have trouble remembering your doctor's name, much less his phone number. To save yourself from fumbling through the phone book when you want to call your doctor, post the following information on your refrigerator in bold print so it's visible not only to you but also to the babysitter, relatives, friends, or anyone else who may be watching the baby:

>> **Your pediatrician's name and phone number:** Even you probably won't remember this information in an emergency.

>> **Your baby's full name and date of birth:** Yes, we're sure you'll remember your baby's name. But today, with hyphenated last names and moms who keep their maiden names, don't be so sure your sitter knows your baby's last name! And it's a pretty safe bet she doesn't know your baby's date of birth, unless she's closely related to you.

>> **Your address:** Believe it or not, people tend to go blank on this kind of information in an emergency. You may not forget where you live, but your mother-in-law may.

>> **Your phone number:** Everyone is on speed dial now; your mother may not even know your phone number!

>> **Your local poison control number:** This is always a good number to have handy.

REMEMBER

Taking the precaution of writing down important information may seem a little silly until you're actually in an emergency and can't seem to remember your own name, much less the baby's birth date.

When you get the doctor or emergency personnel on the phone, speak clearly and slowly enough so she can understand you the first time and not waste time asking you to repeat yourself.

TIP

If you have the presence of mind to do so, jot down a few notes about exactly what happened, because, believe it or not, the actual details get very jumbled in a crisis, which is why eyewitness stories never match.

Open Wide, Baby! Administering Medicine

Getting a baby to take medicine isn't as easy as it seems. Even small babies seem to have an uncanny sense that you've spiked their evening bottle with medicine, and if your partner is breast-feeding, spiking the boob with baby Motrin just isn't going to work.

When drawing up a dose of medication, remember that a kitchen teaspoon isn't always a teaspoon; it can range from half a teaspoon to 2 or more. One U.S. teaspoon equals 5 milliliters or cubic centimeters, usually abbreviated *cc*. Milliliters, known as *ml*, and cc are the same thing. So if the dose for your child's age is half a teaspoon, it's 2.5 ml or cc. To measure these miniscule amounts, you need a specially marked syringe, which pharmacies often provide with medication. If yours doesn't, beg for one.

Because a wrestling match will end up with far more medication on your shirt and on the floor than in the baby, try the following tips when you really need your baby to take medicine:

» **Mix the medicine with a small amount of a sweet-tasting food like baby applesauce.** Unfortunately, even small amounts of medications often change the flavor of the food, so don't put a tiny bit of medicine into a large amount of food hoping to dilute the taste enough so that baby will eat it. Chances are, she won't eat all the food, and you won't know how much medicine she actually got. Mix the medication into just a few bits of food she likes and you may have a fighting chance of getting it into the baby.

» **If you mix medication into formula, don't spike the whole bottle because this will be the first time in your baby's entire life that she doesn't chug down an entire 6 ounces of formula.** Mix it into 1 ounce so she finishes it before she realizes there's something rotten in Denmark.

» **Use a syringe to squirt the medicine into the baby's mouth.** Insert the syringe gently into the corner of her mouth; don't try to force her mouth wide open, unless you want to wear cherry-flavored Tylenol for the rest of the day. Push the syringe plunger down slowly but steadily, gently holding her lips closed, and hope for the best.

» **You can give some medications in rectal suppositories.** This may not sound like a really great solution, but inserting a suppository into the rectum is easier sometimes than getting medicine into a recalcitrant mouth. Just don't put a rectal suppository into the child's mouth, and be sure to push the suppository into the rectum very gently, using just the tip of your finger.

>> **If your child isn't an infant, firmly tell her that she has to take her medicine.** You may not believe this now, but kids often know when you really mean business, and they comply. It's like a miracle when it happens.

Taking a Baby's Temperature

Taking a baby's temperature is much easier now than it was a few years ago. You no longer have to stick a rigid glass thermometer into a flailing child's behind and hold it there for three minutes. You can measure temperatures even in tiny babies much easier today.

Choosing a thermometer

When standing in the big-box baby store looking for items to add to your baby registry, the sheer number of thermometer types may stagger you. Talking to friends who have babies may not clarify the thermometer choices because everyone seems to have a favorite method, and hardly anyone agrees with anyone else. Following is a list of different types of thermometers and their pros and cons:

>> **Digital rectal thermometers:** These are the gold standard for temperature taking, especially for infants younger than three months. Rectal thermometers measure internal temperature, the most accurate way to determine a child's temperature, and they have a flexible tip that gives if your child squirms. They're accurate — have we said that already? — and easy to use on some babies, although others hate them. If yours isn't fond of this procedure, one of you should hold his squirming legs while the other holds the thermometer in place.

>> **Digital oral thermometers:** These aren't practical or accurate until children are 3 or 4 because they can't hold them properly under their tongue and may bite and break them.

>> **Axillary thermometer:** You can use a digital rectal or oral thermometer under the arm as an axillary thermometer, but this method gives the least accurate reading and normally

registers as much as 2 degrees lower than a rectal temperature.

>> **Tympanic thermometers:** These thermometers, shown in Figure 14-1a, are used in the ear canal and aren't appropriate for use in children younger than three months because their ear canals are too small to properly insert the cone-shaped tip. They also may not be accurate for temperatures higher than 102.

>> **Forehead thermometers:** These register temperature as you roll the tip across the forehead, but they're not always very precise.

>> **Pacifier thermometers:** If your baby will suck a pacifier for three minutes, a pacifier with a built-in oral thermometer (see Figure 14-1b) may be the way to go.

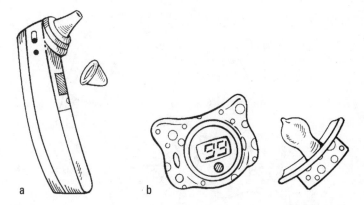

Illustration by Kathryn Born, MA

FIGURE 14-1: A tympanic ear thermometer (a) and a pacifier thermometer (b).

Taking a rectal temperature

Taking a rectal temperature is much easier if the baby is lying face down. Inserting the thermometer while the baby is on her back is possible, but you'll have much more difficulty keeping her from flailing around and possibly hurting herself. To take a rectal temperature, follow these steps and also check out Figure 14-2:

1. Put a little Vaseline or other lubricant on the thermometer to make it less uncomfortable to insert.

2. **Place the baby over your lap, with her head slightly down over your thigh.**

    This brings her rear end up slightly, making the anus, the opening to the rectum, easier to find.

3. **Locate the anal opening visually before you start prodding around with the thermometer tip.**

4. **Hold the thermometer the entire time that it's in the baby's bottom to avoid perforating the rectum.**

Taking baby's temperature with
a rectal thermometer

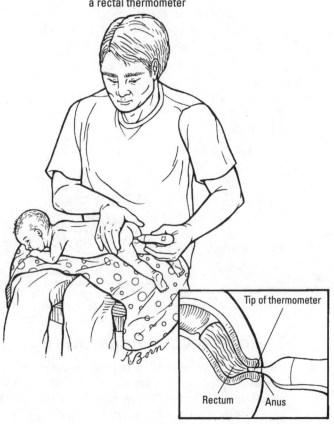

Illustration by Kathryn Born, MA

FIGURE 14-2: Taking a baby's rectal temperature.

WARNING

If you still have an old mercury thermometer lying around the house, get rid of it. Don't just throw it in the trash. The Environmental Protection Agency recommends taking it to a hazardous waste dump. Besides, throwing anything with mercury in it in the trash is actually illegal in some states.

Recognizing fevers

So when is a fever a fever? Knowing can be hard, especially when you're juggling half a dozen methods of temperature-taking in an attempt to get an accurate reading. The following guidelines explain what your medical practitioner means when he talks about a fever:

» **In an infant up to three months, a rectal temperature of 100.4 (or an oral pacifier temperature of 99.5) or higher needs immediate evaluation.** Small babies don't normally run fevers, so even these seemingly low temperatures need attention.

» **Between 3 months and 3 years, you should report a rectal fever of 102 or higher to your medical practitioner.** Although fever is important, the way your child is behaving is equally important. A child with a high fever who is still eating, drinking, and playing happily is less concerning than a lethargic child with a lower fever.

» **An axillary temperature of 99 or higher may be a fever.** Confirm the exact reading rectally, if at all possible.

» **Ear temperatures are roughly equivalent to rectal temperatures.** If you're sure the tip is properly inserted into the ear, call your doctor for a temperature of 100.4 for infants up to age 3 months and 102 for ages 3 months to 3 years.

Treating a fever

Fevers of 100.2 or less don't always need treatment. Fever is the body's way of fighting off infection, so giving your child medication at the first sign of a fever doesn't help his immune system to develop. You can give infants children's acetaminophen or ibuprofen in recommended doses. Don't give aspirin, though, because of the possibility of your child developing Reye's syndrome.

Febrile seizures

Febrile seizures, or convulsions, are extremely scary for parents, although the child probably won't remember them. Most febrile seizures occur when a child's temperature rises suddenly, but the exact degree of fever isn't the determining factor of whether the child has a febrile seizure. Around 3 to 5 percent of children experience febrile seizures, usually between the ages of 5 months and 5 years.

Don't try to do anything while your child is having a seizure, other than trying to cool her off by sponging her down with cool water and turning her on her side so she won't choke if she has something in her mouth. Don't put anything into her mouth or try to restrain her; more damage is done by these attempts to prevent damage.

Move any hard or sharp objects away from the child during a seizure to prevent injury. Remember to move the objects away from the child; don't try to move the child away from the objects.

REMEMBER

Most febrile seizures last only a few minutes, but your child may be limp and lethargic afterward. Follow up with medical personnel immediately after a seizure; your doctor may want you to bring the baby in immediately or may be okay with a visit the next day to determine the fever's cause. Be guided by his advice. Most parents who have just experienced an infant seizure want the reassurance of a visit.

WARNING

If your child's seizure lasts 15 minutes or more, she starts to turn blue, or she remains unresponsive after a seizure, call 911 immediately.

Deciphering Diaper Contents

Some parents are inordinately interested in their offspring's waste products (mostly parents who were raised to be inordinately obsessed with their own). But even parents who are pretty casual about the contents of a diaper can sometimes be concerned about what appears there.

Knowing what's normal

Breast-fed babies normally have frequent stools that are often looser than those of bottle-fed babies. Breast-fed babies' stools are often yellow and seedy, whereas bottle-fed babies' stools may be tan and firmer.

Babies frequently poop after every feeding in the first month or so and then slow down production. Some babies may only "produce" every few days, which is fine as long as the stool is soft. At the same time, they may begin to squirm, cry, grunt, and make faces when pooping, worrying parents that they're having a hard time passing stools. What they're actually doing is becoming aware of their own bodily sensations.

However, if stool is hard or comes out in pellets, or if the baby doesn't go for several days, call the pediatrician for advice.

Checking out color changes

Stool is usually yellowish or tan in babies who are exclusively breast-fed and/or formula-fed. When unusual-colored poop makes an appearance, parents are understandably concerned. Changes in stool color can be perfectly normal or a sign of a problem, so keep the following information in mind when deciding whether to call the pediatrician:

>> If your baby is on iron-fortified formula, he may have green or dark stools.

>> In breast-fed babies, green stools can indicate an imbalance of *foremilk*, the first milk released, and *hindmilk*, which has a higher fat content. Too much foremilk and not enough hindmilk can produce green stools and upset the stomach. Allowing the baby to nurse long enough on one side — ten minutes or longer — to get a good dose of hindmilk corrects the problem.

>> If blood is on the outside of the stool, the baby may have a small anal fissure and may need a stool softener, but ask your pediatrician. Also, make sure baby doesn't have a diaper rash that's causing the blood.

>> Bloody, mucousy stools need immediate attention because they can indicate intestinal problems.

>> Dark, tarry stools may be a sign of intestinal bleeding and should be evaluated.

>> Frequent watery stools — three or more an hour — indicate diarrhea. The diarrhea may look cola-stained, with a mucous ring around the stain.

Teething Symptoms and Remedies

Parents peer into their infants' mouths looking for teeth like gold miners sifting through the silt for nuggets of gold. When it comes to teeth, the best thing you can do is relax. All children, with very few exceptions, get teeth eventually, and prying your kid's mouth open to search for a pearly white doesn't make them come in any faster.

Keeping in mind that these guidelines have many exceptions, you generally can expect teeth to appear in this order and at these times:

>> The first tooth appears between four and seven months.

>> The two lower middle teeth usually come in first.

>> The two upper middle teeth follow next.

>> The back teeth are the last to come, usually around age 2; you probably won't be all that excited by new teeth by then and may not even notice.

>> By age 3, your child will have 20 teeth, 10 on each level.

After you get over the thrill of finding a new tooth, you may be consumed with ways to ease the discomfort of teething. Although alcohol, an old-fashioned remedy for easing the pain of teething, shouldn't be applied to baby's gums, it may help to apply it to *yours*. You can decrease teething discomfort in your baby with the following:

>> Pain medication such as infant's Tylenol or ibuprofen

>> Teething gels applied to the gums

>> Chilled teething rings or other items for baby to bite down on

>> *Teething tablets,* which are popular, over-the-counter mixtures of homeopathic medications — clear these with your baby's doctor before using them

REMEMBER

Teething doesn't normally cause a fever higher than 100 degrees, so a fever still needs investigation, even if your baby is breaking in a full set of choppers all at once. (Not likely, by the way — teeth tend to trickle in in groups of no more than two at a time.) Teething can, however, cause the following:

>> Biting on everything within reach

>> Difficulty nursing or taking a bottle

>> Difficulty sleeping

>> Drooling

>> Irritability

>> Swollen gums

REMEMBER

Whether teething causes diarrhea, vomiting, and rashes other than the rashes associated with constant drooling is debatable. Kids can get sick while teething, so don't assume that teething is responsible for sudden signs of illness.

Reacting to Medicines and Vaccines

Giving a child any type of foreign substance can trigger allergic or hypersensitivity reaction. New foods are actually the biggest culprit, but medications and vaccinations can also cause reactions.

Medications that cause reactions

Any medication can cause allergic reactions, but some are more likely to cause a reaction than others. Antibiotics are more likely to cause an adverse reaction than other medications. Typical offenders include

>> Cephalosporins

>> Penicillin or any of the same family, such as amoxicillin or ampicillin (Interesting fact: Penicillin causes more allergic reactions than any other antibiotic.)

>> Sulfa medications

Drug allergies can cause a variety of skin reactions, including

>> *Erythema multiforme,* a moving bull's-eye-patterned rash with a fever, joint pains, itching, and an overall sick feeling, as well as painful eyes and a sore mouth

>> *Hives,* small welts that move around from one area to another

>> Rashes

Notify your child's doctor if any reaction occurs after taking any medication. Children's diphenhydramine (Benadryl) helps control itching and swelling in most cases, but follow your pediatrician's advice. Severe reactions may require steroids.

Vaccination reactions — yours and your baby's

Many parents have concerns about the number of vaccinations given to infants and worry about which ones their child should have, when to give them, and possible consequences of vaccinations. Remember that vaccines are given to prevent *serious* illness; they're not given to prevent diseases that aren't potentially harmful for your child.

Giving two or three injections at one visit, especially when each one contains more than one vaccine, is concerning to many parents. But the American Academy of Pediatrics stands by the current vaccination schedule recommendations (which you can find in Chapter 11) and states that giving a number of injections at one time doesn't overwhelm the immune system, as some opponents suggest. The AAP states that children are exposed to 2,000 to 6,000 antigens every day, as opposed to the 150 antigens introduced in vaccines during the entire vaccination schedule.

Although there's no proof that vaccines are responsible for the increase in autism and similar issues, vaccines can cause complications in some children. Typical symptoms include fever, pain at the injection site, redness, or rash. Approximately 3 out of 10,000 children experience febrile seizures (described earlier in this chapter) after getting the measles–mumps–rubella (MMR) vaccine, according to the *Merck Manual.*

The debate about how to spread out vaccines and which ones are really necessary could fill books — and undoubtedly has — and every couple has their own feelings about vaccines. The most important factor in deciding on how, when, and what to vaccinate is to find a medical practitioner whose opinion you trust, discuss the pros and cons, and follow her recommendations.

TIP

Because many children do run fevers after vaccinations, some parents premedicate children with acetaminophen or ibuprofen before the doctor visit in an effort to prevent a few hours of misery after the injection. However, one study showed that this treatment may interfere with the vaccine's effectiveness. Ask your own pediatrician for his thoughts on this issue. Fever is usually a short-term reaction, so if your child is still feverish and miserable the next day, let the doctor know.

Some children develop a rash after vaccinations. Again, if it lasts more than a day, ask the doctor about it.

Dealing with Food Allergies

Food allergies affect around 1 in 18 babies before age 3. As with many facets of baby raising, the thinking on solid food introduction and allergies has completely changed since you were a baby, a fact that can result in heated discussions between you and your parents.

Introducing new foods

At one time, introducing solids early was all the rage in parenting, as if having your two-month-old chow down puréed carrots merited some sort of parenting prize. Today, pediatricians recommend waiting until a baby is four to six months old to introduce new foods to reduce the chance of developing food allergies, especially the five most common food allergens:

>> Cow's milk

>> Eggs

>> Peanuts

» Soy

» Wheat

An almost unbelievable 90 percent of food allergies are caused by one of the big five, which is why the American Academy of Pediatrics recommends introducing new foods one at a time. Age at the time of introduction is no longer considered a factor in whether a child develops allergies after six months.

Recognizing allergic reactions

Parents who have food allergies themselves may be looking for signs of allergies in their children, and allergic tendencies do run in families. Some common reactions, such as reddened cheeks after eating tomatoes or citrus fruits, aren't actually allergies. Nor is lactose intolerance, which is caused by a missing enzyme that breaks down milk products, an allergy. Irritability, skin rashes, and intestinal upsets are the most common signs of food allergy in infants.

WARNING

Colic, skin rashes, and stomach upsets such as loose stools are the most common signs of food allergy, but severe anaphylactic reactions with difficulty breathing, hives, and loss of consciousness can also occur, often within minutes of eating the offending food. Get medical help immediately if this occurs.

Having previously eaten a food without a reaction is no guarantee that an allergic reaction won't occur; reactions don't generally occur the first time a person is exposed to a substance. Always call your baby's doctor if a significant reaction occurs and follow his recommendations on treatment.

Preventing allergic reactions

The best prevention for allergy development is exclusive breast-feeding for at least the first four to six months of life. (Some evidence exists for prevention of wheezing in infancy and early childhood by exclusive breast-feeding for the first three months of life.) There's no proof that use of soy formulas prevents allergies compared to cow's-milk-based formulas; in fact, many children with cow's-milk allergies are also allergic to soy.

Cook fruits and vegetables for your infant instead of serving them raw because cooking appears to decrease the risk of allergic reactions. Processed foods, including junior baby foods, contain a number of ingredients, which makes it hard to tell what an infant is reacting to if she develops an allergic reaction.

If your child has severe allergies, your pediatrician may recommend carrying an auto-injector containing epinephrine in case of serious allergic reaction. Fortunately, around 20 percent of children outgrow their food allergies by the time they hit school age.

Chapter **15**

Fun, Freedom, and Finances: The Cost of Having a Baby

E ven before baby arrived, you probably never felt like you had enough time in the day or money in the bank for everything you wanted to do. Money concerns aren't a new worry in the lives of most new parents, but with diapers, baby wipes, and the cutest clothing you've ever seen in your life added to your weekly expenses, even financially sound parents can quickly begin to feel strapped for cash.

The only thing in shorter supply than money may be your time. Sometimes just finding a few minutes to shower may feel like a major accomplishment, but keeping your life and self in order is important for your entire family. Adjusting to a new life in which baby comes first is a challenge, and even the most organized parents find that tasks that used to require minimal effort are now a major undertaking. In this chapter, we take a look at how to juggle your new responsibilities with your old ones — with a little fun mixed in to boot.

Creating a Family/Fun/Work Balance with Baby

Unfortunately, bliss doesn't pay the bills, so unless you're embarking on a new journey as a stay-at-home dad or you win the lottery while on paternity leave, you're going to find yourself back in the throes of work in what feels like the blink of an eye. Don't be surprised if for the first few days you're disinterested, distracted, or bored on the job, especially if your partner is still at home. In the beginning, your mind will be more focused on the amazing event you've just experienced, and the fatigue your brain may be feeling as a result of less sleep won't help any.

When you're working full time again, winding down after a hard day won't be as easy as it once was now that you have to help with baby's bath time, night feedings, diaper changes, and endless chores. Congratulations — you now have another full-time job awaiting you when you get home.

Striking an ideal work/life balance is a major challenge for all parents, and it takes a lot of negotiating, planning, and sacrifice. From work to home to play, everything becomes a little more complicated to juggle. Never fear, though. We reveal how to make the best of a very full plate in the next sections.

Taking time off with paternity leave

Not so very long ago, new dads were expected back on the job the day after welcoming a baby into the world. Sometimes, they worked right through the whole experience! Although American society is still a long way from having equal time off for both mother and father, strides have been made to allow new dads time to bond with their new family.

Looking at possible time-off options

When planning your time off, consider the following options that may or may not apply to your employment situation:

>> **Parental leave:** A benefit offered by many companies, parental leave is time off that may be paid, unpaid, or a combination of both. Companies usually require that you be employed there at least 12 months to qualify. Parental leave

usually applies to maternal, paternal, and adoption leave, and policies vary by company. Speak with your human resources manager to find out your company's policy — or lack thereof.

>> **Family medical leave:** In the United States, the Family and Medical Leave Act of 1993 requires companies that employ more than 50 people to allow up to 12 weeks of unpaid leave in a given year for certain medical reasons, including caring for a new child.

>> **Vacation time:** Is there a better way to use your vacation time than to bond with your new baby? If you don't qualify for either of the preceding time-off options or if the parental leave offered by your company is insufficient for your needs and wants, most companies allow you to use vacation days at the end of the leave to extend your time off. If your company allows you to use vacation days for emergencies and illnesses, be sure to save a few days in case you don't have enough sick time to get you through the rest of the year.

>> **Sick time:** Some companies permit you to use sick time as part of your leave. Using sick time can be especially beneficial to hourly workers and non-salaried employees who don't accrue time-off benefits at a rapid pace or may not be eligible for all of a company's benefits, as well as for employees who haven't worked for their company long enough.

WARNING

Don't use up all your vacation and/or sick time as paternity leave. Babies tend to come down with all sorts of bugs, and some they generously pass on to you. With all the extra responsibilities and late nights involved in parenting, you may find yourself in dire need of a sick day for your own use. Instead of using all your sick time, inquire about the possibility of using unpaid time off so you can save those sick days for when you really need them. Your boss will probably be more willing to give you unpaid time off for baby's arrival than for your stuffy nose.

>> **Flextime:** Perhaps your company really needs you back ASAP. Talk with your boss and HR representative about temporarily working flexible hours or even part time from home. You may be expected to meet daily and weekly goals and complete all your work, but the non-9-to-5 schedule can be helpful for numerous reasons, especially if baby or mom has health concerns that require extra care or help.

Discussing your leave options

TIP

Before meeting with your employers to find out what leave arrangements you can make, speak with other recent fathers in your company about their experiences to get a better idea of what to expect. Their information can provide you an opportunity to craft a plan that meets your needs and adheres to your company's policies. Some great questions to ask other fathers are:

>> What was the company's paternity leave policy at the time you became a new dad?

>> How did your boss react to your paternity leave inquiry?

>> How much time off did the company grant you? How much of it was paid?

>> Did you use the Family and Medical Leave Act, and if so, what was your boss's reaction?

>> How did you structure your paternity leave?

>> Did you ask about using flextime before or after baby's arrival? If so, what was the company's response?

>> How much responsibility did you have to take for covering your job in your absence?

>> What is the one thing you wish you would have done differently in arranging your time off?

When meeting with your boss and/or HR representative, take notes of everything that is said and get any policy-related statements in writing. In addition to asking about some of the issues in the preceding list of questions, be sure to ask about the company's policy regarding additional time off in case of complications with mom or baby. Also, find out whether the leave will cause delays in future raises and how you'll pay your share of health insurance if you're taking unpaid leave.

Getting all your paperwork in order

Be sure to get the necessary time-off paperwork in order prior to heading to the hospital. Don't get defensive if your employer requires a doctor's note regarding your leave — nobody is questioning the fact that you're a new parent, but rules must be followed.

Keep a folder with all the paperwork and forms you need to secure your time off. Following are some of the forms and papers to have on hand:

>> **Family and Medical Leave Act application:** Your HR office can give you a copy.

>> **State-sponsored family-leave applications:** You need these forms only if your state's regulations differ from the federal ones.

>> **Medical time-off verification forms:** Include any forms your family doctor or pediatrician needs to fill out for your HR department.

>> **Your company's family-leave policy:** Maternity and paternity leave should be covered in your company's employee handbook. If not, ask for the policy in writing from your HR department or supervisor.

>> **Copies of all e-mail and letters sent to or received from your boss or HR department regarding your time off:** After you and your boss and HR department have agreed to your time-off request, makes sure you print off a record of the e-mails confirming that time off.

>> **Vacation time request:** This form needs to be approved and signed by your boss and/or HR representative.

Managing sick time when you're back at work

When both parents head back to work, sick time suddenly becomes a hot commodity. Between baby's multitude of doctor appointments, vaccination reactions, fevers, and diarrhea, as well as your sitter's unexpected life moments, expect to leave work more frequently than you used to pre-baby.

Check with your employer several weeks prior to the beginning of your leave to find out whether flextime or work-at-home days are allowed in case of child illness or childcare gaps. If they aren't, stay honest. Don't start coughing and sneezing or fabricate some family emergency as a front to mask the real reason you have to leave.

TIP

Ask for a performance evaluation a month or so after returning from paternity leave. If you've been experiencing bouts of insecurity and anxiety about how you're perceived and performing on the job now that you're a dad, or if you feel intimidated or scared about asking for days off because of the new baby, a performance review gives you an opportunity to address any minor issues that have arisen before they become full-fledged annoyances for your boss. Be sure to let your boss know you're aware that your schedule is trickier than normal and that you appreciate her/his flexibility as you adjust to a new schedule. Letting your boss know that you're open to criticism and want to fix any problems makes you look like the responsible new parent you've become.

Dealing with after-work expectations

Depending on the business you're in, you may be used to participating in after-work activities and commitments. However, after baby arrives, it quickly becomes clear that you no longer have the ability to attend happy hour three nights a week. Although nobody wants to be seen as the new dad who suddenly says no to everything and isn't the same fun, karaoke-loving guy he used to be, a certain amount of reality will dictate your ability to party instead of heading straight home to take care of business and spend time with your family.

Evaluate any after-work requests with the following guidelines to help you determine the appropriate way to handle them:

>> **Mandatory engagements:** Sometimes meetings run late, business dinners take priority, and your boss asks you to work overtime on a very important project. Always say yes to anything that's important to the function and maintenance of your job, and work with your partner to find help for her at home if needed.

>> **Occasionally important dates:** A beer isn't always just a beer. Sometimes going to a bar after work is an important networking opportunity or even where important business decisions and advancement opportunities are made. Try not to commit to quasi-important after-work requests more than a few times each month unless you can arrange for (and afford) childcare during that time.

>> **Optional events:** Sometimes a beer *is* just a beer — and there's nothing wrong with that, as long as you keep in mind that you can say yes only so many times without annoying your partner, and it's best to save those for when it really counts. If you perceive an after-work event to be merely for sport, pass unless you need a mental-health night out. Just remember that every time you say yes, you're giving your partner the opportunity to say yes to an activity of her own down the road. It doesn't take too many commitments to severely diminish that all-important family time.

TIP

Be proactive in scheduling out-of-the-office social events over lunch. If you take the lead, you'll have control over when they're held and won't feel the need to justify your inability to commit to activities after work.

REMEMBER

If a coworker challenges your decisions not to attend after-work events that you perceive to be nothing more than social calls, don't feel the need to defend your decision. Let him or her know that you spend eight hours a day with your coworkers and you like to spend the rest of the day with your family.

Working from home tips to stay productive

Remote and hybrid work arrangements are becoming more popular by the day. Although they provide parents with more flexibility, working remotely is generally not a replacement for childcare. Work is a full-time commitment and so is childcare, and babies don't make it easy to make deadlines, run meetings, or even respond to Slack messages in real time. When you do work from home — whether full or part time — it's important to keep productivity and responsiveness top of mind. The benefits of work from home are robust. You can throw in a load of laundry, play with baby over lunch, and even take time to attend doctor appointments. To stay productive:

>> **Block work hours on your calendar.** This allows your colleagues to schedule meetings during hours that work for you. If your company offers asynchronous work arrangements, this also allows you to work when you're most productive. It also demonstrates to your boss and co-workers that you're putting in a full day of work from home.

» Have quiet time. Babies are unpredictable. Just because you schedule a meeting or set aside 45 minutes to meet a deadline during nap time doesn't mean you're going to get the focus and silence needed. It's important to designate a private, somewhat permanent workspace that offers you all of the amenities you need to do your job well. For virtual meetings, apps such as krisp and Utterly remove background noises from Zoom calls — an absolute must for remote working new dads. If a meeting is casual between you and a colleague, consider putting baby in a stroller or carrier and taking the call on a walk. Just make sure to let your coworker know your plan ahead of time.

» Schedule everything. Did we mention babies are unpredictable? That doesn't end when they grow up, either. The more detailed and planned-out the hours of your day are, the more likely it is you'll accomplish everything on your list. Also, keep track of the times of day you struggle to get work done and the times you are a rock star. Adjust your schedule accordingly.

» Take the thread approach. In the short term, boundaries between work hours and home hours might be blurred. Think of work as a thread you have to weave throughout your day — especially when baby is young and you don't have full-time childcare. If baby is up at night and you are too, take advantage of that time to get work done in case you need a power nap the next afternoon.

» Prepare meals ahead of time — or buy them. Nobody wants to spend all weekend prepping food for the week ahead, but access to pre-made meals can help you take advantage of all of the time you need to get work done. Lunches go by fast, and they go by even faster when kids are in the house asking for your attention and help in between meetings. An easy-to-access lunch will not only save you precious time; it will also reduce daily kitchen cleanup.

» Invest in childcare. Just because you're both home doesn't mean you'll have the mental or physical fortitude — or time — to be parents and employees. It's tempting, especially for couples that both work from home, but any money saved will be lost to stress, exhaustion, and most likely arguing about whose turn it is to watch baby while the other takes a meeting.

Reprioritizing your commitments

With so much on your plate, you may wonder when you'll have time to hit the gym, go to the movies, take your partner on a date, volunteer at the local animal shelter, or engage in any of the myriad activities you enjoy doing. The bad news is that there isn't time in the day/week/month to do everything you've always done on top of caring for baby. The good news is that you'll still have time to have fun despite your overfull schedule.

REMEMBER

First things first: Keep yourself high on the list of priorities because you can't manage work, family, and your social life if you're run-down, sick, or depressed. If you try to do it all, you won't do anything very well because you'll be spread too thin. To have more energy and stave off illness, take your vitamins, get as much sleep as possible, eat healthy foods, and continue to make exercise a priority.

Just as you wouldn't skip a doctor appointment or just not show up at work one day, you have to schedule your personal commitments as well. Whether that's a stroll through the park with your family, sex with your wife, or time to sit and watch a tennis match on TV, don't make your personal time optional or the balance between work and life can easily become off-kilter.

TIP

How do you make the work/life balance stay in balance? Keep a calendar and write down everything, even blocking out time you set aside for fun. Try as best as you can to separate your commitments by focusing on work at work, family during family time, and you during your scheduled personal time. You can't make the most of your time if you're mentally juggling too many tasks and people.

Figuring out what's most important to you

Because thinking about everything you need and want to do at the same time is impossible, make a list of all your commitments and activities, then ask yourself, "If I could only give my attention to one thing in life, what would that be?" After you pick the most important thing in your life, choose the next four until you've designated your top five priorities. As your child grows and your life changes, frequently revisit this priority list. What's important to you now may not be as important four months from now.

Deciding what can go, at least for now

After you set your priorities, drop any unnecessary activities from your to-do list — at least the ones that require a major time commitment. Sure, a twice-weekly pool league may be a fun getaway, but is it really vital to your well-being and that of your family? How much TV can you cut out of your week and still feel entertained? Any activity that eats up copious amounts of your time without much reward should be removed from your regular routine.

Work with your partner, as well as babysitters and family members, to help you adhere to your priority list. Couples often tag-team to great effect: Mom watches baby while dad attends guitar lessons, and dad watches baby while mom goes to yoga. And when your friends and family members offer to baby-sit, try not to always use that time for errands. Instead, take your partner out for a night — or an afternoon, which is sometimes easier with babies — on the town.

Readjusting When — or if — Mom Goes Back to Work

Not every mother (or father, for that matter!) decides to go back to work. Others have to do so for financial reasons even when their hearts and tear ducts tell them otherwise. And some mothers and fathers are excited to get back to the daily routine and job they love. Everyone's experience is different, but regardless of what choice you and your partner make, the transition is challenging.

Making going back to work easier on mom

Mom gets far more time off work after baby is born than you (usually 6 to 12 weeks), which only makes the going-back process more difficult and emotional for her. There may be tears, running mascara, threats of quitting her job — lots of them — and it's your job (on top of everything else!) to support her through this difficult transition.

Mom's innate protective instincts will be at an all-time high the moment she's forced to put her 3-month-old baby into full-time day care for 40-plus hours every week. When you went back to work, you had the benefit of transitioning back when baby was at home with the only other person you trust as much as yourself to care for your child. Under most circumstances, mom doesn't get that luxury, and taking the leap back into business-as-usual won't be easy for her. Try these techniques to ease mom's return to work:

>> **Get comfortable with childcare.** Trusting someone else to care for your fragile baby isn't easy, but the sooner you start, the easier it will be when that care becomes more frequent. Start letting friends and family take short shifts watching the baby, and even ask your future childcare provider to take on a shift before your partner goes back to work. Also, feel free to ask your provider for time to observe his or her interaction with your child on-site.

>> **Plan ahead for morning.** Mornings are tough for everyone, so don't leave anything other than showering and getting dressed for the a.m. because you now have to factor in getting baby ready for the day and travel time to the sitter. Take time the night before to make lunches, pick out clothing, pack baby's diaper bag, and so on to create a calmer mood in the morning.

>> **Practice in advance.** Getting out the door won't ever be the same again, and the last thing you want is a panicked, rushed mom on her first day back. Much like you did with the trial run to the hospital before baby's birth, take the time to go through a trial run for mom's first day back to work. It will benefit you, too, because you'll be involved in the process of getting baby fed, clothed, and delivered to the sitter *and* still making it to work on time.

>> **Provide mommy alone time.** It's not so unusual for new moms to cling to their newborns, and in some cases, going back to work is your partner's first separation experience after giving birth. Start slowly by giving your partner blocks of time to be alone on the weekends or evenings during which she can practice doing things without baby around.

>> **Stagger the return.** Going from full-time mom to full-time employee overnight can be a major shock to the system. Have your partner talk to her employer about the possibility of a staggered return. If the first week back she only works one day, and then the following week she works three, and so on, the transition will be much smoother.

If your partner is threatening to quit her job the first day back, don't panic and certainly don't try to change her mind. The best thing to do is listen to her concerns and give her all the bonding time she needs with baby upon returning home from work. Tell her to take it day by day, and that at the end of every week the two of you will reevaluate the situation. There's nothing wrong with her making the decision to stay home, but making the decision when her emotions are heightened isn't a good idea.

Following are some thoughtful ways to improve your partner's emotional state during the transition back to work:

>> **Digitize baby.** Buy your partner a digital picture frame for her desk at work or even a pocket-sized device if she works in a non-office environment. Add new pictures every day to give your partner a daily, visual baby update, which will help her feel more connected.

>> **Don't try to fix it.** Let her cry and validate her experience, even if you don't understand why it's so hard. Mothers give birth to babies, and as deep as the bond between fathers and kids can run, it's still different for mom. Call her throughout the day to check in and let her know that what she's experiencing is normal.

>> **Give her chore-free nights for bonding.** Though you won't want to shoulder the chore burden all by yourself forever, consider giving your wife a get-out-of-jail-free card during her first week back. Allow her to spend every waking moment with baby to give her the opportunity to reconnect with her child and not feel like she's missing out on everything.

>> **Shower her with gifts and praise.** You don't have to go overboard, but some flowers on her first day back may go a long way toward making her smile, at least for a second, during that first week back. Also, tell her how well she's doing at adjusting to the changes and that you think she's a wonderful mother.

Deciding to be a stay-at-home mom

Making the decision to be a stay-at-home mom can be the fulfillment of a lifelong dream for some parents and a total surprise to others. If you and your partner make the decision that she'll stay at home to care for the baby, thus begins another exciting, challenging chapter in your new parenthood experience. However, it isn't a decision that you should take lightly. If you've been used to income from both yourself and your partner, losing half that income will make a profound difference in your lives, and you and your partner need to carefully consider whether you can make it work.

Considering whether you can afford for your partner to stay home

Some women know in advance that they don't want to go back to work after having a baby, and some come to that decision after baby arrives. For example, your partner may have loved her job before, and you may have thought the routine you'd established as a family was working fine. If you can make it work financially and your partner is refusing to budge, do your best to make arrangements for her to stay at home that work for both of you. Although you don't always need to understand why your partner feels the way she does, it's vital that you respect her right to feel that way.

Take plenty of time to talk it over and make sure staying home is really a feasible option. When choosing to stay at home, you must consider many costs beyond salary. If your insurance coverage comes from your partner's employer and she decides to stay home, you'll have to opt-in to your company's plan, which will reduce the size of your check. Also, most companies have an open season at the end of each year during which you can enroll for insurance. Having a baby is considered a change-of-life circumstance, which gives your family the opportunity to change an existing policy. However, if the decision is made outside of the open-season period, you'll either be without insurance or be forced to pay for private insurance until that time arrives.

Looking at options when you can't afford to lose the income

Sometimes the desire to stay home won't subside, and you and your partner may be at odds as to what's best for your family. If your financial situation doesn't allow for your household income to be reduced by tens of thousands of dollars annually, stand your ground. Be understanding of her concerns and desires, but don't put your livelihoods at risk to make her happy. Most important, don't rule it out forever. Make a savings plan that you both can work toward to achieve her goal of staying at home. Encourage your partner to seek out work-at-home opportunities. Work with your partner to create a tangible goal that will keep your finances in the black and eventually allow your partner to stay home.

Sometimes both parents want to quit their jobs to stay home and care for the child. Unless you and your partner are independently wealthy, this isn't an option. As unfortunate as it is, the decision will probably come down to money. If you can only afford for one person to stay home, the logical choice is for the person with the larger salary to continue working. It's possible, however, that the person who makes more money is working long hours and traveling frequently. Sometimes the decision is better made from a work/life balance standpoint rather than salary. In this case, you have to make lifestyle changes to make up for the loss of salary, but it can be done.

Increasingly, companies are adapting to the push for flexibility by allowing new parents the opportunity to spend some or all of their work hours at home. This arrangement can ease your partner's pain if she really wants to stay at home with baby but you can't afford to lose her income. However, working at home doesn't eliminate the need for childcare; you still need someone in the home to help while your partner gets work done, unless your partner is willing to work nights and weekends while you take over childcare duties. Even then, having babysitters at the ready is a must for busy times, meetings, and phone conferences.

If you and your partner can both work from home, you may be able to stagger your work hours so that you take turns caring for the baby. These kinds of alternate work arrangements can vary widely; your company may have guidelines in place for such arrangements or you may have to renegotiate your own plan. Ask your boss or human resources manager about this option if you're interested.

Helping mom adjust if she doesn't go back to work

The adjustment to being a stay-at-home mom can be just as challenging as heading back to work, only in different ways. As wonderful as it is to have the opportunity to raise your own child during the day, it can be an isolating experience. Some women find themselves a bit stir-crazy from all the indoor time and begin to crave adult interaction.

Here are some ways to help your partner transition to staying at home:

>> **Repeat after us: Raising a child is a job.** Sure, staying at home may seem at times like a dream gig — access to the TV all day, no more commuting — but resist the thought that she's got it made. As you know full well by now, taking care of a baby is exhausting. Babies require full-time attention and are the most demanding bosses on earth.

>> **Remember that her office is your home.** If your partner suddenly has higher standards for the cleanliness and tidiness of your home, help her keep it that way. She's now in the house all day, every day, and as strange as it may sound, you need to treat your home as her office, too.

>> **Encourage hobbies.** Mental boredom is inevitable, no matter how much you love your child. Stacking blocks, reading books, and taking long walks can be fun, but urge your partner to take up a hobby that's just for her that works her mind and gives her something to focus on other than baby.

>> **Give her personal time.** When you get home from work, you'll both need some time to decompress from a long day. Make sure to give her as much time off from baby duty as she needs. Plan relaxing surprises for her, such as a massage, every once in a while to make sure her emotional needs are being met. Work together to create an evening schedule that allows both parents ample baby-free time. Alternate being responsible for bath time, reading, the bedtime routine, and so on, to give both of you free time to relax. Just because you're away from baby all day doesn't mean you should be the sole caregiver when you get home.

>> **Ask her about her day.** Just because she's not in meetings and dealing with bosses doesn't mean she won't need to talk about the challenges and events of the day. Be sure to ask how she's doing — it's easy to do, but easy to forget.

>> **Don't think of her as your maid/errand girl.** Just because she's home all day doesn't mean picking up your dry cleaning, making dinner, grocery shopping, and vacuuming are all her responsibilities. She has more time to do things around the house, but don't give her a list of things to do for you. Being a stay-at-home mom doesn't mean you're her boss. Thank her profusely for everything she does do, which benefits the both of you every day.

TIP

Some days you hate your job, and the same rings true for the stay-at-home parent. Imagine how you'd feel if you never got a day off from your job. A stay-at-home parent works every day, and nights and weekends, too, so if your partner reaches the boiling point, don't hesitate to offer her a day off. Either take a vacation day to stay home with your child or encourage her to find alternate childcare for the day.

You may be surprised how much stress will be removed from your life when your partner transitions to full-time childcare and can take care of some of the chores and tasks that eat up your precious weekend, but don't have unrealistic expectations. Taking care of a baby is a full-time job as it is. To help both of you adjust to her stay-at-home schedule, sit down together and work out what her new role will look like to ensure the two of you expect the same things. Create a "job description" that will benefit the entire family and help avoid frustration down the road, and be open to modifying it if she discovers that, say, doing all the laundry and cooking in addition to her childcare duties is exhausting her.

Becoming a stay-at-home dad

By no means is the stay-at-home dad a norm in our society. As of 2016, dads make up 17 percent of all stay-at-home parents in the United States, a number that has grown slowly in the past decade. If you decide to stay at home, remember that the rules outlined for the stay-at-home mom are no different from the rules for you.

Following are some special considerations for the stay-at-home dad:

» **Fight for your right to "daddy."** If you've never experienced sexism in your lifetime, get ready for an onslaught. As a stay-at-home dad, at every turn you'll be confronted by people who are surprised at your choice, concerned that you don't know what you're doing, and judgmental of your decision to "throw away" your career. Strangers, especially women, will fawn over you and even say that it's so nice of you to "baby-sit" for mom. Be confident in your decision and let the world know that you're excited about your new career and that men are capable of more than changing a diaper. Taking care of a baby is a lot of hard work, but it's not rocket science — you can do it!

>> **Make friends with other parents.** Be it moms at the park or daddy play groups, reach out to other stay-at-home parents in your neighborhood even before the baby comes. You'll need friends to lean on for advice and last-minute babysitting, and the more you help out your new-parent friends and neighbors, the more options for help you'll have when you need it.

>> **Turn off the TV.** It's tempting to keep ESPN on in the background all day, but too much TV isn't good for babies and children. Babies learn language by being talked to, so narrate your day instead of letting your favorite show provide the soundtrack. Limit your TV time to two hours or less a day while baby is awake. Nap time is all yours.

>> **Utilize your unique skills.** Babies are mesmerized by everything, so use your stay-at-home time as an opportunity to play guitar, further your baking skills, or even start an out-of-the-home business. Having a daytime activity provides you a much-needed creative outlet, and down the road, your kid will learn to appreciate (and mimic) your skills.

Exploring the Expected (And Unexpected) Costs of Baby

One of the first things you'll hear from other parents is how expensive it is to have and raise a child in today's high-cost world. According to the U.S. Department of Agriculture, raising a child to the age of 18 will cost a middle-income family more than $284,000 — and possibly more depending on location and inflation.

Some costs of having a child are fixed and can't be avoided. Babies need food, clothes, diapers, wipes, and a safe, warm place to sleep. Babies don't need an entire closet jam-packed with enough designer-label clothing to make Harper Beckham weep with envy, though. You and your partner need to control the urge to shower your baby with every possible toy or accessory.

The following sections help guide you in spending your money wisely on only the things baby truly must have.

Deciding what baby really needs

Experts estimate that baby's first year of life, including day care, diapers, clothing, and medical expenses just to name a few, will cost you between $20,000-50,000. Costs are higher in cities, where childcare costs are far more exorbitant. You'll find quickly that the choices you make with your cash have to count. Some costs arrive early: The average hospital delivery costs between $7,000 and $11,000, and even with a great insurance plan you'll still be getting hit with a portion of the bill.

TIP

Contact your insurance company in advance of baby's birth to verify what's covered and up to what cost. This information gives you a rough idea of how much of the medical bills will be your responsibility and may even help you make some decisions based on what you want versus what's covered.

After you bring baby home, his needs are rather modest, but the costs will add up quickly if you don't stick to the basics. Before you run out and buy the baby bouncy chair, swing, play mat, and so on, spend some time getting to know what your baby likes so you won't be stuck with a lot of unused toys that cost you a lot of dough.

Most towns have a vibrant baby resale shop or, if not, a hopping garage sale culture. One thing you'll learn quickly is that the life span of baby goods long outlasts the amount of time your child will actually use them, and there's nothing wrong with buying used items rather than new ones. Just make sure that what you buy is clean, in good condition, and meets current safety standards. Buying secondhand is a great way to get inexpensive clothing, toys, and strollers — particularly because your baby will grow out of all of them before you know it.

TIP

Network with the other parents you know, especially those with older babies or toddlers born in the same season as your baby. Many parents will happily pass along or sell you the things they no longer use, which frees up space in their home and cuts down on the cost for you.

Whenever possible, before you buy anything, give your child the chance to try it out. Pull down the floor sample or take it out of the box to make sure your child is engaged with what you're about to buy. You may think all bouncy chairs are the same, but your baby inevitably will like one more than another. To make sure you get your money's worth, buy what your baby shows interest in.

Bracing yourself for the costs of must-have baby supplies

Babies don't need a lot of stuff, but what they do need tends to be a bit on the expensive side. If your partner isn't breast-feeding, you'll have to spend a great deal of money on formula, which is quite expensive. Parents opting to use only organic, chemical-free goods for their baby will find the costs increase as well.

Every choice you make will change the weekly amount you spend, but here's a basic look at what to expect:

>> **Diapers and wipes:** If you develop an allegiance to a national brand of disposable diapers, you'll spend $15 to $20 every week. Many big-box stores offer their own brands, which can cut the cost in half. Baby wipes present the same conundrum, with the name-brand options costing $12 to $16 for a month's supply.

TIP

For both diapers and wipes, the cost-per-unit goes down when you buy a larger-sized box. You're going to be using wipes for the foreseeable future, but baby will outgrow diapers, so don't buy a box that may go to waste. Also, buy only what you have room to store — it's worth a little extra not to have a house overfilled with diapers and wipes.

Upfront costs are higher for cloth diapers than disposable, but you'll save money in the long run. Expect to pay about $600 for the first year of cloth diapers — including liners, detergent, and energy costs. (All-in-one styles grow with baby up to 35 pounds and cost approximately $20 per diaper.) Cloth diapers increase your energy and water use as well as the amount of baby-safe laundry detergent you must buy. The total cost for baby's first two years in cloth diapers will be about $1000. Bonus: You can use the same cloth diapers for any subsequent children you have, which makes the cost extremely low. Cloth diaper services are also available, which provide fresh, clean diapers in exchange for your dirty ones. It cuts out the hassle of cleaning but does increase the cost.

>> **Feeding supplies:** Whether your partner breast-feeds or uses formula, you'll have costs to meet.

- **Breast-feeding supplies:** Breast milk may be free, but you still need supplies, especially if mom is going back to work. Aside from a decent breast pump (a one-time cost of $150 to $400), you need freezer storage bags ($8 to $12 for a two-week supply), as well as nursing/breast pads ($8 to $12 for a two- or three-week supply) and freezer bags or reusable containers (prices vary), as well as additional parts for the pump, such as pump horns and extra bottles.

TIP

  Some insurance plans, including some that are part of the Affordable Care Act, allow women to get a free breast pump because it is, indeed, a medical supply. Make sure to check your insurance allowance for a pump before buying — it could save you hundreds of dollars.

- **Formula:** Expect to spend between $150 and $200 per month on formula, depending on the brand and formula you choose to purchase. Specialty formulas, including those for sensitive tummies and organic brands, cost even more. Also, if you use bottles with liners, expect to spend another $15 to $20 per month.

>> **Insurance and medical expenses:** Adding baby to your insurance plan increases the monthly amount withdrawn from your paycheck, generally by $50 to $100 per month, depending on the quality and cost of your insurance plan. You must complete the change in policy within 30 days of baby's birth. Account for one doctor visit per month in the first six months to be on the safe side, with the only cost being the amount of your copay.

>> **Clothing and laundry:** Make sure to use a dye-free or baby-safe laundry detergent, which costs more than the standard fare. And, seeing as babies grow at a rapid pace, you need to allot anywhere from $50 to $100 per month on clothing, which includes hats, shoes, sleepers, coats, socks, onesies, and outfits so cute they could make a puppy bark with jealousy.

TIP

Some parents opt to use dye-free detergents, such as Tide Free or All Free and Clear, which are intended for adult use. Using these detergents for the whole family simplifies the laundry process and saves you money. Make sure to read the label of any product to make sure it's nontoxic. Also, for babies with sensitive skin, use ½ cup of vinegar in the wash cycle in lieu of fabric softener.

You can save money on clothing by checking out consignment shops and garage sales and asking for hand-me-downs from friends with older children. All babies outgrow clothes before they're worn out, so you can find a lot of perfectly nice used items at a fraction of the cost of new.

TIP

College may seem a long way away, but it's never too early to start saving for your kid's education. However, if you don't have a retirement fund or an emergency fund for your own future survival, start there. You have to take care of your future first, and that responsibility sets a good example for your child. And if you can't pay for that college education someday, well, that's what student loans are for!

Comparing childcare options and costs

Paying someone else to care for your child 40 to 50 hours each week will become your new number-one expense. In fact, depending on where you live, it very well may cost you more than your mortgage or rent. Taking care of a baby is big business, but it's also a huge responsibility, so it comes with an equally huge financial burden.

Like when shopping for cars, you have many options when choosing childcare. Depending on whether you're looking to buy a luxury car (an in-home nanny) or a two-door compact (your neighbor's in-home day care) or something in between, the costs will vary depending on the services you're promised.

TIP

Regardless of which childcare option you choose, create a contract (unless the provider has one of his own) to make sure you're getting what you expect and that you won't have unexpected costs when you pay the bill. Go over the following questions with your day-care provider and get the answers in writing:

>> Are you licensed to provide childcare in this state?

>> What training have you received in childcare and education? What about your staff?

>> Are you insured in case of accident?

>> Who is providing the food?

- **»** How often and on what day are you expecting payment?
- **»** Do you need my permission to take my child in a car?
- **»** How much notice do you need to give in order to terminate the agreement?
- **»** Do you frequently have visitors? Are they allowed to interact with the children?
- **»** Am I allowed to drop by unannounced to observe you with my child?
- **»** Will my child always be under your care or will your spouse/child/friend/family member be helping?
- **»** Do I have to pay when my child is sick or when we're on vacation?
- **»** How do you discipline children?
- **»** What do you charge for days I need to drop my child off early/pick her up late?
- **»** What security provisions are in place?
- **»** Are you certified in both infant and child CPR?
- **»** Will you work with cloth diapers?

Outlining your expectations in writing reduces your fears and helps prevent any unexpected surprises or litigation down the road.

If after you check out the costs of day care you're reconsidering quitting your job (or having your partner quit her job) and staying at home, be sure to carefully weigh the points outlined earlier in this chapter. Staying at home is expensive in its own way and isn't a decision to be made lightly.

The following sections describe the three most common options for childcare.

Private in-home day care

A friend, neighbor, or local day-care provider who operates a facility out of the home likely will be your cheapest option, depending on the sophistication level of the facility. Expect to pay between $150 and $300 per week depending on your location. Many providers who work in their own homes are also watching their own children, which can reduce the cost to you.

Be sure to visit this type of day care on a regular weekday during business hours to see how things function during "high-volume times." Some states require certifications for any day care providing care for a certain number of children, and you should research the regulations in your state and make sure the provider is compliant.

Day-care center

A day-care center, also sometimes called *corporate day care,* is any facility that accommodates many children and employs multiple staff members to care for a wide age range of children. Depending on the facility and the qualifications of the people it employs, this service can cost between $200 and $500 per week. For instance, if the day care has child-development specialists on staff and a play facility that pulls out all the punches, costs will be higher than at a basic facility.

REMEMBER

Make sure the child-to-adult ratio at the facility meets accepted guidelines. The U.S. Department of Health and Human Services recommends a 3:1 ratio for babies age 0 to 24 months; 4:1 for 25 to 30 months; 5:1 for 31 to 35 months; 7:1 for 3-year-olds; and 8:1 for 4- to 5-year-olds.

Your own in-home nanny

Paying someone to come into your home to provide full-time childcare for your child and your child alone is a custom and very expensive option. For many parents, the peace of mind involved in this setup is worth every penny, especially when you factor in the time, gas, and stress saved by not having to take your child to the sitter every day. Costs typically range from $400 to $800 per week, depending on your location, expectations of the care provider, the provider's experience level, and the number of hours the provider is expected to be in your home.

Managing Your Money

Regardless of your financial situation, you'll feel the impact of a baby early and often. Aside from the frightening amount of supplies, toys, doctor visits, and clothing, the enormous cost of childcare will leave you with a lot less cash — and financial freedom — than you had in the past. Depending on where you live and the option you choose, you may be paying your childcare provider the same amount you'd pay for a car payment — every week!

So perhaps your days of three-dollar lattes are behind you. Maybe you'll be buying one less album online each month. Regardless of your vices and other financial obligations, you need to get your spending habits in tip-top shape to absorb the high cost of having children.

Prioritizing your needs

The difference between what you want and what you need is a gulf roughly the size of the Grand Canyon. The same can be said for what you want for your baby and what your baby actually needs to thrive. As a parent you have to get the needs of your entire family in check to secure a financially sound future for all.

TIP

Every family's situation and needs are different, but one rule is universal: Make a budget. Start by taking a realistic look at where your money goes. Visit your credit card company's website for an analysis of how you spent your money in the past year (some companies send you this statement automatically each year), and look at your bank statements from the same time period. If you struggle to make cuts, consider meeting with a financial planner. Figuring out how to spend, save, and survive is a big job, and you don't have to go it alone.

Factor in the monthly costs of housing, food, transportation, investments, insurance, and any medicines you take regularly. You also have to plan for the unexpected, and with a baby in the equation you'll have a lot of unexpected. Starting an emergency fund is easier said than done, but it's a must. When you have a kid, absorbing an unexpected job loss, income reduction, or family emergency can be debilitating. Try to slowly work your way up to having six months' expenses set aside just in case life throws you a curveball.

REMEMBER

As unpleasant as thinking about tragedy is, now is the time to make sure you have sufficient life insurance coverage for you, your partner, and your baby. Work with a reputable insurance agent to make sure your family will be provided for if the worst were to happen. Also, make sure you have short- and long-term disability coverage through your employer. If not, consider buying your own policy. Missing even one paycheck can spell disaster for some families, so try to be overprepared for emergencies. (Head to Chapter 16 for more on insurance and disability coverage.)

Determining where to cut costs

Giving up things you love isn't easy, but it's a must now that you have someone to provide for. Consider cutting costs in the following areas:

>> **Convenience purchases:** Sure, buying lunch is simpler than getting up early to make it in the morning. Same goes for coffee. If you find yourself a constant consumer of takeout food, taxis, dry cleaning, bottled water, and other nonessential items that simply make your life easier, cut back. Even one fewer purchase per month can make a major impact on your bank account.

>> **Entertainment:** Take a look at the last six months of expenses and try to cut or reduce the monthly cost of these nonessential items, which are the biggest expendable category for cost savings. Cable isn't a utility, and if you're struggling to make ends meet, consider cutting your package down to basic or even getting rid of cable altogether, even just for a little while. If you have both cable and a mail-based movie subscription, do you truly need both? Baby will automatically limit the days you can go out to dinner, catch a movie, or attend a football game, but monitor and limit these expenses, too, especially if you have to pay for a babysitter when you go out.

>> **Food:** Prepackaged and/or snack foods tend to be expensive. Items such as chips, ice cream, candy, beer, frozen dinners, and soda are not only bad for your body but also bad for your budget. You may not be willing to give them up altogether, but try to cut down on the number of purchases of these high-cost, low-nutrition foods. Also, consider making a big casserole or stew to eat for numerous meals, which will reduce both your time in the kitchen and your grocery bill.

>> **Utilities/bills:** Take a long, hard look at your monthly expenses. Do you need both a cellphone and a home phone? Can you downgrade any of your plans to a lower-cost option that still suits your needs? If you live in a cold-weather climate, can you go on a monthly payment plan to evenly spread out the costs of heating your home throughout the year? Are you in good standing with your credit card company? If so, ask to reduce your interest rate. Call every insurance company you do business with and see whether you can get a lower rate. Don't be afraid to ask all the companies that you do regular business with for a financial break.

Check out Chapter 16 for more pointers on budgeting and cutting costs.

IN THIS CHAPTER

» Organizing your finances and putting safety nets in place

» Considering saving options for your child's education

» Buying life insurance for worst-case scenarios

» Choosing the right health insurance for baby

» Creating a will and designating a guardian for your child

Chapter **16**

Ensuring a Bright Future for Your New Family

During this time of immense joy, you probably resist worrying about the ifs, ands, or buts that could bring all that happiness to a screeching halt. You may also think it seems a bit premature to begin squirreling away cash for your baby's education when she hasn't even mastered the art of sitting up. But, as the time-honored cliché goes, they grow up so fast.

Planning for the future, whether for planned events or unexpected ones, is the least enjoyable part of being a parent because it reminds you just how fleeting life can be. And people don't want to think about what would happen if they die, especially with a newborn just beginning to enhance life. However, now is the time to make sure your child will be taken care of, regardless of the circumstances.

Planning for a Financially Sound Future

New parents are saddled with an enormous uptick in caretaking responsibilities. In fact, your role as caretaker now involves getting your financial life in order so you can properly care for your child today, tomorrow, and even after you and your spouse die. Organizing your finances isn't the cheeriest item on the new-parent to-do list, but it's one of the top priorities.

In the following sections, we share some financial tips that will help to ensure a bright (and green!) future for your entire family.

Prioritize your expenses

Singling out purchases that you can — and should — live without can be a real buzz kill. Giving up the little things in life can be a difficult adjustment, especially for new parents who are already sacrificing sleep and freedom. For most first-time parents, the financial strain of having a child means looking at where you can cut down on your own expenses. If you fall into this category, this section helps you make some tough choices.

Your fixed costs are food, housing, electricity, heat, and transportation. The rest is a mix of choices that you and your spouse make about how to live your lives. There are no hard-and-fast rules about what to axe from your life, but depending on your particular needs and your income, the following areas are good places to cut back:

>> **Entertainment:** This category includes movie tickets, concerts, streaming services, magazine subscriptions, books, vinyl, hobbies, sporting events, and so on. With baby occupying most of your free time, time constraints will help you cut way back on sporting events, movies, and concerts. And instead of spending money on some of the other items, get a free membership to your local library; most have extensive movie and music collections as well as books and magazines. Borrow movies from your friends, too, or host a movie night and share in the rental and food expenses. Remember, although streaming services are generally less expensive than cable, subscribing to Netflix, Disney+, HBO Max, Hulu Plus, and more can cost as much or more than a traditional cable package. If money is tight, pick one or two favorites and cancel the rest — for now.

» **Food:** Whether you eat out often, rely on DoorDash and ÜberEats, always dine in, or regularly grab coffee, you can make a change in your food spending. Look at your past expenses and find places to save. Even choosing to order food delivery one fewer time each month or spending $10 less per week at the grocery store will save you big over the long haul.

TIP

To replace the fun of eating out, host a dinner party or start a rotating dinner club with a group of friends. Assign each attendant a different course so you can drink and dine in style at a fraction of the cost.

» **Interest rates:** If you have high interest rates on your credit cards, mortgage, or other debt, you're essentially spending money on nothing — clearly a spending habit you won't mind changing! Refinancing your home can save you a bundle in the long run, and if you have good credit, try to negotiate down your interest rate with your credit card company. Doing so isn't always easy or possible, but it's always worth a call to find out whether — and how — you can save.

» **Luxury:** Trendy clothing, the latest phone, expensive haircuts, high-end skin-care products, and costly jewelry are a few items that you can downgrade, reduce, or perhaps ax altogether.

Create (and stick to) a budget

After you put your expenses under the microscope and find places to cut back, make a plan and stick to it. Knowing what you plan to spend each month allows you to explore savings options, such as setting up a college account for your baby. Saving money can be a fun game. The more you save, the more thrilling it becomes to push yourself further and watch your personal worth rise.

TIP

If you find yourselves struggling to spend only what you've designated for each item in your monthly budget, use cash. If you take $100 to the grocery store, you have exactly that much to spend. Calculating what you can buy takes more time, but before long you'll be able to eyeball what you can and can't afford.

To make a budget, start by breaking down your finances into the following categories, placing a monthly spending allotment next to each:

» Mortgage/rent

» Home/rental insurance

» Electricity

» Gas

» Water, sewage, and trash

» Phone

» Internet

» Home maintenance

» Car payment, insurance, and gas

» Childcare

» Groceries

» Entertainment, cable, and streaming services

TIP

Many excellent software programs, books, and websites can help you make and maintain a monthly budget. Quicken is one of the most popular computer programs for managing your personal finances and even paying your taxes, and www.mint.com offers a popular (and free!) online and app-based service.

Pay down your debt

Not all debt is equally bad. Some debt, such as student loans and real estate mortgages, tends to have low interest rates and build future value. Bad debt is anything with a high interest rate — mainly credit cards, and especially credit cards used to purchase unnecessary or disposable goods and subsequently not paid off every month.

There are two schools of thought on paying off debt. One is to build success by paying off the smallest debt first and then moving on to the next smallest to build a series of wins. The other, more common advice is to pay off your high-interest debt first, which is most likely your credit card bills, and to do so as aggressively as your finances allow.

REMEMBER

Don't use your credit card until all your debt is paid down, and after that, only use your card for emergencies and essential expenses, such as groceries. Using it for limited essential items (that you've budgeted for) ensures that you can pay off the balance every month. Pay for nonessential items with cash or you'll end up paying even more for them if you don't pay off your balance each month.

After you pay off your credit cards, start paying off your debt that has the next highest interest rate — likely a car loan. Also, paying one additional mortgage payment every year can take years off the length of your loan. Remember, this financial approach isn't about getting rid of debt altogether. Everyone has debt, and debt actually helps build your credit score. The goal is to get rid of unnecessary and high-interest debt.

PARENTING ON THE CHEAP

People tell you that babies are expensive, and, for the most part, they're right. All the things that babies need to survive add up quickly, especially over time, which is why buying only what you need is of the utmost importance.

Baby stuff is cuter and more expensive than ever before, and more and more parents are buying high-end goods. If you don't have the money for the $1,000 stroller that all the other parents in your neighborhood seem to have, don't buy it. Your baby doesn't need — and won't remember having — an expensive crib, stroller, or bassinet, and he certainly doesn't need nicer clothes than you wear.

Create a monthly budget for your baby expenses. Buy the essentials first and use any leftover money to buy secondary items, such as new toys. Babies don't need a lot to play with; in fact, your tot will probably like the packaging the toy came in better than the toy itself.

Local resale and consignment shops aren't just for hipsters and low-income families. Buying lightly used goods saves you a fortune, and, considering that babies grow in and out of clothes, toys, and furniture very quickly, you're likely to find exactly what you want at a fraction of the cost. You can also utilize online sites such as Craigslist, eBay, and Freecycle to get what you need for cheap or even free!

Create an emergency fund

An emergency fund can be a lifesaver for a number of reasons. Job loss happens when you least expect it. Family members get sick and require your time and attention. Houses and cars break down all too often. Whatever life throws at you, it's going to cost you some dough. The rule of thumb changes all the time, but most experts advise saving enough money to cover anywhere from 6 to 12 months of expenses.

If you managed to read that and not faint, take heart — most people don't have that much money tucked away, and a lot of folks never will. However, you have to start somewhere, and the less you spend, the more you can save. And now that you have a baby to care for, being able to handle the unexpected expenses is more important than ever.

Make a plan that works for you and your family. For some, having a set amount or percentage of salary automatically moved into an account each month is easiest. To begin saving, try putting 5 percent of your paycheck into a separate savings account. If after a few months you find you still have extra money in your primary checking account, start saving more.

Buy disability insurance

Most companies provide employees the option to buy short- and long-term disability coverage, which generally pays 60 percent of your salary in the event that you're injured and unable to work. If you haven't signed up for that coverage, do so immediately. You're far more likely to get injured than die, and the loss of a salary can sink your family into financial ruin in no time. Short- and long-term disability can provide a source of income for around two to five years if you're unable to work.

If you're self-employed or your company doesn't offer coverage, contact a local life insurance representative or financial advisor to help determine the right amount of coverage for you. Having a policy that can cover your family's expenses if you're out of commission is essential.

Contribute to a retirement account

REMEMBER

Taking care of yourself first means ensuring that your kids won't have to take care of you in the future. It's vital that new parents begin saving for their own retirement. As your kids grow, so will your financial needs, which means you need to start saving when you're young to have enough to live the way you want to when you retire.

If your work has a 401(k) or similar program, make sure you contribute the maximum amount allowed each year, especially if your company matches that amount. Consider opening a Roth IRA account, which allows you to contribute a certain amount of your earnings to the account each year while making tax-free withdrawals when necessary.

Work with a financial advisor

If numbers make your head spin or if you're not sure you have the right kind or enough of the savings, insurance, and retirement accounts you need for your lifestyle, you may benefit from working with a financial advisor. Consultations are free, and the advisors work on commission from sales (of life insurance, investments, and so on), so meeting with one doesn't cost you anything except your time.

WARNING

If your advisor unnecessarily pressures you into buying her company's wares, beware. Her main role is to help you prosper financially, and if you aren't interested in or aren't in the position to buy something she's pushing, seek counsel from someone else. Yes, she has a job to do, but don't get suckered into something you don't want. Always take a day or two to think about a financial advisor's advice before committing to anything and, when possible, seek a second opinion.

Mind your credit score

If the only scores you keep track of involve the doings of professional athletes, you're probably long overdue for a check of your credit scores. Your credit score affects the interest rates of every line of credit you have, and a mistake may be costing you on your mortgage, car payment, credit cards, and student loans. Credit scores change all the time, so periodically check to make sure that yours is on track and that your credit history has no mistakes.

Credit scores range from 350 to 850. A very low credit score is any number below 600. An average credit score is between about 650 and 700. An excellent credit score is anything above 700. Your credit score is reported by three different agencies that provide three different scores. Checking all three is important so you can clear up any mistakes. You can request your free credit report once a year from each of the following:

>> Equifax: www.equifax.com

>> Experian: www.experian.com

>> TransUnion: www.transunion.com

Saving Money for Your Child's Future

Every parent wants his child to get the best college education money can buy. Not all parents, however, can afford that education, nor do they want their children to accrue massive amounts of student loan debt.

If you have the luxury of being able to save some money for your child's education, here are a few common savings options:

>> Parents can invest money in a Coverdell Education Savings Account (CESA), which allows you to save $2,000 a year tax-free. However, CESA funds are considered student assets and can reduce the amount of student loans available to your child.

REMEMBER

>> Every state offers at least one 529 plan, a state-sponsored college savings plan that allows you to choose the amount of money you want to invest and how aggressive you want that investment to be. Your investment grows tax-free, and it only requires you to fill out an easy form, usually available on your state's website. After you file the paperwork, you begin depositing money according to the plan you chose. The investments are even managed by a professional. Plus, you can begin saving before your child is born.

>> You can save in a personal investment account — that is, a savings, stock, bond, or mutual fund account. These accounts give you more control to add or remove money,

and you earn capital gains, interest, or dividends. You pay taxes on the income each year you earn it, but these accounts give you more freedom to use the savings when and how you see fit. Depending on what level of access you want your child to have to the money, set it up as a trust that can be accessed with conditions or simply pay the tuition bills yourself.

For parents looking to save for college, first make sure you have an emergency fund in place. Make sure your own future is secure with retirement savings. Don't prioritize your kids' education above these other crucial savings. After all, you don't want your money tied up in a college savings account if your house burns down, and although there's no such thing as a retirement loan, generations of college students have been taking out student loans to pay for higher education.

If you don't want a college fund to go to a child if she decides not to attend college or if you don't want her to coast through high school knowing she doesn't need scholarships, set up a personal investment account in your own name. If your child doesn't go to college, you can dispense the money at your discretion or keep it for yourselves. If she does go to college, you can reward your child for her hard work when the time arrives.

If you value gap years, travel, or allowing your child to follow their dreams no matter whether that includes college, consider setting up an investment account in their name. Not every kid is going to have or want a job that requires college. Whether your child wants to become a professional musician or start a business, this gives them the chance to dream big without going into (as much) debt.

Getting the Lowdown on Life Insurance

Purchasing life insurance policies in the event that you or your child dies couldn't be more outside the spirit of happiness that comes with welcoming a newborn. However, tragedy can strike in many ways and at any time, and although it's not pleasant to think about, life insurance is a must.

Obtaining adequate life insurance for mom and dad

Priority number one has to be making sure your child is well cared for in the event of an emergency, which means confronting your own mortality. Buying life insurance for both you and your partner provides a security policy that allows your family to continue living the life you're all accustomed to without financial ruin in the event one or both of you were to die. Now that you're a parent, it's your responsibility to make sure you can pay bills and put food on the table — even in the event of your death.

Policy needs vary based on your financial circumstances, but the amount you buy should be enough to cover not just funeral costs but also a few years of your current income and expenses, as well as funds to pay off any bad debt you currently have. This safety net keeps your family financially sound while they deal with their grief.

Considering a policy for your baby

Buying life insurance for your baby is a controversial and unsavory topic. Many financial experts say it's a waste of money because a life insurance policy is necessary only when the death of the individual causes financial stress on a family. For many lower- and middle-income families, however, a policy that would cover the funeral cost is well worth the monthly payment.

Whole-life coverage versus term

Not all life insurance policies are the same. Some policies are "rentals," covering a child through a certain age and then offering no more benefit. If you elect to go the "buying" route for a policy, it will start your child on the right track to financial security for retirement. You can choose between two basic types of policies that determine the price, coverage level, and longevity of the policy:

>> **Whole-life coverage:** As the name implies, a whole-life policy stays with your child for his entire life. This permanent insurance has a fixed premium that never increases as your child ages and offers the policy owner a guaranteed cash value against which the owner can borrow money in case of emergency.

The coverage is generally between $25,000 and $150,000. Buying whole-life coverage for your baby usually doesn't require a medical checkup. One of the more popular plans is available through Gerber, but most life insurance providers offer competitive plans, too. We advise speaking with a professional before purchasing, though. You can't cash out the whole-life policy at any time for full value, and depending on your financial situation, saving money in an interest-yielding account may be a better idea. That way, you can always access the money you've invested.

>> **Term coverage:** Term insurance is sometimes referred to as a "rental policy" because the named person on the policy never owns it like one does with whole-life coverage. Think of it as a magazine subscription with huge financial benefits: As long as you have a subscription, you're covered; when the subscription runs out — that is, when the policy expires — you stop getting coverage.

The money you invest is simply going toward "what if" protection. The cost is generally a fraction of the price of whole-life coverage, which is why it's such an attractive option for some parents. Plans generally come in 10- to 30-year terms, with coverage ranging from $25,000 to $150,000. However, premiums aren't fixed and do increase as your baby ages.

How much coverage is enough?

Determining how much coverage you should buy depends on your budget. Buy only what you can afford. The more payout benefit you purchase, the more you pay each month. If you're purchasing term insurance, you don't need to buy a policy that exceeds the costs of a funeral and, perhaps, any wage losses due to unpaid leave during your grieving period.

Talk with a financial planner to determine whether a whole-life policy is actually the best investment for your child or whether another form of savings would yield bigger rewards for him down the road — and still provide you a safety net in case of death.

Health Insurance Options for Newborns

Navigating the health insurance mélange has always been a bit of a headache. HMO, PPO — what does it all mean? For the most part, your insurance won't be any different after you have a baby. The only thing that definitely changes is the cost. For those parents without insurance — or those who can't afford it — the process is a bit more complex.

Adding baby to an existing work-paid plan

Don't worry if baby doesn't arrive during your company's insurance open season. Whenever a major life event occurs, such as the birth of a baby, you're allowed to change your insurance coverage. Check with your HR department to get the proper paperwork for adding baby.

You won't actually add baby until after she's born. Your insurance company will need her name, sex, and birth date in order to issue a policy. However, baby's medical expenses are covered according to your current plan's postnatal coverage. Policies are retroactive back to birth but don't continue to cover baby's expenses forever. Most plans require you to add baby within the first month of life or your child won't be covered under your plan.

REMEMBER

The most important thing to consider when adding a baby to your insurance is the cost of plans. If you purchased your company's top-notch insurance plan, the cost may skyrocket out of your price range with the addition of a child. Don't just add baby to your existing plan without first looking at the price of all the family plans your company offers. A different plan may save you hundreds of dollars every month.

Look for the plan that offers the highest level of coverage you can afford. Also, be sure to choose a plan with a reasonable copayment because your child will be going to the doctor frequently.

TIP

Be sure to call your insurance company to add your child to your plan as soon as possible. Some companies give you as little as 30 days to make the change following the birth of a baby, and because you'll be going to the doctor multiple times in those early weeks, you want to get the changes made ASAP so you aren't on the hook for some huge expenses. When you add a child to a plan, the insurance company usually has a time limit for submitting proof of birth, such as a copy of the birth certificate, to make it official. Check with your insurance company for the deadlines and paperwork specific to your plan.

Buying coverage just for baby

Statistics show that around 31 million Americans live without health insurance. That number includes 5.6 percent of American children. If you're living without health insurance and about to have a baby, you're facing the high costs of labor and delivery, but the money hemorrhage doesn't stop after baby arrives. Your child must have wellness checks and vaccination appointments frequently, which means you'll be shelling out a large portion of your hard-earned cash to your child's pediatrician.

If you're enrolled in a plan through the ACA, make sure you completely understand your coverage dates and what your plan provides. If you're switching plans, you have no cause for alarm — your insurance will still cover your childbirth as laid out in the plan you're purchasing, even if you subscribe after you're already pregnant.

Regardless of your stance on the ACA, consider buying a health insurance policy for your child. Even if you can't afford to buy coverage for you and your partner and must pay for labor and delivery out of pocket, coverage for your baby is essential. Policies generally start around $100 per month, and, ultimately, you'll spend much less than if you pay 100 percent of the bills yourself.

Obtaining free and low-cost care for uninsured kids

If you don't have a work-sponsored health insurance program and can't afford to buy a policy for your child, yet you earn too much to qualify for Medicaid, explore the free or low-cost coverage options provided by both the federal and state governments. Your child may qualify for coverage if you meet certain low-income standards. Visit www.insurekidsnow.gov to see whether your family qualifies for federal coverage and to find a provider in your state.

If you don't meet the low-income guidelines, many state-sponsored programs offer coverage. For the contact in your state, visit the National Association of Insurance Commissioners' website: www.naic.org/state_web_map.htm.

Taking Care of Legal Matters

Arranging legal matters is an important step in ensuring your child's well-being in the case of your early death. As unpleasant as the topic may be, you need to sit down with your partner as soon as possible and make decisions about what will happen to your assets and who will take care of your child if you die, and what should happen if either of you is incapacitated. Then make those decisions legally binding by creating a formal will and establishing power of attorney. These tasks aren't fun, but the peace of mind you'll have is worth it.

WARNING

Although most of the forms you need to make these decisions and declarations are available for free online, the only way to make sure your forms are valid and written in accordance with state and federal laws is to have a lawyer review them. Doing so is an added expense, but it's worth the money to know your family will be taken care of in the event you're no longer around.

Creating a will

Drawing up a will doesn't have to be as macabre as reading a Stephen King novel. As a soon-to-be or new parent, having a will can bring you peace of mind by leaving no question about what will happen to your possessions (and children!) when you die. A will includes three provisions:

>> **Who will inherit your bank accounts, real estate, vehicles, and personal property when you die:** Most dads have simple wills that leave everything to their partners and, in the event they both die, to their children.

>> **Who will be your child's guardian in case you and your partner are incapacitated or die:** This is your chance to make sure your child is cared for by the person of your choice and not put into foster care.

» **Who will manage any property and money you leave to your child until he reaches a designated age:** Most people name a single executor of their will who's charged with carrying out their wishes. However, some people are more comfortable having the person responsible for carrying out the will's commands be separate from the person who controls the money.

A will doesn't trump the beneficiaries listed on life insurance policies. Make sure to contact your life insurance company to make the desired changes to those policies, such as adding your new child as a beneficiary.

Making your will

You don't have to go the lawyer route to make a will. Several do-it-yourself computer programs and books (such as Aaron Larson's *Wills & Trusts Kit For Dummies* [Wiley]) provide simple step-by-step instructions for arranging what happens after you die.

Filling in the blanks and hitting print doesn't automatically offer you the protection you need. Any will not made with a lawyer still has to be notarized to be valid in the eyes of the law. Leave a copy of your will with your executor and one in a safe-deposit box.

Make a separate will for each parent. A joint will is binding after the death of even one person, and that makes it difficult for the surviving parent to make changes that may better suit his changed circumstances. Separate wills are especially important when kids are involved because finances change, and you want your partner to have access to funds to care for your kids. Name your spouse or partner as the sole beneficiary to ensure she has 100 percent control of your assets, and have concrete, detailed discussions about how you want the dispersing of money and property, as well as your funeral and burial, handled in the event of your untimely demise.

Appointing guardians

If you have children, you should address guardianship when you create a will. If you work with a lawyer, she can help you fill out all the necessary paperwork. However, if you use an online form or a software program, be sure that it includes the appropriate form for your state.

If you're unsure of the legal requirements, consult your state's courts website to find the necessary forms. Most forms require a signature from both parents and the appointed guardian as well as notarization.

A will allows you to designate temporary guardianship until the new guardian arrives, in cases where your named guardian lives a few states away or can't come for your child immediately. This temporary situation keeps your child out of the foster care program and in the loving home of your choice.

QUESTIONS TO ASK YOURSELF WHEN CHOOSING A LEGAL GUARDIAN

When deciding who would make the best guardian for your child in case of your death, consider the following questions:

- Does the person love my child?
- Is the person good with children in general?
- How important is it that my child's guardian be family?
- Will my child be uprooted from her home to move in with the guardian?
- Does the person have the same parenting philosophies I have?
- Is the person going to raise the child with the same religious beliefs?
- Does the person have any medical conditions that would prevent him from being a long-term, able-bodied guardian?
- Will my child cause too big of a personal, professional, or financial strain for the person?
- Does the person have a stable home life and career?
- Will this person guarantee my child has access to family?
- Does this person value the same things I do (education, music, community, and so on)?

Guardianship is a huge responsibility for the person you ask. When approaching him, keep in mind that you may not get an immediate yes. In fact, if the person you ask needs some time to think it over, it's a good sign that he understands the responsibility and won't make rash decisions he may later regret. This person will not only be in charge of your child but will also have to cover any of the financial gaps not covered by the money you set aside to be used for your child's upbringing.

If the person you ask declines, ask for more information about why he refused. Perhaps you have information that can assuage any fears he may have about the job. However, if the person you ask (even after further discussion) isn't up for the job, find someone else. Yes, it will be disappointing, but respect that person's honesty and forthrightness in admitting he's the wrong person for the job. And when it comes down to it, finding the right person is most important.

Appointing an executor

The person you appoint as executor is in charge of *executing* your will — making sure taxes and debts are paid and your estate is distributed according to your stated wishes. Avoid appointing someone as an executor who's also a beneficiary of your will. You can name coexecutors if you want one person to manage your money and the other to manage, say, your property. Appointing coexecutors can give you backup if one person drops the ball.

You designate an executor using the same online or software program you use to make a will or when creating a will with your lawyer. Of course, make sure the person you designate is willing and able to perform the role. Most forms that designate an executor for your will require you to provide one or two contingency executors in case the first named executor can't perform the job. Some states only recognize executors who live in the same state as the deceased. Check your state's rules before you designate.

When there's no will

State laws vary, but if you don't have a will, less than half of your property and money goes to your spouse, and the rest is divided among your children. If your children aren't 18, all money and property is managed by a state-appointed trustee until that time arrives, which means your partner won't have access to your money in order to raise your children.

In the event that both parents die without a will, the state designates a guardian for the children, which is likely the most closely related family member willing to accept the job. While guardianship is arranged, your child will enter the state's foster care program.

Establishing power of attorney

Granting *power of attorney* to someone gives that person the power to make decisions — both legal and medical — in the event that you're incapacitated. The person you name can make important decisions about life support and control of your bank accounts.

Knowing your options

You can designate four main types of power of attorney. Not everyone appoints a person for each, and appointing the same person to serve in multiple roles is common:

>> **Durable power of attorney:** Granting someone this power means his authority ceases to be recognized by the law after you pass away, except in the areas in which you give him control.

>> **General power of attorney:** The American Bar Association refers to this person as your *agent,* and she has the power to act on your behalf in every capacity that you did prior to your incapacitation. This person literally becomes you in the legal sense until you're capable of handling your own affairs once more.

>> **Healthcare power of attorney:** This person is empowered to make important medical decisions but has no control over your finances.

>> **Limited power of attorney:** The person you designate is allowed only to act on your behalf for a specified amount of time. This, most likely, won't be helpful when creating a will that covers the care and guardianship of your children.

Appointing a power of attorney

Generally included as part of the will-making process, appointing power of attorney takes only a simple form that usually must be signed by you and the named power of attorney and then notarized.

Experts suggest choosing someone you trust but who isn't a close friend or family member. After all, even if you've made it clear that you don't want to be on life support for an extended period of time, your spouse or someone in your family may have difficulty pulling the plug. Select a person whom you can trust to follow through with your wishes.

The power of attorney should follow what you outline in your will, so go over your will with that person to make sure he's comfortable following your orders. If not, find someone else or complications may arise that can cause added stress for everyone involved. What's most important is finding a person you can trust who will be informed about your wishes and make sure they're followed.

Growing together as a couple

Right now it might seem like you and your partner are on top of the world. A new baby can fill your life with a sense of hope and wonder, and it might even make you feel like nothing could ever go wrong again. Unfortunately, life doesn't work that way, and the stresses associated with major life changes can be quite damaging to relationships. Things are going to change after you become parents and it's important to acknowledge as much. As previously discussed, there will be less time and more responsibilities. It's easy for the baby to become the focus of your lives and for the care and feeding of your relationship to fade into the background.

There's no road map for growing together, but solid, proactive communication is key. Learn how to communicate your feelings, needs, and wants with your partner in a nonaccusatory, blame-free manner. Also, learn how to be a good listener and validate your partner's needs, wants, and feelings, too. Consider taking a communication course to ensure you know how to handle conflict and your emotions when the pressure is on. It'll come in handy when you're tired, crabby, and you need to negotiate who's going to do the laundry.

Also, your relationship will continue to change throughout its lifespan, especially after kids. You're parents now, in addition to being a couple. Talk openly about what you both want and need from each other. Plan date nights, relationship check-ins, weekends away, and so on. Keep your relationship in focus even when baby takes center stage. Remember — unexpressed expectations lead to disappointment and, too often, arguments. Expect change and encourage each other to grow.

TIP

Find a couples therapist or counselor before you feel like you need one. Parenting is stressful. Transitioning from a carefree early relationship to a mature family is stressful. Don't go it alone. Therapists provide a safe third-party point of view to help you both work through any issues you might not feel comfortable talking about alone. If you're telling yourself you don't need therapy, think again! All of those little things that annoy you now tend to snowball into bigger issues down the road. Protect your relationship and family by being proactive.

Learning how to be parents on the same team

Everyone was raised in a different way. If you and your partner haven't already figured this out, you will after baby arrives. Differences in parenting styles are great when it comes to the little things like play styles, but when you're talking about sleep routines, feeding issues (Juice or no juice? Kid food or eat what the family eats?), issues pertaining to safety, and — eventually — how you deal with the heavier issues such as reprimands and punishments. One of the most important things to remember is that you'll want to be on the same page ahead of time so you and your partner feel like you have each other's support.

TIP

Real-time feedback for your partner is fine in potentially dangerous or damaging situations, but if you have the opportunity to have a conversation after the fact instead of a judgment in the moment, the two of you will feel closer and more like a team.

Investing in your mental well-being

Mental health is key to being a good parent. Not only will your limits be tested, but you will be put in new, constantly changing situations on an almost daily basis. Chances are you'll feel overwhelmed, stressed, anxious, and even depressed. If you have preexisting mental health issues, make sure you and your doctor have a game plan for how to manage the stress of an expanding family.

Although busy new parents might not feel like they have time to invest in self-care, online therapy and meditation apps can be useful tools that get you the skills necessary to manage stress. Simple moments like taking a walk, going to the gym, or taking a bath are also easy, low-impact ways to improve your mindset. Make sure to have mental health check-ins with your partner, too. If you know each other well enough to have a baby, then you will be the best person to spot changes in the other person's mood or behavior.

5

The Part of Tens

Get involved with the pregnancy and birth in the best ways possible. No, you can't take over the most odious parts or experience the most exciting, like actually giving birth, but there are lots of other ways to let your partner know how important this pregnancy is to you.

Bond with your baby right from the start. For example, even though breast-feeding is out of the question for you, you too can go skin-to-skin with baby.

Chapter **17**

Ten Must-Do's to Compensate for Not Having to Give Birth

During the course of your partner's pregnancy — and many months thereafter — she'll expect myriad tasks, words of comfort, and loving gestures from you without her having to ask for what she wants. Sadly, you weren't born with advanced psychic aptitude, and therefore you'll have to infer a few must-dos to keep peace around the house. Follow these ten simple tips to make sure your partner gets everything she needs.

Say Nice Things

Face it — you'll never know what it's like to give up your body so that someone else can grow inside of you. That said, it probably isn't too hard to remember the last time you got a new haircut or lost 10 pounds and then waited around for someone to tell you how nice you looked.

Going fishing for compliments is never a fun or fruitful excursion, so try to spare your partner from going to that length. When her hormones and ever-increasing waistline are waging a full-fledged attack on her insecurities, remind her early and often exactly how beautiful she looks. And the best part is, you won't have to lie. It may be hard to imagine finding your partner gorgeous when she's carrying around 30 to 40 extra pounds, but pregnant women glow, and knowing that she's having your baby can be extremely attractive.

REMEMBER

When she asks you how she looks or whether she has gotten fat (and she will ask you!), flatter her to no end and thank her for her sacrifices.

Start a Baby Book

Baby books — whether digital or physical — with their endless pages of blank space calling out for someone to fill in the missing data, can be a daunting undertaking, especially when chronicling the journey is left solely to the mom-to-be/new mommy. Most women won't admit it, but during pregnancy they're looking for constant signs that you're just as committed to raising a child together as they are. Filling out a baby book together can be the perfect way to put into words just how ready you are for baby.

A great way to exhibit your commitment and excitement to the baby she's carrying is to find the best baby book on the market that suits your styles. If you and the mom-to-be are the long-form journaling types, pick one that offers lots of space to write about how you're feeling during each trimester and your thoughts about becoming a parent. If you fall into the less-is-more crowd, choose a book that adheres to a mostly fill-in-the-blank format. If you both would rather spend time chronicling your baby's life on your smartphones, opt for a book with a corresponding app or digital environment. Many themed books are available, running the gamut from religious to hipster chic, so choose one that represents both parents.

Make Exercise Fun

Exercise is of the utmost importance to both baby and mommy, but try telling your partner to get up off the sofa and go for a walk without having something hard thrown at your head. Getting a loved one involved in fitness is never easy to do without hurt feelings, so instead of telling her she needs to exercise, help her exercise without making it personal.

TIP

Turn fitness into a social activity: Plan walks with friends and family members or schedule errands together that require you to get up and move around. Plan a "treasure hunt" date to local baby stores to scope out the latest gear or even a hunt with a romantic bent. Even a trip to the mall can be good exercise — as long as you steer clear of the food court.

If your partner has a particular interest in a certain type of exercise, give her a free pass as a gift. Be it yoga, spinning, or running, most fitness clubs or personal trainers offer prenatal versions of their classes. Many classes welcome partners, too, and by making it a couples' affair, it won't send the message that you think she's fat.

Listen . . . Don't Try to Fix It

Let your partner complain about her job, her body, the mere fact that she's pregnant, or whatever. Also, don't take her complaints, gripes, or outbursts personally. We're not saying you should give her free reign to be a raving lunatic just because she's pregnant. Rather, we're encouraging you to avoid trying to solve her problems with your sage wisdom unless she specifically asks for it. Listen to her and validate what she's feeling, but don't tell her how to fix it.

Attend Prenatal Appointments

REMEMBER

Repeat after us: Prenatal appointments aren't just for the mothers. Yes, she is carrying the baby, but that baby didn't get there on her own. You're in this together, and if she has to make time in her schedule to attend countless appointments, ultrasounds, and tests, so should you. Doing so demonstrates to her that you're a team in the raising of this baby, and you'll be much more excited and invested in the process by being just as involved as your partner.

Childbirth is an empowering experience for both mother and father, and the more appointments you attend, the more knowledgeable you'll be about the entire process. Being an involved father starts long before the baby arrives. In fact, if you plan on being a 50-50 partner in the raising of your child, it won't just happen overnight. You wouldn't play a baseball game without practice, and you shouldn't enter into parenthood without practicing the type of dad you want to be.

If your work schedule doesn't allow for you to attend every appointment, go to as many as possible. Follow up with her immediately after each appointment you miss and ask her for a recap. Ask lots of questions; your partner will be grateful to know you care. Many important decisions and discussions occur during prenatal visits, and even if you can't be present, you can remain part of the discussion.

Book a Mini-Vacation (Babymoon)

After baby arrives it won't be easy to abandon ship and head for the hills when you need a relaxing reprieve from life. And as the long wait for baby drags on and you both begin to realize how much is going to change in your personal lives after he comes, you may find yourselves looking for one last couples retreat.

Take the lead and plan a trip. Keep in mind that the later she is in her pregnancy, the closer to home you'll want to be in case she goes into labor. Also, her body (and especially her bladder) won't be up for sitting in a plane or in the car for long periods of time. Wherever you go, make the trip romantic, personal, and quiet. Make it a time to focus on your relationship — just the two of you — because that won't be the focus of your lives for some time to come.

REMEMBER

If you plan something during the third trimester, keep in mind that many airlines have restrictions about how close to her due date your partner can travel. Check with your airline before booking tickets because many require a medical practitioner's note for travel.

Register for a Prenatal Class

The days of prenatal parenting classes that focus solely on breathing and birthing techniques are over. Today's classes offer opportunities for parents-to-be to explore birthing options, relationships, the type of parents they want to be, CPR, and infant care. Find a class that's welcoming to both mother and father and register, either through your local hospital or birthing center or by searching online. Today's couples can even choose virtual classes and attend from the comfort of home.

TIP

Many communities have fatherhood experts that offer a new brand of class just for fathers-to-be that explores the myths of fatherhood, what it means to be a father, and male bonding exercises. It allows men to confront their fears of fatherhood and any issues they have regarding their own fathers. Putting in the work before baby comes only increases the odds that you'll be the best dad you can be.

Get Smart about Baby

Clearly, if you're reading this book, then you've already done the majority of your homework. Congratulations — you're going to be a great dad. Now don't be afraid to toot your own horn. Not every dad-to-be is as equipped and awesome as you, and you deserve credit. Make a point of telling your partner how much you've found out in these pages. Ask her, "You probably already know this, but I just learned . . .?" and "We should consider . . .?" Who knows, you just may expose her to a new idea that will work for your family. And is there any better feeling in the world than feeling accomplished?

At the very least, you'll set a good example of your own involvement in the future of your relationship. In the past, fathers weren't expected to know anything about pregnancy, and not too long ago, the majority of men stayed out of the delivery room and returned to work the day after delivery. The more you know, the more your partner will trust you to care for the baby. Trust is earned, and by getting educated about babies, you're earning that trust that many fathers of the past forfeited.

Master Prenatal Massage

Pregnancy puts stress on all the body's joints and ligaments as muscles (and even bones!) shift and expand, causing mothers-to-be to walk, stand, sit, and sleep in ways that often are at odds with their normal movements and positions. Add an additional 30 to 40 pounds hanging off her front, and it's no wonder that your average pregnant woman gets achy, tired, and downright sore.

Learning the basics of massage can help you help your partner alleviate many of those aches and pains and make you her hero after a long day of carrying around your child. Many hospitals and birthing centers offer prenatal massage classes. Doulas often are trained in light massage, and if you hire one, be sure to learn techniques from her. If you can't find someone to learn from, stream a prenatal massage course or buy a book that offers ample illustrations so you'll know what to do.

While you're at it, consider learning the ins and outs of infant massage. Research shows that infant massage can help babies digest foods and sleep better, and helps prevent and treat colic. Check with your hospital or birthing center for more information.

Keep the House Neat and Tidy

The closer you get to delivery time, the more likely your partner is to desire a clean, tidy home. Limited by a rather large belly and an unflinching tiredness, your partner won't always feel like cleaning or be able to do it. Areas that fall below your partner's knee level and things out of her reach are particularly difficult for her during the latter stages of pregnancy.

But her limitations don't mean that you have to clean everything all by yourself. In fact, the exercise involved in cleaning can be beneficial for her. However, assign yourself the job of picking up everything from the floor on a frequent basis. Clutter-free floors and walkways prevent her from falling and keep her from pulling a muscle in her back trying to reach down.

TIP

While you're down there, you have a good view of what baby will see when she's crawling around your home. You can always begin baby-proofing your abode; the extra time you give yourself lets you get used to the new limitations and restrictions.

Though it's a myth that a pregnant woman will strangle the baby if she raises her arms above her head, it may be a rather uncomfortable experience. Take the lead on cleaning the blinds, putting away dishes in the cupboards, changing light bulbs, and dusting.

Chapter **18**

Ten Ways to Bond as a New Family

When it comes to parenting, what you don't know won't kill you, but it sure can keep you from making the most of the greatest, most joyous time in your life. After nearly a year of waiting for baby to arrive — or longer in some cases — don't forget that now is the time to have fun. Yes, bringing a teeny, tiny baby into your home evokes a great deal of worrying, but babies aren't as fragile as you may think. If you want to be a super family, try to follow these tips on how to be a confident, loving, and tight-knit family from day one.

Don't Be Afraid . . . Be Awesome

Babies can sense when their caretakers are uncomfortable. If you or your partner is afraid of holding your baby, you probably aren't providing a solid, sturdy base for her, and she'll fuss and cry until somebody who is confident takes over the reins. The same holds true for diapering, feeding, and cuddling. Repeat after us: I'm not going to break my baby.

Take deep, steady breaths and hold your baby in the same casual-yet-protective way you grasp your $1,000 iPhone. Don't fumble with the baby as you lift her up onto your shoulder. Use firm, fluid movements. The more you act like you know what you're doing, the more the baby will like what you're doing. Work with your partner to perfect your moves — the more you work together to understand your baby's needs, the closer you'll all be as a family.

Trust Your Instincts

Lucky for you, babies are designed to be cared for by people who don't have any education in the raising of children — which also means that you have no choice but to follow your instincts. Babies have been around since, well, the dawn of humans, and all the parents since that time have raised them their own way. We're born with the instinct to care for our children, and as long as you don't have mental or emotional impediments (such as postpartum depression), you'll just know what to do.

Just remember that nobody can know your baby better than you and your partner do, and despite the seeming lack of faith others may show toward your judgment (how warmly you dress him, how often you feed him, how you hold him, and so on), the only truly vital task of the parent is to ensure safety. Trust yourself and educate yourself and you won't steer your little one wrong.

Spend Time Skin-to-Skin, Eye-to-Eye

Mothers get an amazing opportunity to spend skin-to-skin time with baby while breast-feeding. This sensory bond is so important that mere moments after the baby is born, the doctor or midwife will often place her on mom's bare chest. Studies show that skin-to-skin contact increases the bond that both mother and child feel and the soothing feeling babies experience from listening to mom's heartbeat. Also, a newborn's eyesight is just powerful enough to see the distance from the breast to mom's eyes.

You won't be breast-feeding, so you have far fewer opportunities to experience the same closeness. Yes, baby's head will rest on your hands and arms, and you can get close and make eye contact, but that doesn't provide the same bonding feeling. When baby is only in her diaper, take off your shirt and place her on your chest. It may sound a little cheesy, but it's an important bonding experience for every parent, not just mothers, and it gives you and baby the opportunity to meet skin-to-skin and eye-to-eye for the first time.

Check Frustrations

Admit it — your son or daughter is the most beautiful sight you've ever seen. As you stare into the wondering eyes of your newborn, you may think it impossible to ever feel anything but absolute adoration for this child. However, babies often are exhausting and unmanageable beings that wake you up in the middle of the night, cry endlessly without giving you a clue as to what's wrong, and require 100 percent of your attention.

Feeling frustrated is okay, because parenting, especially when you're brand-new at it, can and will be a frustrating experience from time to time. In fact, bonding over how frustrating it all is can be a very healthy thing for new parents. Sharing frustrations with each other allows both of you to know how the other is feeling, which means you won't feel alone.

TIP

Here are some simple ways to manage your baby-related frustrations:

>> **Blow off steam.** Whatever it is that puts your mind at ease, make sure you take time to continue engaging in it. If you find yourself getting frustrated, spend five minutes doing your favorite activity. Even a walk around the block can be a great way to hit your reset button.

>> **Control the controllable.** Don't waste your time trying to solve problems that aren't really problems. If your baby has a clean diaper, a full belly, and a gas-free stomach, yet still continues to fuss, just put on some noise-canceling headphones and let him cry. Unless something is wrong, don't worry about him.

>> **Lean on your support system.** When the going gets rough and you feel like you need to get out of Dodge, do it! Call a sitter, a friend, or a family member to fill in for you, even if

it's just for an hour so you can run to the grocery store in peace.

>> **Monitor baby's routine.** Keep a log of when baby sleeps, wakes, eats, poops, and pees. Understanding his routine takes a lot of the guesswork out of determining what he needs at any given time.

>> **Sleep in shifts.** If baby is constantly waking during the night, both you and your partner will quickly lose patience in the wee hours of the morning. Though it's not the ideal situation, try taking turns sleeping for blocks of time in the night and throughout the day while on leave (or the weekends). You need to get as much sleep as possible, even if those hours aren't consecutive. The key to keeping your frustrations in check just may be two hours of peaceful slumber. Make sure you and your partner get the time away you need to function.

Embrace Your Goofy Side

By now you've probably made a list of all the things you're not going to do as a parent. For many too-cool-for-school dads, that list includes such things as baby talk, funny faces, and the pure lunacy of dress up, tea parties, and dancing that requires dads to check traditional masculinity at the door in favor of fun.

Do all the things on that list. Better yet — don't make a list at all. Don't feel stupid and don't feel restrained by how you think men should behave. Babies (and kids, for that matter) love expressive faces, singing, and goofy voices, and while acting silly may leave you in a shroud of self-consciousness, you'll get over it the instant your baby laughs or smiles at your goofball antics. Allow yourself to have fun and you'll reap the rewards for life.

Steal Away for a Date Early On

Going to work doesn't qualify as getting out of the house. Yes, it may be a nice change of pace to spend time doing things that don't require baby wipes and a Pee-Pee Teepee, but the kind of getting out you need is of the date variety.

TIP

You may be surprised to know that getting out of the house is easier when your baby is younger. Make sure to schedule a date within the first month of baby's arrival. Start slowly — new moms (and many dads) find it hard to leave baby for the first time. Ask a trusted friend or family member to watch baby while you grab a quick bite at your favorite restaurant.

Ground rules? Don't talk about the baby. You may not achieve this almost impossible goal, but shoot for the stars. You need to connect as adults again, not just as parents, and that brief time away will remind you why you love your partner so much. And, upon returning home, you'll have a welcome reminder of just how much you love that baby.

Teach Baby New Tricks

You may think babies discover the world of their own volition, but the truth is that you need to give your little one a push. In fact, the more time you put into teaching and nurturing your baby, the prouder you'll be when she learns to roll over, clap, wave bye-bye, or play with a toy. Bonding happens daily with babies, and a child's way of thinking is practically set in stone by age 3. You can have a huge influence on the rate at which your child develops, but more importantly, you can have a huge influence on your child's entire life by getting involved in playtime and the open expression of love.

Following are some milestones you can help baby achieve in the first six months:

>> **Crawling:** Studies show that the way babies' brains react during crawling (the right brain controls the left side of the body and vice versa) is an important milestone that can help reduce behavioral and mental disorders in children. Help ensure your child can crawl by putting a coveted toy just out of reach and waiting for her to come and get it.

>> **Making sounds:** Babies have their own language that you don't understand, and the more they hear it repeated back to them, the more they'll talk, which aids in language development down the road.

>> **Peekaboo:** Babies will laugh as you disappear and reappear time and again, all while beginning to understand the idea of cause and effect.

>> **Reaching and gripping:** Dangle colorful toys and baby-safe objects in front of your child and wait for her to reach for them. Encourage gripping by wrapping baby's hand around the object and letting go.

>> **Rolling over:** Lay your baby on her back on a play mat or a colorful rug to encourage her to turn over and begin to explore. When she can support her own head, give her plenty of tummy time on her belly, which develops the stomach muscles and allows her to roll over.

>> **Tracking objects:** Slowly move a colorful object back and forth and up and down in front of baby's eyes. This activity helps the brain begin to follow movement.

Roughhouse the Safe Way

Though we don't want to engage in gender stereotyping, fathers are often more likely to get physical during playtime with their kids. And although you probably won't be wrestling with your newborn (please, don't wrestle your newborn!), go ahead and swing him in your arms, hold him up high over your head, rub your scratchy face into his belly, tickle him, and chew on his feet. Mom may think it's too much, but more than likely, baby will think it's hysterical. As long as you're being safe, have fun.

Read Daily

Read to your baby every single day. Not only will she love the sound of your voice, but she'll also learn to speak from hearing the constant repetition of speech patterns. It doesn't matter what you read to her; what matters more is that you do it. The more you read to baby, the more likely it is that she'll develop a strong vocabulary and the ability to speak at a younger age.

Say Goodbye to Mommy

Unless you're fortunate enough to be a work-at-home parent, you need to make sure that both you and your partner block off some one-on-one time with your baby. Finding your own way as a parent and learning your capabilities are important steps in feeling empowered as a new dad, which means mom needs to go away for a while.

Book an appointment at the spa for your partner and spend the afternoon doing everyday things with your baby. Take him for a walk, feed him, change him, or even go out to the coffee shop and read the paper with him. Regardless of the activities you do together, this time establishes one-on-one intimacy with your child and proves to yourself and your partner that you're capable of taking care of your child on your own.

Index

A

abdominal pain, as a medical issue, 159

abnormal ultrasounds, handling, 138–140

acceptance stage, of grief, 289

accepting limitations, 85

access, for hospitals, 173

accidents, common, 303–306

acetaminophen, 301, 313

active labor, 202

activity, during third trimester, 156

administering medicine, 308–310

admission process, ensuring a smooth, 164–165

Affordable Care Act, 107, 150, 229

after-work expectations, 328–329

agencies, working with, 58

alcohol
  after birth, 258
  development problems and, 83
  during pregnancy, 15–16, 37

The Alexander Technique, 106

all-natural method, 181–182, 211–212

alpha feto-protein, 99

amenorrhea, 38

American Academy of Adoption and Assisted Reproductive Technology Attorneys (AAARTA), 57

American Academy of Pediatrics (AAP), 241

American College of Nurse-Midwives, 178

American Congress of Obstetricians and Gynecologists (ACOG), 132

amniocentesis, during second trimester, 98–100

amniotic fluid, leaking
  as a medical issue, 159
  myths about, 104
  during third trimester, 156

anabolic steroids, 37

androgens, 34

anemia, as a health risk to mom with multiples, 149

anencephaly, statistics on, 139

anesthesia, in hospitals, 173

anger
  controlling, 15
  as a stage of grief, 289
  as a symptom of postpartum depression, 285

ankles, swollen, during third trimester, 158

announcing arrival of baby, 193–194

anovulation, 34

antidepressant medications, 161, 287

anxiety, with breast-feeding, 228

appetite loss, as a symptom of postpartum depression, 285

appointing
  executors, 365
  guardians, 363–365
  power of attorney, 366–367

arm bones, checking on ultrasounds, 101

aspirin, 301, 313

attending
  births, 192
  first prenatal visit, 74–75
  first ultrasound, 75
  prenatal appointments, 375–376

autism spectrum risks/prevention, 84

avoiding trigger foods, 86

axillary thermometers, 310–311, 313

B

babies
  announcing arrival of, 193–194
  determining the needs of, 340–341
  development during first trimester, 75–78
  development during second trimester, 92–94
  development during third trimester, 153–156
  health problems in, 279–284
  helping after birth, 205–206
  naming, 127–130

Babinski reflex, 225

baby bathtub, 124–125

"baby blues," 267, 285–286

baby books, 250, 374

baby carrier, 123–124, 238–239

baby DVDs/CDs, 125

baby monitors, 119

Baby Namer, 129

Baby Names Country, 129

baby registry
  about, 118–119
  baby monitors, 119
  determining what you don't need, 124–125
  determining what you need, 121–123
  online-*versus*-local, 123–124
  research for, 119–120
  travel systems, 120

baby showers
  about, 125–126
  gender reveal parties, 126–127
  naming babies, 127–130
  virtual parties, 127

babymoon, 376

baby-proofing, 117–118

The Baby Name Wizard, 129

"Back to Sleep" campaign, 241, 283

diethylstilbestrol (DES), risk of
preterm delivery from,
140–141
difficulty bonding, as a
symptom of postpartum
depression, 285
digestion
colic, 244–245
gas, 246
reflux, 246
digital oral thermometers,
310
digital rectal thermometers,
310, 311–313
dilatation and curettage
(D&C), 80
dilation, 206
disability insurance, buying,
354
discomforts, first trimester,
84–89
disinterest, as a symptom of
postpartum depression,
285
doctors
about, 176
calling, 307–308
DONA International, 180
dotted newborns, 224
douching, 37–38
doulas, 179–180
Down syndrome
about, 280
checking for on
ultrasounds, 101
statistics on, 139
drawing up contracts, 59
drop (baby), during third
trimester, 156
drugs, recreational, 15–16, 37
durable power of attorney,
366
DVDs, 125

E

ear infections, 299
ear temperatures, 313
early labor, 201–202
eating healthier, during
pregnancy, 15, 95–96
e-cigarettes, 82
ectopic pregnancy, 29, 80–81
Eddleman, Keith (author),
Pregnancy For Dummies,
62

egg donation, 55–56
eggs
about, 25–26
donors of, 54–56
freezing, 48–49
producing mature, 26–27
eighth month, baby's
development during,
154–155
elective procedures,
insurance and, 108
emergency funds, creating,
354
emotional changes, during
third trimester, 160–161
emotional outbursts, 85
encephalitis, 301
endometriosis, 34
engorgement, during breast-
feeding, 262
enhanced formula, 231
ensuring smooth admission
process, 164–165
entertainment
for bed rest station, 137
cutting costs and, 347, 350
epididymis, 36
epidurals, 181–182, 212–215
episiotomy, 184, 205
Equifax, 356
ergonomic bouncy chair, 123
errands, running, 255–256
erythema multiforme, 318
establishing power of
attorney, 366–367
estradiol, 26
estriol, 99
evaluating
growth during ultrasounds,
100–101
health before conception,
32–38
examining newborns,
223–225
executors, appointing, 365
exercise
about, 38
after birth, 256–257
for bed rest station, 137
regimen for, 16
tips for, 374–375
exercise balls, for colic, 245
expectations, with preemies,
143–144
expenses, prioritizing,
350–351

Experian, 356
external monitoring systems,
during labor, 209–210

F

fallopian tube, sperm
journeying through the,
28–29
falls, 303–304
Family and Medical Leave Act
(1993), 325, 327
family medical leave, 325
family members
announcing pregnancy to,
69–70
discussing baby name
choices with, 129–130
grandmas, 270–271
handling overbearing,
168–169
involving in nontraditional
fatherhood, 57
sharing birth plans with,
190–191
family resemblance, of
newborns, 225
family/fun/work balance,
creating, 324–332
fatherhood. *See also*
nontraditional
fatherhood
about, 8
fears of, 9–10, 71, 164
myths about, 10–13
reacting to, 9
fears
of fatherhood, 9–10, 71, 164
handling in third trimester,
162–163
febrile seizures, 314
feeding
bottle-feeding, 230–233
breast-feeding, 227–229
cost of supplies for, 342
determining what you need
for, 121–122
newborns, 226–233
problems with preemies,
144
feet, swollen, during third
trimester, 158
female health issues,
affecting conception,
33–35
female infertility, 45

U

ultrasounds
  attending first, 75
  handling abnormal, 138–140
  risk of during second trimester, 98
  during second trimester, 100–103
umbilical cord, cutting, 185–186
unexpected pregnancies, 19
unplanned Cesarean (C-section), 217
unsolicited advice, managing, 51, 271
urination
  as a side effect of epidurals, 214
  during third trimester, 156, 158
uterine abnormalities, 80
uterine issues, 43
uterus
  implantation in the, 28–29
  during third trimester, 158
utilities, cutting costs on, 348

V

vacation time, 325
vacation time request, 327
vaccinations
  infectious diseases and, 300
  reactions to, 318–319
  scheduling, 247–250
The Vaccine Book (Sears), 249
vacuum extraction, 184
vaginal bleeding, as a medical issue, 159
vaginal discharge, during third trimester, 158
vaginal exams
  at first prenatal visit, 75
  during labor, 206
varicoceles, 47
varicose veins, during third trimester, 158
venting room, for bed rest station, 137
vernix, 224
vibration, for colic, 245
virtual parties, 127
visiting policies, of hospitals, 173

visitors, planning ahead for, 192–193
visualizing ideal experiences, for birth plan, 183–185
vitamin D, 257
volume, of sperm, 46
vomiting, 86, 214, 299–300, 304

W

wake-sleep patterns, during third trimester, 156
walking epidurals, 182
Warning icon, 3
water, requirements for after birth, 258
water birth, 182–183
water breaks, 198, 208–209
websites
  American Academy of Adoption and Assisted Reproductive Technology Attorneys (AAARTA), 57
  American College of Nurse-Midwives, 178
  Baby Namer, 129
  Baby Names Country, 129
  The Baby Name Wizard, 129
  Bradley Method, 181
  Cheat Sheet, 3
  Consumer Reports, 120
  DONA International, 180
  Equifax, 356
  Experian, 356
  health insurance marketplace, 109
  International Board of Lactation Consultant Examiners, 263
  International Lactation Consultant Association, 263
  La Leche League International, 263
  Midwives Alliance of North America, 178
  National Association of Insurance Commissioner, 362
  Social Security Administration's Popular Baby Names, 129
  TransUnion, 356

week 2, baby's development during, 76
week 3, baby's development during, 76
week 4, baby's development during, 76
week 5, baby's development during, 76
week 6, baby's development during, 76
week 7, baby's development during, 76
week 8, baby's development during, 77
week 9, baby's development during, 77
week 10, baby's development during, 77
week 11, baby's development during, 77
week 12, baby's development during, 77
weepiness, as an emotional change during third trimester, 160
weight gain, 87, 94–96
weight loss, 15, 37
wheezing, 298–299
white blood cells, sperm and, 46
whole-life coverage, 358–359
wills, creating, 362–366
wipe warmer, 124
wipes, cost of, 341
womb, 54–56
women, with previously diagnosed diabetes, 134–135
work, announcing pregnancy to, 71
working-from-home, tips for, 329–330
workplace toxins, 36
workspace, for bed rest station, 137
wraparound slings, 238–239
wrinkled skin, of newborns, 224

Y

yoga ball, 124

About the Authors

Matthew M.F. Miller is a husband, a father of two, a youngest brother, and an only son. Matthew was a member of the University of Iowa undergraduate writer's workshops in poetry, fiction, and nonfiction, and is a graduate of the University of Southern California's Master of Professional Writing program. His infertility blog, Maybe Baby, was the catalyst for a book of the same name. Matthew lives in Chattanooga, Tennessee and is editor-in-chief at a fully remote tech company.

Sharon Perkins has never been a dad, but she's had lots of experience on the mom side of parenting, with five children and three grandchildren. More than 35 years as a registered nurse in fertility, labor, and delivery; neonatal intensive care; and pediatric home health have also taught her a thing or two about pregnancy and babies. Sharon lives in New Jersey but would live in Disney World if it were legal.

Dedication

From Matt: This book is dedicated to my wife, Constance, and my two little girls, Nola and Daphne. Our family is pretty much everything to me, and I'm grateful and humbled daily. Thank you for this charmed life.

From Sharon: This book is dedicated to my three grandchildren — Matthew, Emma, and Jessica — who keep me current on what's going on in the world of kids.

Author's Acknowledgments

From Matt: Writing about family takes a deep, rich understanding of what it means to be loved, and I'm grateful to my parents, Marlan and Joy Miller, and sisters, Angie Plagman and April Miller, for always loving me. Much appreciation to my agent, Grace Freedson, who brings amazing opportunities my way. Sharon Perkins is the best coauthor a guy could ever hope for — you are a joy both as a creative partner and a person. Finally, thank you to my wife and, most importantly, our two daughters Nola and Daphne, both of whom were born via IVF. If you ever wonder exactly how much your mom and I love you, know that we struggled for years and spent a small fortune just to have the chance to love you both every day of our lives. And we do love you every second of every day — intensely.

From Sharon: Matt Miller and I are so in sync with writing that when we're finished, neither of us can recognize our own writing! Thanks, Matt, for being a great coauthor. My agent, Jessica Faust and the Wiley acquisitions editors have kept me supplied with work for the last 20 years. I'm grateful to you all!

And last but not least, thanks to my family for supplying all the raw material over the years. Yes, I know you're sick of seeing your most embarrassing childhood moments in print, but you'll thank me someday, when your memory starts to go!

Publisher's Acknowledgments

Acquisitions Editor:
Elizabeth Stilwell

Project Editor: Christopher Morris

Copy Editor: Christopher Morris

Technical Editor: Lynn Shinn

Production Editor:
Tamilmani Varadharaj

Cover Image:
© Africa Studio/Shutterstock